Developing Clinical Practice Skills for Pharmacists

Kimberly A. Galt, Pharm.D., FASHP

Professor of Pharmacy Practice
Department of Pharmacy Practice
Creighton School of Pharmacy and Allied Health Professions
Omaha, Nebraska

American Society of Health-System Pharmacists®
Bethesda, Maryland

For more than 60 years, ASHP has helped pharmacists who practice in hospitals and health systems improve medication use and enhance patient safety. The Society's 30,000 members include pharmacists and pharmacy technicians who practice in inpatient, outpatient, home-care, and long-term-care settings, as well as pharmacy students. For more information about the wide array of ASHP activities and the many ways in which pharmacists help people make the best use of medicines, visit ASHP's Web site, www.ashp.org, or its consumer Web site, www.SafeMedication.com.

Any correspondence regarding this publication should be sent to the publisher, American Society of Health-System Pharmacists, 7272 Wisconsin Avenue, Bethesda, MD, 20814, attn: Special Publishing.

Produced in conjunction with the ASHP Publications Production Center. The information presented herein reflects the opinions of the contributors and reviewers. It should not be interpreted as an official policy of ASHP or as an endorsement of any product.

Drug information and its applications are constantly evolving because of ongoing research and clinical experience and are often subject to professional judgment and interpretation by the practitioner and to the uniqueness of a clinical situation.

The authors and ASHP have made every effort to ensure the accuracy and completeness of the information presented in this book. However, the reader is advised that the publisher, authors, editors, and reviewers cannot be responsible for the continued currency of the information, for any errors or omissions, and/or for any consequences arising from the use of the information in the clinical setting. The reader is cautioned that ASHP makes no representation, guarantee, or warranty, express or implied, that the use of the information contained in this book will prevent problems with insurers and will bear no responsibility or liability for the results or consequences of its use.

Acquisitions Editor: Cynthia Conner
Senior Editorial Project Manager: Dana Battaglia
Production Manager: Johnna Hershey
Design Manager: David A. Wade

RS 100
.G3
2006x
86329434

ISBN: 1-58528-085-2

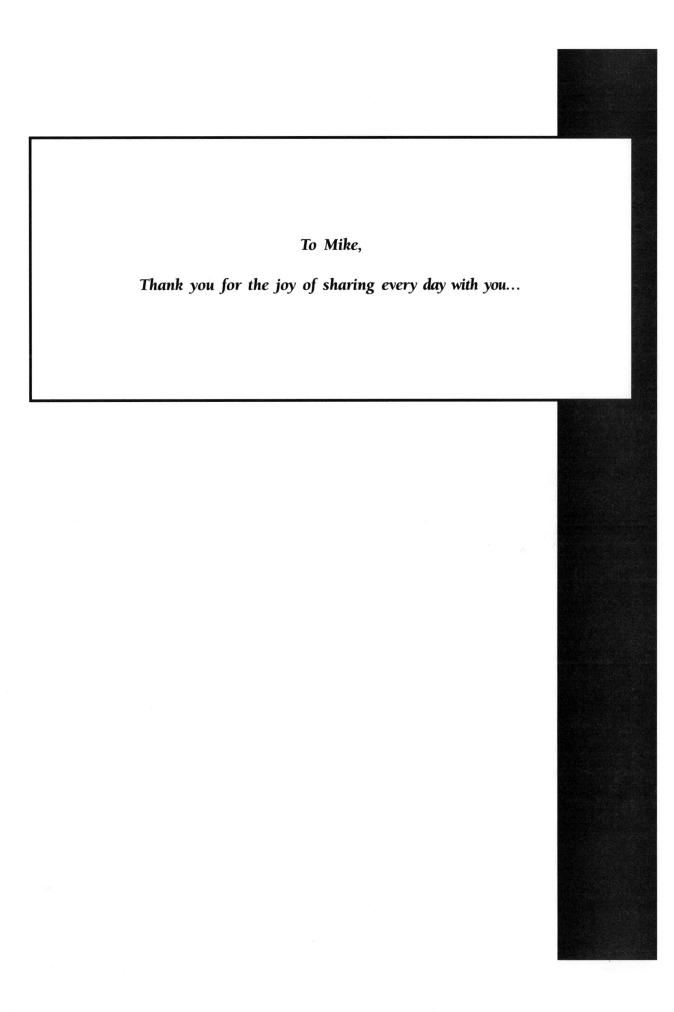

To Mike,

Thank you for the joy of sharing every day with you...

TABLE OF CONTENTS

What is it about your patient care services as a pharmacist that makes you valuable to society? The answer to this question is revealed in understanding society's demands and needs. The following discussion highlights key areas that are driving the pharmacist's role to be patient centered and to be expanded to fully develop the patient–pharmacist encounter to include clinical assessment, evaluation, and treatment.

Dramatic changes in health care technologies over the last several decades have caused both an increase in use of these technologies and a substantial increase in complexity of systems for delivering care associated with their use. Many of the technologies are new forms of medications or medications and devices combined. With the advancement in technology often comes the potential for error either in the use of the technology or its overall outcomes. A survey of 2,012 adults recently found that one in three people say they or a family member experienced a medical error at some point in their life. One-fifth of all Americans indicate that a medical error that they are aware of had serious health consequences; these consequences are categorized as death, long-term disability, or severe pain. Almost half say that they are concerned about safety of the medical care received.[1]

Society has recognized the need for professional expertise to manage these complex technologies both safely and effectively. The most recent evidence supporting this is the passage of the Medicare Prescription Drug, Improvement, and Modernization Act of 2003.[2] From this legislation has emerged the formalization of reimbursable therapeutic drug management services for patients. Pharmacists are becoming a primary provider of these services because their technical expertise is well matched to the specific technologies.

It is not a question in most Americans' minds whether we can provide high-quality health care to our citizens. We know this is done and possible. The bigger concern is in the high variability in quality that is experienced, leading to an overall lower quality of health care than it should be in this country. This is commonly referred to as the "quality gap," and is considered so large that it was retermed the "quality chasm."[3] The primary reason for this quality gap is due to poorly organized and coordinated care delivery. Necessary care processes frequently don't occur because of lack of knowledge, inadequate access, inadequate monitoring, and inadequate documentation and communication.

The need for human caring by patients is evident in all that you observe in health care. The absence of caring produces evidence about how caring is core to your work as a health professional.[4] It is this caring that makes you relate to patients in a way that brings them comfort and peace. It is what makes you continue to advocate for a patient's needs when usual avenues of assistance have been exhausted. It is what motivates you to be a lifelong learner, striving for continued growth and expertise development. Patients recognize the great value you bring at an interpersonal level when caring is at the core of your interactions.

The clinical skills you are introduced to here are essential to providing patient-centered, safe, high-quality, and caring health care to your patients. The initial eight training books in the successful *Advanced Pharmaceutical Care Clinical Skills Program* served as successful groundwork. This first edition of *Developing Clinical Skills for Pharmacists* develops further the clinical care concepts required for an effective patient–pharmacist relationship. It further advances the explanations and teachings needed by pharmacy students and pharmacists who are training to apply clinical skills to patients in a comprehensive way. Concepts of scope of practice and work environment, patient health concepts and behaviors, health literacy and adherence, caring behaviors, clinical reasoning skills, patient safety, and culturally relevant care are examples of areas of inclusion. The context of your work as a pharmacist within the work environment and scope of practice govern the teachings. You are introduced to four pharmacists and four patients who have ongoing care relationships, each in different professional practice settings and with varied scopes of practice. The book follows these four patient care stories, using them as a framework to develop your knowledge and contextual application of clinical skills.

Patients need the care that you can provide with technical and information expertise, clinical expertise, and your caring approach to their concerns. It is our hope that this book is a tool that assists you with accomplishing it in your work.

Kimberly A. Galt
2005

References

1. Kaiser Family Foundation. U.S. Agency for Healthcare Research and Quality (AHRQ) and the Harvard School of Public Health's *National Survey on Consumers' Experiences with Patient Safety and Quality Information*. Menlo Park, CA: Kaiser Family Foundation; July 5, 2004.

2. Medicare Modernization Act of 2003.

3. Institute of Medicine. Crossing the quality chasm: a new health system for the 21st century. Washington DC: National Academy of Sciences; 2001. At: www.nap.edu.

4. Galt KA. Need to define care in pharmaceutical care: examination across research, practice and education. *Am J Pharm Educ.* 2000; 64(3):223–33.

ACKNOWLEDGEMENTS

My heartfelt thanks go to Donna Balado, who provided me with this opportunity, and to Dana Battaglia, whose project management skills, openness to ideas, and editorial prowess was instrumental to my progress.

This work would not be completed were it not for the hard work and constant support of Wendy Taylor, a long-time colleague and friend.

My deepest gratitude goes to my husband Mike and children Christine, Ryan, and Jenee for sharing their precious gifts of time, humor, and love. You are each remarkable and talented individuals who enrich the lives of others around you.

REVIEWERS

Amy G. Bigus

Lucy W. Chaio

Nancy Kawahara

Eric C. Kutscher

Miriam Mobley-Smith

Developing Clinical Practice Skills for Pharmacists
Continuing Education Program

How to Earn Continuing Pharmacy Education (CE) Credit

To obtain continuing pharmacy education (CE) credit for this program, **Developing Clinical Practice Skills for Pharmacists ACPE Program Number: 204-000-05-089-H01**, you must successfully pass the online test on the ASHP CE Testing Center at http://www.ashp.org/ce/homepage.cfm. If you score 70% or higher, you will be able to immediately print your CE statement. You will have two opportunities to pass the CE test. Also you can start, save, and exit the test at any time and be able to return to submit your final answers.

Use your 8-digit ASHP Member/Customer ID to log on (be sure to include any leading zeroes). Your member/ Customer ID can be found on your membership card or on the mailing label of your copy of *AJHP*. To log on, click on "Enter the CE Testing Center" and type your ID number and password. Follow the instructions (below) to pay the CE Exam Processing Fee and also to select the CE test for **Developing Clinical Practice Skills for Pharmacists.**

If you are not an ASHP member or don't have a customer ID, you have two options to get one:
- Click on the link to obtain an ASHP Customer ID at http://www.ashp.org/ce/homepage.cfm
- Make a purchase at our shopping cart https://shop.ashp.org/timssnet/products/tnt_showprdsplash.cfm. An ASHP Customer ID and password would automatically be created for you.

Cannot remember your password?

Click on the "forgot password" link at http://www.ashp.org/ce/homepage.cfm

Program Title: Developing Clinical Practice Skills for Pharmacists
ACPE Program # 204-000-05-089-H01
CE credit: 14 hours (1.4 CEUs)

CE Exam Processing Fee: There is a nominal fee to access the test on the CE testing center. The fee for ASHP members is $20.95, and for non-ASHP members it is $30.95.

Go the ASHP Shopping Cart (http://shop.ashp.org/timssnet/products/tnt_showprdsplash.cfm) and select "Continuing Education." Click on "Add to Cart" icon and checkout. You can access the CE Testing Center immediately after your purchase to begin to take the CE test.

Questions: Call ASHP Customer Service Center toll free at (866) 279-0681.

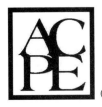

The American Society of Health-System Pharmacists is accredited by the Accreditation Council for Pharmacy Education as a provider for continuing pharmacy education.

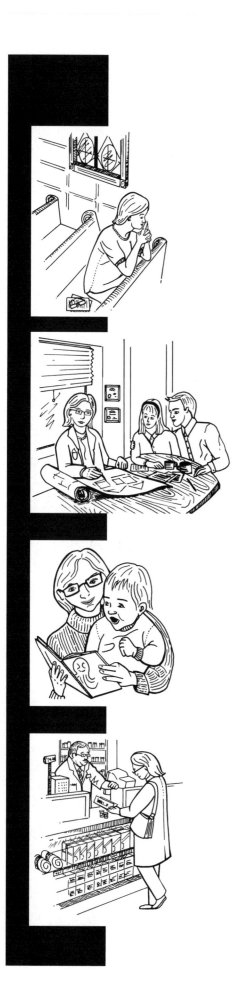

CHAPTER 1

The Patient

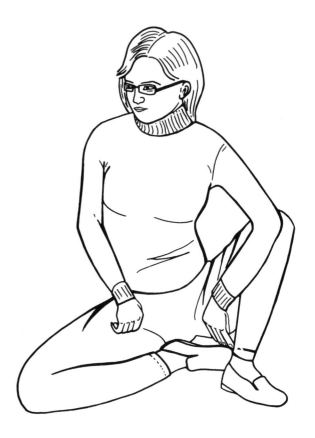

*"Kindness is a language which the deaf can
hear and the blind can see."*

Anon

Chapter Outline:

- ❖ The Patient
- ❖ The Patient as a Person
- ❖ The Patient's Concept of Health
  Conceptual Factors
    Cultural Influences
    Values and Beliefs
    –The Health Beliefs Model
    –Patient Relationships

Medication Use
–Health Behavior
Types of Patients
- ❖ The Patient–Pharmacist Relationship
  Expertise and Trust
  Understanding the Pharmacist as Healer
  Understanding the Pharmacist as Merchandiser

Objectives / To gain knowledge of:

1. the patient as a person;
2. health and illness from the patient's perspective;
3. the importance of the person's values, preferences, and beliefs about health and the care he or she desires or needs;
4. the imperative to provide care, either directly or as an advocate, that is consistent with the patient's values, preferences, and beliefs;
5. the need to be sensitive to the patient's community and culture; and
6. the importance of addressing the special needs of some patients who can be considered part of a special population (e.g., pediatric, geriatric).

Purpose: The purpose of this chapter is to assist you in developing a concept of the patient that is personal, rich, and human. Your understanding must be in the context of the patient's life and how he or she experiences it. From this perspective, clinical skills development will be taught. You will be introduced to four patients in this chapter. Their lives will be followed as we explain the concepts and skills applications important for your development as an expert pharmacist.

THE PATIENT

I once cared for a man who was 79 years old. He was frail, quiet, and solemn; he rarely smiled. His family made him come to the clinic. He had difficulty with his medication management. The last time he skipped his digoxin, his atrial fibrillation became worse and he wound up in the hospital. After three visits, the physicians who evaluated him decided he was not mentally competent. As the clinical pharmacist, I was asked to "get his medications in order." We talked. At first we talked about his medications. I talked, and I learned little. Then I asked him what he liked to do. He assessed me with a keen look—the first engaging look I'd seen. He decided that I really wanted to know. He spoke of his painting, sculpture, and ceramics. Of his love for Native American art. Eventually he told me that he felt he was a burden to his son.

He stopped taking his medications because he thought it was time to let nature take its course. We talked about his medications again. This time he told me all about them, and I listened. He knew what each one was, what it was for, and how he was supposed to take it. He told me that he knew they were giving him a test (MMSE—mini-mental status exam) to see if his brain worked fine. "I know how to make it look the way they want," he said. I administered the MMSE to him again, and he scored a 29 out of 30. He agreed to let his son and physician come in and talk.

Kim Galt, 1994

THE PATIENT AS A PERSON

Who is this person who comes to you as a patient? What does this person want? What does this person need? We must understand the patient as someone who possesses certain strengths, vulnerabilities, preferences, worries and fears, hopes and joys. By virtue of our humanity, we possess the same fundamental dignity and value as any other human being. It is this viewpoint that is needed to serve all patients.[1] The patient is the central reason for your work and the only reason for a health profession.

Our values, beliefs, attitudes, and concepts define us as people. These things create our frame of reference about how we approach life and the world around us. This critical frame determines the patients' beliefs about their health and health-related needs. You, as a pharmacist, provide services and care that the patient perceives as wanted or needed. This understanding also frames the context for the remainder of the work you will do as a pharmacist. **Figure 1-1** shows a model for understanding the patient in the context of having a personal health concept. Whenever we refer to the patient in this book, this model will serve as the conceptual frame.

THE PATIENT'S CONCEPT OF HEALTH

Let's begin by understanding the ways that health professionals and patients conceptualize health. Health thinking, from the health professions' perspective, has historically been based on a disease concept founded in the traditional biomedical model (see *Glossary*). Disease is described in terms of negative symptoms combined with the directly related physical pathology that causes those symptoms. In this model, the concept of health is represented by "the absence of disease."[2]

Patients, on the other hand, come to us with a diverse set of concepts, ideas, beliefs, and values about what health is and what it means. Many patients understand their health in a way that is considered consistent with Western medicine where body, mind, cognition, emotion, and spirituality are seen as discrete

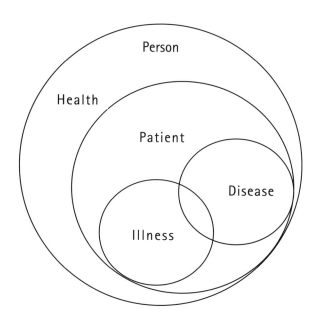

Figure 1-1. The Patient: A Health Context

entities. In contrast, they may also participate in Eastern philosophies of Buddhism, Taoism, or traditional Chinese medicine. These philosophies adopt a holistic conceptualization of an individual and his or her environment. In this view, health is a body–mind–spirit concept perceived as a harmonious equilibrium that exists between the interplay of "yin" and "yang."[3] Several traditions are practiced within our communities, such as Chinese herbal medicine, indigenous North American medicine, and chiropractic, acupuncture, homeopathy, and naturopathic medicine. The same patients who use these alternative approaches also participate in the mainstream Western philosophies. Although we as health professionals may attempt to provide professional care within a singular primary model of health, patients may find no need to actually choose among models. They sometimes participate in multiple, seemingly inconsistent, health care models.

Differences in these understandings of health have led to a broader examination of the concept and its possible meanings. For example, one shift in recent years included the concepts of functionality and well-being in the overall concept of health. Historically, Western measures of health did not include a patient's perception of well-being. Measures of health are changing today to reflect this shift. Increasingly, we see writings about recognition of 1) diversity, 2) the value of the whole person and the richness of life, 3) broad concern about the person, and 4) the need for inclusion of spirituality.

Given the breadth of patients' beliefs and behaviors, why try to have a health model defined at all? Models help *us* frame our ability to serve the needs of patients by proscribing a context to the care they seek and we provide. Models help us behaviorally define *our* actions to be consistent with the beliefs and expectations consistent with the models that represent our patients' expectations. Recently, a review describing four prominent models for defining health was published (see **Table 1-1**). Not all concepts of health are represented to our satisfaction. However, these models recognize the various ways in which patients define health. If we know the model that best fits a patient, we can offer professional care that meets those needs and acknowledge the influences that modify one's expectations of care.

Conceptual Factors

How do you know what concept the patient has of health? Each of us has our own concept, but it is formed by many factors. Let's briefly examine factors that may influence one's concept of health. In future chapters, we will practice the skills needed to solicit and understand the patient's health concept.

Cultural Influences[4,5]

Culture is described as a property of society.[4] There is no such thing as a pure culture, because there is diversity, often recognizable as subcultures. Within a

Table 1-1. Models of Health

Health Model Definitions[15]	Your Model	Your Patient's Model	Organization Model
Medical Model: *The absence of disease or disability.*			
World Health Organization Model: *State of complete physical, mental, and social well-being and not merely the absence of disease or infirmity.*			
Wellness Model: *Health promotion and progress toward higher functioning, energy, comfort, and integration of mind, body, and spirit.*			
Environmental Model: *Adaptation to physical and social surroundings: a balance free from undue pain, discomfort, or disability.*			

large ethnic group, substantial variation may exist in education, socioeconomic status, and practiced religions. America continues to become a more ethnically diverse population. Currently, 74% of the population is Caucasian. This percentage is expected to decrease to 64% by 2010. Asians will represent 5%, African Americans 13%, and Hispanics 15%. The population's average age is rising, with female life expectancy averaging 86 years and male life expectancy averaging 76 years by 2010. By 2005, 55% of the U.S. population over 25 years of age will have the equivalent of one year of college. Access to care will continue to be segregated into three identifiable groups: 1) empowered consumers who have resources, use technology, and want to share in health decisionmaking; 2) worried consumers who have health insurance but no choice in plan; and 3) people who are excluded because they have no form of health insurance or method of payment other than out of pocket.[5]

Pharmacists should view health and illness from the patient's perspective. How can we understand a person's culture in a way that helps to meet his or her health care goals and needs? One way is to learn the values and attitudes considered important enough to pass down from one generation to the next. Understanding a patient's cultural view of illness will be helpful in meeting the person's needs.

This approach requires a reasonable understanding of the culture as a whole before you can confidently apply this knowledge. In your initial assessment of an African American woman, you may automatically assume she is from the United States. As you begin to listen to her, you may realize that her dialect resembles a British accent. One of her cultural frames is actually from an area in Britain. You realize that you were applying your own cultural bias over hers.

This example illustrates the problem of ethnocentricity or the interpretation of one culture using the norms of another, usually your own. It may cause you to make errors in interpreting what a patient means. It may also cause you to communicate information that is misleading to the patient because he or she interprets the meaning one way and you deliver it with a different intention. Understanding another person through critical cultural norms unique to that person's community is important. Competence in cultural interpretation matters and is certainly true of health beliefs that dominate cultures. To illustrate this point, examples of health beliefs in two common cultures are provided.

Latinos will represent the second largest segment of the U.S. population by 2025. Research on 189 Latino cultures around the world has demonstrated all but four have a cultural belief that illness is caused by supernatural or spiritual agents.[6-8] Illness among Latinos appears to be influenced by moral and religious implications. It is also common to find that Latinos use folk healing. As Latinos integrate into U.S.

cultures, their emphasis on these beliefs weakens but is never entirely gone.

People of Vietnamese descent are our fastest growing population within the Asian/Pacific Islander population. One strong cultural belief is the profound respect for authority, leading individuals to not question health care providers. Another belief is avoidance of promoting one's self, making it difficult for some Vietnamese to acknowledge their pain or suffering. This belief results in delays in seeking care. A common practice of this culture is to use traditional and Chinese medicines (**Figure 1-2**).[9]

There is a great deal to know about the cultural context of the patients you serve. Health professionals should become culturally competent through the ongoing process of integrating cultural awareness, knowledge, skill, encounters, and desire. Campinha-Bacote described this model of cultural competence in health care delivery as a framework for developing and implementing culturally responsive care.[10] The model assumes that cultural competence is a process, not an event. It recognizes that there is more variation within ethnic groups than across groups. It assumes that the provision of culturally responsive care is directly related to the health professionals' level of cultural

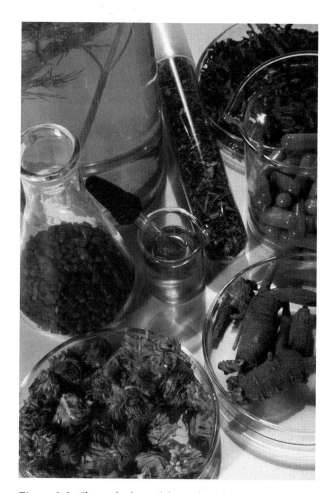

Figure 1-2. Chinese herbs used for medicinal purposes.

competence in the context of each patient. The model defines the concept as follows:

1. Cultural awareness is the self-understanding of one's own cultural and professional background.
2. Cultural knowledge is the process of seeking and obtaining an educational foundation about different cultural and ethnic groups.
3. Cultural skill is described as the ability to collect relevant cultural data about the patient's problem as well as performing a culturally based physical assessment.
4. Cultural encounter involves the health professional engaging in cross-cultural interactions with individuals from diverse backgrounds. This interaction is almost impossible when the patient and health provider speak different languages, the patient has a limited English proficiency, the patient is speaking from a different perspective, or the provider has a limited proficiency in the patient's language. Occasionally, cultural tradition may preclude a patient speaking directly to a provider. For these reasons, an interpreter is sometimes needed.[11]
5. Cultural desire is the motivation of the health care provider to engage in the process of culturally responsive care.

A culturally competent pharmacist will consciously adapt care for the patient in a way that is consistent with the patient's need from the context of a cultural framework.[12] How does one become culturally competent? One way is to live within the group. For most people, this is not a realistic approach. Alternatively, learning can be accomplished through reading, convening focus groups, and participating in community activities. It is most important to remain open to learning from the patient what is culturally important and relevant.[13] Cultural competence is the discovery of the way in which a health care provider can move a relationship with the patient from parallel to mutual through increasing the provider's knowledge, skills, and understanding.[14]

Values and Beliefs

The Health Beliefs Model

To fully serve the person as a patient, you must understand his or her values and beliefs in relationship to the person's concept of health. It is a common theme in health profession literature to highlight the difference between the professional's understanding of the patient's disease and the patient's interpretation of feeling unwell. In this distinction, we see the patient's need for more than a scientific formulation and treatment of problems. Patients generally want to feel understood and valued and to be involved in making sense of their health problems. Additionally, many patients want to be involved in decisions about care management.

A common model for understanding this phenomenon is the health beliefs model (**Figure 1-3**).[15] It explains specific factors that may increase the likeli-

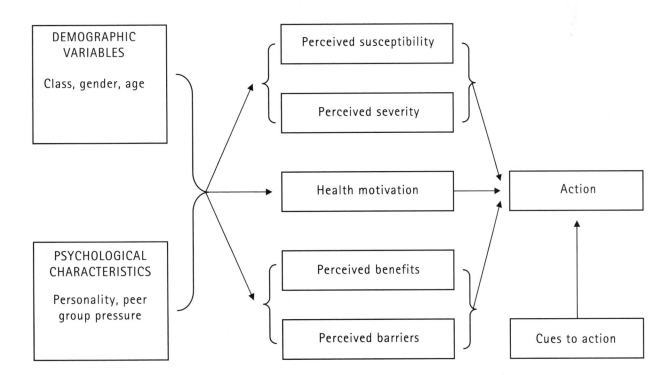

Figure 1-3. Health Beliefs Model

hood of a person taking action to try to positively affect his or her health. Individual factors include perceived susceptibility to illness; perceived seriousness of illness; perceived barriers to action; and perceived benefits of action, motivation, and self-efficacy. Modifying factors include past personal and family experiences, information and advice from family and friends, age, knowledge, fitness levels, and the external influence of the media. The person intuitively decides if he or she is ready to take the health action perceived as necessary by weighing its costs and benefits. Moreover, the model recognizes that a person will finally act when a cue of some type occurs—usually a profound negative event (e.g., stroke after uncontrolled hypertension, hospitalization after uncontrolled hyperglycemia secondary to uncontrolled diabetes). This model has proven to be a practical representation of patient beliefs and holds up to both cultural variation and differing definitions of health.

Patient Relationships

You also need to know who other decisionmakers are in relationship to your patient. A spouse may actually be the decisionmaker in care or may have great influence. A patient may make decisions through the family members as a unit. Both of these relationships are observed as routine in some cultures. The patient may have a caregiver, either voluntarily from relatives, friends, and neighbors, or formally through the health system. Finally, other people important to the patient may play a role in influencing him or her.

Medication Use

What does this person believe about the use of medication as a form of treatment? Many studies indicate that perceptions of the role of medication use are highly varied—as varied as the characteristics that affect concepts of health. Multiple studies have shown that patients from different ethnic and cultural backgrounds use alternative medicines or home remedies, while also participating in a formal health care system approach.[16–18] Your knowledge of the patient's beliefs and his or her evaluations of treatment options should be considered when developing therapeutic plans and monitoring patient outcomes.

Health Behavior

Health-relevant behavior and attitudes are products of culture and are viewed in the overall cultural context in which they occur. Fundamental to this new paradigm of practice is understanding behavior, its relationship to health, and methods by which it can be altered. Current concepts of health behavior have been heavily influenced by social learning theory, self-efficacy theory, and a biopsychosocial view of health and disease. The way that patients behave in relation-

ship to treatment depends on a complex interplay of many psychological, social, and environmental variables. To assist them in reaching their goals, you must understand how behavioral techniques may be used.[19] Patients with less positive health practices are more likely to be health illiterate.[20] Furthermore, the stronger a person's perceived capability to carry out behavior, the more successful he or she is in doing so.[21]

In recent years, self-care has become a prominent aspect of patient behavior. Self-care may sometimes be observed as an individual taking responsibility for both identifying one's problem and determining the preferred treatment. The over-the-counter product market is one example where a person can, without ever consulting a health professional, self-diagnose and treat. The range of self-care products is broad and varied, including such things as herbal remedies, neutraceuticals, vitamins, minerals, and other dietary supplements.

The concept of self-care extends to patients in hospitals. A recent study showed that 90% of hospital pharmacy departments allowed "own use" medications to be brought in by patients.[22] Prior literature has shown that between 35 and 64% of patients bring their own medications to the hospital, averaging three medications per patient.[23,24] Patients often do so to reduce anxiety and loss of self-control while being hospitalized.[25]

Individuals also "self-help" by identifying with self-help groups (e.g., Alcoholics Anonymous). These groups offer people both emotional support and practical advice about a common problem they share. The groups are almost always member run, voluntary, and fairly inexpensive. An estimated 15 million Americans are members of self-help groups, which often lead patients to seek health information. With 70,000+ web sites disseminating health information, more than 50 million people are seeking health information online. Online information is frequently inaccurate, and people in general have poor information-evaluation skills. However, the fact that 50 million people use the Internet for this purpose illustrates the potential of the source as part of a larger health communication system. An investigation and understanding of the Internet's influence on health beliefs and behaviors is needed.[26] As a pharmacist, you are in a unique position to be accessible to the public yet have a high degree of expertise. Patients will seek you out to verify the accuracy of health information and obtain your advice.

Types of Patients

To optimally care for a patient, you need to determine what type of "patient" the patient is. Your goal should be to recognize and respect the patient's autonomy and support him or her in the determination of needs.[27] In this context, you might view the patient as coming from three different possible points of view:

- *The patient as a consumer.* The patient views you (the professional) as a competitor who has something he or she wants or needs, but views you as willing to give as little as possible for the most amount of money. In this case, the consumer shops around for the commodity (i.e., health care services, pharmaceuticals).
- *The patient who is dominated by the professional.* The patient views him- or herself as powerless in decisionmaking and hands over in a highly dependent way the decisions to be made to you (the health professional).
- *The patient as autonomous and interdependent with the professional.* The patient views him- or herself as vulnerable and seeks care in an interdependent fashion. The patient wants to trust the professional's expertise. However, he or she wants to participate in, rather than hand over, decisions to the professional.

As a pharmacist, you will encounter all three types of patients. Understanding them can help you to determine how to best meet their needs. Your professional responsibility remains the same in all three cases. The way you meet your responsibility will vary.

THE PATIENT–PHARMACIST RELATIONSHIP

Does the patient have a concept of the pharmacist as a care provider?

Expertise and Trust[28,29]

Some research suggests that from a patient perspective, pharmacist expertise is the main factor necessary for establishing quality relationships between pharmacists and patients. Also, mutual disclosure is critical for building trust in pharmacist–patient relationships. In a study of 200 patients who came to the pharmacist for prescriptions, 80% expressed the importance of confidence (professional trust), while only 58% thought that knowing and liking (personal trust) the pharmacist was important in their selection of a pharmacy. For a nonprescription remedy, 72% stated they would accept the pharmacist's advice. For prescription medication, 57% were willing to accept advice. A strong interrelationship exists between personal and professional trust in both selecting a pharmacy and accepting advice from a pharmacist.

Understanding the Pharmacist as Healer

Some patients view you as a healer. Pharmacists occupy a specialized community role, holding the social status as a healer by the use of medications as treatments. Pharmacists are recognized as experts who hold the capacity to cure as well as harm. In general, as with other healers, the pharmacist is a trusted and respected member of the community. This status is granted by patients who give the pharmacist this power. When a patient seeks a pharmacist for advice, he or she is placing trust in the intention and skill of the pharmacist. Many patients understand the pharmacist has knowledge that is specialized for this purpose. For the patient who invests in relationships, a hand hold or touch to the forearm has meaning from you as a healer, every bit as much as the medications you dispense, monitor, and educate about.[30]

Understanding the Pharmacist as Merchandiser

Some patients may view you as a merchandiser, recommending a drug product from the point of view of sales. The 2001 National Pharmacy Consumer Survey found that 30% of patients view pharmacists as their first choice for information regarding medications, and only 4% view pharmacists as their first choice for information regarding diseases.[31] These results suggest that individuals may have pre-formed ideas about the role and value of a pharmacist without ever having a direct experience with a pharmacist. A patient's perception of the pharmacist is formed by interacting with you. To change perceptions, you must change the patients' experiences by helping them realize all of the health care value you can provide.

Patients usually come to pharmacists to receive services, products, and/or care. It is usually their choice. However, as illness progresses or acute events require intervention, the patient's choices become limited. When patients come to the hospital to get care, they don't choose you. You are assigned or provided. Similarly, when patients are referred to home care services or long-term facilities, pharmacist services are assigned. As choice is eliminated, the patient becomes more dependent on the pharmacist's attributes as a care provider who advocates for patient needs.

SUMMARY

The patient is a unique individual who brings the influences of culture, ethnicity, education, socioeconomics, spirituality, family and friends, values, beliefs, and attitudes. As we consider how to give care, we must establish a knowledge of our patient as a person with a full life whose care includes management of illness. We will label this knowledge as the Patient Database, listing in detail all of the components in **Table 1-2**. The database consists of both what the patient tells us through our interactions and basic information needed to provide care on his or her behalf. We will refer to this Patient Database throughout the remainder of the book.

Table 1-2. Pharmacist's Patient Database Model

Demographic	Behavioral/Lifestyle	Administrative
Name	*Health beliefs*	*Physicians/prescribers*
Address	*Concepts of Illness*	*Other health providers sought by*
Date of birth	*Diet*	*patient*
Gender	*Exercise/recreation*	*Pharmacist(s)/pharmacy(ies)*
Religion and religious affiliation	*Tobacco/alcohol/caffeine/ substance use*	*Room/bed numbers (hospital/long-term*
Occupation	*Sexual history/orientation*	*care)*
	Personality type	*Consent forms*
Social/Economic	*Daily activities*	*Patient identification number*
Social history		
Family members	**Medical**	**Drug Therapy**
Significant relationships with others	*Family history*	*Prescribed medications*
Living arrangement	*Genetic history*	*Nonprescription medications*
Ethnic background	*Acute/chronic medical problems*	*Medications prior to admission (if*
Cultural influences	*Current symptoms*	*hospitalized/long-term care)*
Primary language/secondary language	*Vital signs/other bedside monitoring*	*Home remedies/folk remedies/herbal*
Financial/insurance	*information*	*products/other types of health*
	Allergies/intolerances	*products*
	Past medical history	*Medication regimen*
	Laboratory information	*Adherence with therapy regimen*
	Diagnostic/surgical procedures	*Medication allergies/intolerances*
		Concerns or questions on therapy
		Assessment of understanding of therapy
		Pertinent health beliefs

Modified from Mason NA and Shimp LA. The pharmacist's patient information needs. In: Mason NA and Shimp LA. Building a pharmacist's patient database, module 2. Bethesda, MD: American Society of Hospital Pharmacists, Inc.; 1993:7.

INTRODUCTION TO FOUR PATIENTS' CASES

We will follow the lives of four patients and four pharmacists throughout this book as they work together in a pharmacy practice setting related to the patients' care needs. Let's meet the patients:

Patient 1—Lauren Smith

Ms. Lauren Smith is a 23-year-old Caucasian woman who seems too angry for her young age. She is from a privileged socioeconomic neighborhood just outside of Detroit, Michigan. She completed college to be an interior designer, with a minor degree in fine arts. Ms. Smith grew up with an unlimited amount of spending money, as her generous parents were two people who became successful business owners feeling that they should "give the children everything they never had."

Lauren was raised with a Lutheran upbringing, but she dropped any involvement in a church when she started college, telling her friends that "she wasn't sure she believed in a superior being." She is living in her own apartment, first year paid by her parents. Most of her social life is centered on some college friends. She has a varied cultural background, mostly a mixture of Irish, Polish, and German descent—a third generation American. Employment is a challenge for Lauren, as she tells her parents "she just hasn't found quite the right job yet … she is getting around to it." Her parents continue to pay for her medical insurance and any additional expenses incurred. She avoids doctors, and mostly treats her own illnesses by shopping for over-the-counter products if she thinks she needs them. We will get to know Lauren's other health issues a little later.

Patient 2—Eduardo Montanez

Mr. Eduardo Montanez is a 68-year-old Latin American man originally from Matamoros, Mexico. He moved to San Antonio, Texas, 5 years ago because his son, daughter-in-law, and their five children wanted to take care of him. He has limited English skills but is able to navigate his way reasonably well. His son is a schoolteacher and has excellent health benefits. Mr. Montanez is a dependent; therefore, he is eligible to receive the full benefit of his son's health insurance plan.

All of his life, Mr. Montanez has been a deeply religious person. He was raised in the Catholic Church and went to a Catholic school in Mexico. His mother raised him to believe in the church as a spiritual basis for everything in his life. He also has traditional Mexican beliefs about the spiritual nature of illness. Mr.

Montanez believes that any illness he develops is related to a failing or wrongdoing on his part. He was raised with folk medicines administered by his mother and spiritual healers. We will hear more about his condition later.

Patient 3—Huong Tran

Huong is an 8-year-old Vietnamese boy who arrived in the United States 4 years ago with his mother and father. He speaks English well; however, his mother and father are quite limited in their command of the language. Huong attends public school in Omaha, Nebraska. He is doing very well with all of his subjects. His schoolteacher and a friend in his neighborhood help him to learn his lessons because his parents are not able to correctly interpret the assignments in English. Huong interprets for his parents when they do life chores, such as purchasing items at the hardware or grocery store. He is their "window" to the English-speaking world. His parents frequent a shop that sells Chinese medicines.

Patient 4—Samuel Robinson

Mr. Samuel Robinson is a 76-year-old African American male who has resided in Biloxi, Mississippi, since he was 12 years old. He and his wife, Georgia, were married for 40 years. Georgia died 1 year ago. He is having a difficult time keeping his life in order now that he lives alone. He has always been a self-sufficient man. However, Mr. Robinson had a deep love and interdependency with Georgia, as did she with him. She would prepare remedies when he did not feel well, exchanging and discussing several of the traditional comfort remedies with her friends. These remedies were not written down anywhere, and Mr. Robinson cannot help himself with it. He finds this discomforting. Georgia frequented a pharmacist in town regularly. She took care of her husband's needs with the pharmacist as far as he was concerned. Now he is forgetful and often distracted. Mr. Robinson attended Baptist church with his wife. He has only gone to church twice since she died—at her funeral and at the six-month anniversary of her death.

Mr. Robinson is on Medicare, his only form of health insurance coverage. He retired from being a farm worker 9 years ago with a very small pension and no supplementary health coverage. He has several health problems that will be presented a little later.

CASE-SPECIFIC QUESTIONS

Instructions: Complete the answer to each of the following questions.

1. Patient 1—Lauren Smith. Identify the health behavior that best describes Lauren's approach to health.

2. Patient 2—Eduardo Montanez. What challenges do Mr. Montanez's traditional Mexican culture pose to his participation in the U.S. health care system?

3. Patient 3—Huong Tran. Describe two cultural beliefs that Huong Tran's parents are likely to hold that will influence how he receives care in the future.

4. Patient 4—Samuel Robinson. What roles might the pharmacist who is familiar with Mr. Robinson's history play in his care, based on the history that is provided?

GENERAL ASSESSMENT QUESTIONS

1. How do health professionals and patients differ in their concepts of health?

2. Distinguish between "illness" and "disease."

3. What is ethnocentricity? Why is it a problem in clinical care?

4. Why is it important to understand the patient's health values and beliefs?

ASSIGNMENT

Instructions: Review the definitions of the models for health shown in Table 1-1. Use Table 1-1 to complete this assignment. Select the one that best represents your own health beliefs. Next, select the one that you think represents most patients' health beliefs likely to be in your care. Finally, if you work in a pharmacy setting, select the one that best represents the concept of health that prevails in that organization, as represented by organizational programs, services, and decisions about care provision. If you are working with other health professionals, discuss each other's perceptions about this matter. What do you think should be done to successfully provide care to the patient when there are differences among these models?

REFERENCES

1. Gormally L. Definitions of personhood: implications of the care of PVS patients. *Ethics and Medicine.* 1993; 9(3):44–8.

2. Woodhouse M. The concept of disease in alternative medicine, in eds. Humber JM, Almeder RF. What is disease? Humana Press Inc; 1997.

3. Chan C, Ho PS, Chow E. "A model in health: an Eastern approach." *Social Work and Health Care.* 2001; 34(3-4):261–82.

4. Sensky T. Eliciting lay beliefs across cultures: principles and methodology. *British Journal of Cancer.* 1996; 74:S63–5.

5. Institute for the future. Health and healthcare 2010—the forecast, the challenge. San Francisco, CA: Josey-Bass Publishers; 2000.

6. Murguia A, Zea MC, Reisen CA et al. The development of the cultural health attributions questionnaire (CHAQ). *Cultural Diversity and Ethnic Minority Psychology.* 2000; 6(3):268–83.

7. Garcia V. Hispanic health beliefs. *Texas Pharmacy.* 1999; Jul:14–5.

8. Williams DP, McPherson HA. Providing culturally sensitive care to Hispanic patients in Arkansas. *The Journal.* 2000; Jan (96):312–4.

9. Garcia V. Vietnamese health beliefs. *Texas-Pharmacy.* 1999; 118 (Jul):18–9.

10. Campinha-Bacote J. The process of cultural competence in the delivery of health services: a model of care. *Journal of Transcultural Nursing.* 2002; 13(3):181–4.

11. Enslein J, Tripp-Reimer T, Kelly LS et al. Interpreter facilitation for individuals with limited English proficiency. *Journal of Gerontological Nursing.* 2002; Jul:5–13.

12. Purnell L. The purnell model for cultural competence. *Journal of Transcultural Nursing.* 2002; 13(3):193–6.

13. Leonard B, Plotnikoff GA. Awareness: the heart of cultural competence. *AACN Clinical Issues.* 2000; 11(1):51–9.

14. Ehret D. Devising and nurturing effective cross-cultural relationships between patients and caregivers. *Patient Care Management.* 2001; 16(12):8–9.

15. Rosenstock IM. The health belief model and preventive health behavior. In: Becker MH, ed. The health belief model and personal health behavior. Thorofare, NJ: Charles B Slack Co.; 1974:27–59.

16. Johnson RE, Pope CR. Health status and social factors in nonprescribed drug use. *Medical Care.* 1983; 21(Feb): 225–33.

17. Brown CM, Segal R. Effects of health and treatment perceptions on the use of prescribed medication and home remedies among African American and white American hypertensives. *Social Science and Medicine.* 1996: 43(6):903–17.

18. Boyd EL, Taylor SD, Shimp LA et al. An assessment of home remedy use by African Americans. *Journal of the National Medical Association.* 2000; 92:341–53.

19. Kehoe WA, Katz RC. Health behaviors and pharmacotherapy. *Annals of Pharmacotherapy.* 1998 Oct; 32(10):1076–86.

20. Christensen AJ, Moran PJ, Wiebe JS. Assessment of irrational health beliefs: relation to health practices and medical regimen adherence. *Health Psychology.* 1999; (18)2:1969–76.

21. Aljasem LI, Peyrot M, Wissow L et al. The impact of barriers and self-efficacy on self-care behaviors in type 2 diabetes. *The Diabetes Educator.* 2001; 27(3): 393–404.

22. Norstrom PE, Brown CM. Use of patients' own medications in small hospitals. *Am J Health Syst Pharm.* 2002; 59:349–54.

23. Kostick J, Chidlow J, Plihal T. A program for controlling mediations through to the hospital by patients. *Am J Hosp Pharm.* 1973; 30:814–6.

24. Breau DJ, Nickerson AL. Utilizing home medication supplies for hospital patients. *Can J Hosp Pharm.* 1997; 50:224–8.

25. Hones L, Arthurs GJ, Sturman E. Self-medication in acute surgical wards. *J Clin Nurs.* 1996; 5:229–32.

26. Cline RJ, Haynes KM. Consumer health information seeking on the Internet: the state of the art. *Health-Educ-Res.* 2001 Dec; 16(6):671–92.

27. Ozar DT. Patients' autonomy: three models of the professional-lay relationship in medicine. In: theoretical medicine. D. Reidel Publishing Company; 1984:61–8.

28. Worley MM, Schommer JC. Relationship quality between pharmacists and patients. APhA-Annual-Meeting: 1996; 143(Mar):6.

29. Riley DA, Baldwin HJ. Confidence in the pharmacist and acceptance of the pharmacist's advice. *Contemp-Pharm-Pract.* 1980; 3(1):18–23.

30. Thorne S. Health belief systems in perspective. *Journal of Advanced Nursing.* 1998; 18:1931–41.

31. Stergachis A, Maine LL, Brown L. The 2001 National Pharmacy Consumer Survey. *J Am Pharm Assoc.* 2002; 42:568–76.

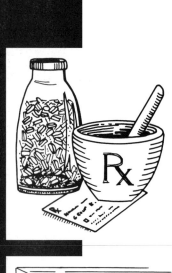

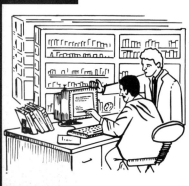

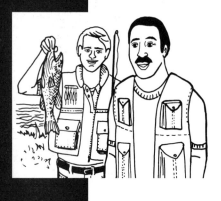

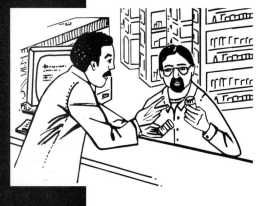

CHAPTER 2

The Pharmacist

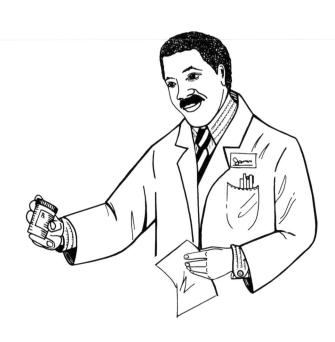

"Only an open heart will allow you to float equally between everyone."[1]

Chapter Outline:

Objectives / To be knowledgeable about:

1. how a philosophy of practice governs our professional life;

2. the influence of the pharmacy profession's culture on our ways of caring for patients;

3. our own values, the patient's values, and the structure-based values governing systems of health care for patients;

4. the foundation knowledge, skills, and behaviors for a patient-centered practice;

5. the skills of clinical reasoning: empathy, moral reasoning, and metacognition;

6. the roles of pharmacists as generalists and specialists;

7. the range of responsibilities pharmacists may perform in the medication-use process; and

8. expertise—the goal of a professional.

Purpose: The purpose of this chapter is to understand how pharmacists are influenced by their own values and practice skills development in relationship to patient needs and pharmacy practice. You should have a clear idea of how the pharmacist deals with the patient, his or her own employer, and society's expectations at large. This chapter describes what it means to be a pharmacist.

THE PHARMACIST

Pharmacists are defining what business they are in and want to be in during the years ahead. Pharmacists occupy many possible roles, including a caring health professional, pharmaceutical product formulator and compounder, dispenser, counselor, consultant, prescriber, merchant, and entrepreneur. The choices of "role" have continued to increase as we have moved into the twenty-first century.[2] In these various roles, how will you choose to conduct yourself towards patients?

To be a pharmacist who can fill these roles, as well as continually adapt to changes, you need to start with a basic framework for your own development. This framework is a solid foundation that includes a philosophy of practice, professional knowledge, skills, behaviors, and clinical reasoning. Governed by values and beliefs, this framework requires you to know your own values and beliefs that support this practice foundation. **Figure 2-1** shows a visual representation depicting the various components that construct "the pharmacist." This chapter emphasizes the importance of defining yourself as a pharmacy practitioner who is shaped and influenced by the components identified in this figure. *If you embrace your professional identity in this way, you will be able to make the right decisions in your professional development and future actions as a pharmacist.*

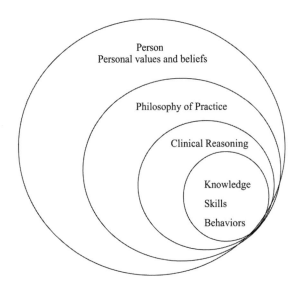

Figure 2-1. The Pharmacist: A Health Context

Pharmacy Practice

The Pharmacy Profession's Culture and Pharmaceutical Care

Literature from various disciplines has shown us that professions are advancing thoughtful models of health.[3] What is the pharmacy profession's position on health? The culture of pharmacy has chosen to adopt a patient-centered approach described in the definition of pharmaceutical care.

Definition of Pharmaceutical Care

Pharmaceutical care is the responsible provision of drug therapy for the purpose of achieving definite outcomes that improve a patient's quality of life. These outcomes are 1) cure of a disease, 2) elimination or reduction of a patient's symptomatology, 3) arresting or slowing a disease process, or 4) prevention of a disease or symptomatology.

Pharmaceutical care is a necessary element of health care that should be integrated with other elements. However, pharmaceutical care is provided for the direct benefit of the patient, and the pharmacist is responsible directly to the patient for the quality of that care. The fundamental relationship is a mutually beneficial exchange in which the patient grants authority to the provider and the provider gives competence and commitment (accepts responsibility) to the patient. The goals, processes, and relationships of pharmaceutical care exist regardless of practice setting.[4]

As part of pharmaceutical care, a pharmacist cooperates with a patient and other professionals in designing, implementing, and monitoring a therapeutic plan that will produce specific therapeutic outcomes for the patient. This, in turn, involves three major functions: 1) identifying potential and actual drug-related problems, 2) resolving actual drug-related problems, and 3) preventing potential drug-related problems.

Which model of health is most consistent with this definition? The definition of pharmaceutical care most closely matches the World Health Organization model (see Chapter 1); however, the outcomes identified in the definition are consistent with the biomedical model. In this sense, the definition is broader, but the outcomes expected are more limited than what a patient might anticipate and what you might expect to achieve with patients. As you advance in practice, you will find that these outcomes are core to your work. If you choose a patient-centered approach, you will relate to patients about how they perceive their illness and the beliefs that are influencing them. You will likely provide emotional comfort that generates a sense of security for the patient.

In a recent survey, pharmacy students were surveyed about which health model most closely matched their personal belief system.[5] The results are shown in **Figure 2-2**. These results illustrate that few of the profession's future pharmacists have a personal concept of health which is as narrow as that ascribed to by the traditional biomedical model. Experienced pharmacists were more likely to select the wellness model, which includes interpretation of the mind, body, and spirit in defining health. As you make patients central to directing their own care decisions, you will discover that the biomedical model is increasingly inadequate in describing the comprehensive care believed to be pharmacy practice. This model does not recognize comfort and well-being as health goals, even though they are paramount to what you will do as a pharmacist.

Patient-Centered versus Disease-Centered Care

Patient-centered care places the care plan development around the patient's concerns and needs. In contrast, disease-centered care focuses around the signs, symptoms, and outcomes of a particular disease and assesses how well the patient is progressing toward reduction of the disease impact or cure. Patients are not diseases, and their concerns are within a frame of illness and discomfort. No matter how hard you try, you can't assign a diagnostic label (e.g., ICD-9-CM code—see *Glossary*) to everything!

Common patient interview questions such as, "Hello Mr. Robeson, how is your asthma responding to the inhaler? And your blood sugar?," rather than, "Hello Mr. Robeson, how are you feeling today?," illustrate the point. If you are only concerned with the disease label, your patient will know it. In turn, the patient may not invest in you and the relationship you have to offer. The patient understands that you are not necessarily interested in his or her concerns, but, rather, progress with

regard to a particular condition. To provide care that addresses Mr. Robeson's concerns, you have to ask questions that indicate to him that you care about his needs as he perceives them. This approach does not suggest that specialized care programs are inappropriate. Nor does it suggest that specific questions about a patient's response to drug therapy are wrong. These questions are critical to understanding the drug response aspect to the patient's disease, and it is your job to ask them. The distinction is in the emphasis. If you only emphasize the disease, you missed the opportunity to respond to the patient's perceived needs. You must first find out about the patient's needs and then advocate for those needs to be addressed.

Patient-Centered versus Pharmaceuticals-Centered Care

In contrast to patient-centered care, pharmaceuticals-centered care focuses on dispensing or selecting and recommending the pharmaceutical for treatment. It pays no attention to the patient nor does it apply clinical reasoning skills or involve direct communication with the patient.

Pharmaceuticals can be dispensed in a patient-centered way. Patient-centered approaches include applying clinical reasoning skills at the time of evaluating the prescribed medications, compounding and dispensing the medications accurately for drug interactions, and communicating with the patient about purpose, expectations, proper use, and followup plans. The pharmacist is the expert on the product. Without a doubt, no one else has the same knowledge as the pharmacist about products. It is both critical and uniquely valuable that the pharmacist builds a practice philosophy around this point. However, the pharmacist who will help patients

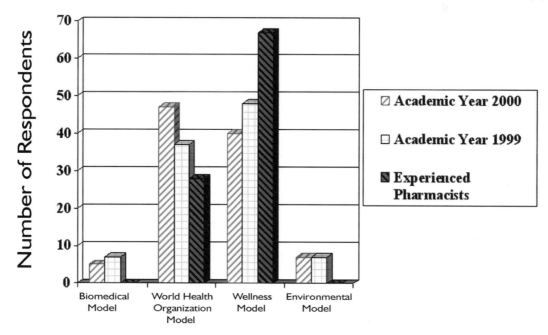

Figure 2-2. Health Models of First Professional Year Doctor of Pharmacy Students and Experienced Pharmacists (Adapted from Galt KA. The need to define care in pharmaceutical care: an examination across research, practice and education. Am J Pharm Educ. 2000; 64:223–33.)

make the best use of their medicines is one who provides patient-centered care with this expertise.

Types of Practice

Pharmacy Practice Related to Direct Patient Care

The numerous roles you occupy as a pharmacist that we describe as "practice" sometimes do not involve the direct interaction and involvement of a patient. For purposes of this book, the term *pharmacy practice* will specifically apply to the roles you have as a pharmacist that directly involve patients. You will use the philosophy, knowledge, skills, behavior, and clinical reasoning to be effective in all roles. However, the concept of practice in the clinical context means the direct care of patients.

To know the ways you can use your clinical skills, you must understand your role for its potential breadth and depth of responsibilities as well as the expertise required to meet them. Your practice will take on characteristics that likely classify you as a *general pharmacy practitioner* or as a *specialized pharmacy practitioner*.

General Pharmacy Practice

As a generalist, you are expected to have extensive knowledge about pharmaceuticals and treatments. Your role is to serve the varied and many—and respond to the multiple needs of patients quickly and simultaneously. In general, the practice responds "on demand." And, in this sense, it *is* demanding. Your scope of knowledge about pharmaceuticals and treatments is vast, and your ability to use drug information resources to continuously provide competent care must be well developed. The generalist represents most of us in practice. Examples of generalists include an inpatient hospital pharmacist, a community pharmacist, a nursing home consulting pharmacist, a home care pharmacist, or a clinical pharmacist.

Specialized Pharmacy Practice

As a specialist, you are expected to have depth about a narrower area of pharmaceuticals and treatments. Specialists are needed to serve those who have highly complex treatment needs. This complexity may be related to the clinical reasoning applied to product use, ongoing care processes related to product use, and/or complexity of product preparation, delivery, and administration. Examples of specialists include a hospital pharmacist whose primary focus is critical care, nutrition, or oncology. A pharmacist may run a specialty care clinic in anticoagulation, asthma, diabetes, or dyslipidemia in a health system or community pharmacy.

Role in the Medication-Use Process

The medication-use process starts from the time that a medication is determined as needed through the time that a patient has taken it and is being monitored for its effect on outcomes. The process is commonly described in five major steps: prescribing, preparation, dispensing, administering, and monitoring. Pharmacists accept direct responsibility for some or all aspects of the medication-use process and indirect responsibility for all steps. Pharmacists may accept responsibility for prescribing, either because state laws have designated a class of prescription drugs that pharmacists have authority to prescribe, or because the pharmacist has entered into a collaborative drug therapy management agreement and accepted delegated authority from a licensed prescriber.

Pharmacists also administer medication in all states unless prohibited by state law. Nationally, pharmacists administer oral, topical, and parenteral products, and in all practice settings.

Role of Dispensing

Both categories of practice may or may not involve the dispensing of pharmaceuticals, however, the majority of pharmacists' duties include dispensing as a basic responsibility. When dispensing takes place, it may be performed by the pharmacist or by a pharmacy technician or pharmacist intern directly under the supervision of a pharmacist. Functional models vary. In general, if your position is responsible for dispensing or its oversight, you have the broadest opportunities for care input, problem identification and resolution, problem prevention, and care delivery. If your position does not involve dispensing, then your ability to effect and implement changes to the care plan becomes one of recommending and following up (much like a quality assurance check).

Your primary role as a pharmacist is always to ensure patient safety first. It is a minimum practice in which you must engage. Patient safety related to medication use is a primary concern of our nation. Medication errors is in fact one of the most prominent health issues known today. Root causes of medication errors are usually in systems of care delivery.[6]

The first process step that takes place in the medication-use system is prescribing.[7] A 1992 study of 89 community pharmacists in five states documented the frequency and type of prescriber errors in the community setting.[8] The results revealed that for 1.9% of 33,011 new prescription orders, the pharmacists intervened to resolve a prescriber-related problem. Errors of omission, commission, and interactions accounted for 60.5% of these prescriber-related problems. Illegibility accounted for 6.4% of the errors identified. Expert evaluators concluded that 28.3% of the prescribing problems identified during the study could have caused patient harm if the pharmacist had not intervened to correct the problem.

Legibility of prescriptions is a widely recognized cause of medication errors.[9] Inability to correctly read a medication name, dose, or regimen has resulted in injuries and death. The issue is of such importance that the American Medical Association (AMA) studied the legal implications resulting from poor legibility of medication orders. The AMA publicly reported that misinterpretation of physician prescriptions was the second most prevalent and expensive malpractice claim listed on 90,000 malpractice claims filed over a 7-year period.[9] Through computer entry and printing, these errors can potentially be avoided. They resolve the difficulty of translating illegible orders and greatly reduce the need for duplication through transcription to enter information into the ambulatory care patient record.[10]

The increasing use of pharmaceuticals by our young adult population coupled with the concurrent increase in median population age will probably lead to rapid growth in pharmaceutical use. Our health care delivery systems need to improve to accommodate the demands that this will place on the pharmacists' expertise. One response will likely be to increase the use of pharmacy technicians in preparing, compounding, and dispensing. Pharmacy technicians are now organized as a group who seek training and certification to meet minimum standards of their profession. At your place of employment, you will be responsible for the direct supervision of these employees and for the accuracy and completeness of their work.

Collaborative Drug Therapy Management

The delegation of prescriptive authority to pharmacists has been successfully applied in acute care, long-term care, and ambulatory care settings. In public health and military settings, pharmacists have frequently been delegated prescriptive authority under protocol. This authority has been and continues to be a natural extension of the pharmacist's professional duties.

The professional pharmacy can be recognized as part of the solution to the three most significant problems in health care: escalating costs, insufficient access to medical care, and inconsistent quality of care. Pharmaceutical care provides several benefits, including the following: 1) patients receive care in drug therapy management from the most appropriate health professional, 2) efficiency of physician-directed care is enhanced by shifting appropriate drug therapy management functions to the pharmacist, and 3) more patients receive required medical services by increasing the amount of physician time available. Use of the pharmacist in this manner extends the availability of primary patient care service, enhances the overall quality of care, and is cost effective. In general, receiving delegated authority involves the following:

1. Authority granted to a pharmacist is delegated by a physician based upon the demonstrated knowledge and competence of the pharmacist;
2. Pharmacists and physicians voluntarily enter into professional arrangements resulting in prescriptive authority under protocol; and

3. The purpose of these arrangements is to improve the general public health by extending a higher quality of health care services to more patients than is currently available.

Health care services in which pharmacists' prescriptive authority under protocol is practiced demonstrate equivalent or higher levels of health care services and outcomes than when pharmacists were not involved in providing these services.[11,12] Prescriptive authority ranges from therapeutic interchange to complex functions such as initiating drug therapy, ordering laboratory tests, and performing physical assessments to determine a patient's response to therapy. Other examples include performing pharmacokinetic dosing consultation, modifying doses based on patient specific characteristics, writing discharge prescriptions, and authorizing medication refills. **Box 2-1** describes the usual arrangements for prescriptive authority privileges for a pharmacist.

The Pharmacist as Practitioner
Philosophy of Practice

Your philosophy of practice is your set of values and beliefs that determine the behaviors you demonstrate throughout your career. You will adopt a philosophy that transcends the many varied roles you will fill as a professional. What should your philosophy be?

> *"As the old man walked along the beach at dawn, he noticed a young man ahead of him picking up starfish and flinging them into the sea. Finally catching up with the youth, he asked him why he was doing this. The answer was that the stranded starfish would die if left in the morning sun. 'But the beach goes on for miles and there are millions of starfish,' countered the other. 'How can your effort make any difference?' The young man looked at the starfish in his hand and then threw it to safety and said, 'It makes a difference to this starfish.'"*
> —*Anonymous*

William Zellmer, one of our contemporary leaders in the profession of pharmacy, suggests that the life management advice of Steven Covey be followed. Covey recommends that we begin with the end in mind.[13] In other words, when you look back on your life as a pharmacist, what do you want to see and feel?[14] Will you adopt the three habits suggested to lead you down the road of being a fulfilled person in your chosen profession? The habits of being empathetic with your patients, making complex things simple enough to be effective for patients you serve, and caring enough to act on obvious things can make a difference for a patient.[14] Will you adopt a philosophy of caring, always having personal concern for the well-being of your patient?[5]

Box 2-1. Implementation of Prescriptive Authority

Implementation of prescriptive authority usually involves the following:

1. A protocol between the physician and the pharmacist which clearly defines the arrangement with respect to the delegated prescribing authority.
2. These protocols are generally readily retrievable from either of the parties involved in the arrangement. Individuals are generally not required to submit these protocols to any governing body for prior approval although this varies by state or practice setting.
3. Core elements of the protocol should include the following:
    a. a written statement specifying that prescriptive authority of the stated physician or physician group practice is delegated to the pharmacist(s);
    b. the prescribing activities that are delegated must be clear to both the physician(s) and pharmacist(s);
    c. the scope of practice for the pharmacist should be defined for each protocol;
    d. limits are identified beyond which the physician must be contacted in order for the pharmacist to proceed;
    e. procedures are clearly defined for documenting the pharmacist's practice decisions and care provided;
    f. a time limit for each protocol arrangement should exist, beyond which the protocol should be reviewed and revised, if necessary;
    g. a system should exist in which the physician and pharmacist periodically evaluate the quality of care provided to patients who are treated using the protocol treatment guidelines; and
    h. pharmacists must demonstrate and maintain knowledge and competence needed to meet appropriate standards of practice.

In general, the minimum qualifications of a pharmacist to practice prescriptive authority under protocol is a pharmacy license.

Personal Beliefs and Professional Judgments

All of your professional judgments are based on the beliefs and values held by you from a personal frame of reference. It is important to be aware of your own concept of health, your own values about what is appropriate and not appropriate with treatments, your own cultural beliefs, and your own beliefs about what your behaviors should be in response to a patient's needs. We all have boundaries that govern our beliefs and actions. Sometimes these boundaries conflict with the patient's own beliefs and needs. You may have ethical beliefs that conflict with the patient. In some circumstances, you may believe what the patient wants is wrong and you cannot participate in this aspect of care. If you have beliefs that prevent you from being able to serve a patient's preferences, you have a responsibility to inform the patient.

Identifying the Patient's Health Care Needs

Are you and the patient a good fit? Do you offer what the patient needs? For the patient's preferences to be incorporated into the delivery of care, he or she must be able to express preferences. Your role is to support the patient's concepts of health and his or her values and beliefs. As a pharmacist, you must be prepared to care and advocate for, to the best of your ability, people from diverse backgrounds. Within this context, you should determine the following:

*   Is the patient able to understand the information you provide about treatment?
*   Does the patient demonstrate the ability to appreciate how that information applies to his or her situation?
*   Does the patient have the ability to reason?
*   Does the patient have the ability to make a choice and express it?

You must ensure that the patient is able to act on his or her own behalf, to an optimal capacity, given circumstances that will allow. If the patient is not capable of any of these four items, then it is the pharmacist's responsibility to work with a representative (e.g., interpreter or proxy) to best serve that patient's needs.[15]

Clinical Practice Skills

In addition to both your practice philosophy and health beliefs, you will integrate a unique set of practice-based knowledge, skills, and behaviors with clinical reasoning to practice pharmaceutical care. The knowledge, skills, and behaviors may be described as follows: clinical assessment, drug information, communication, professional behavior, and caring behaviors. Clinical reasoning is built on three skills: empathy, moral reasoning, and metacognition. The practice of pharmaceutical care involves management of the medication-use process within a patient-centered approach. Let's briefly review each area.

Clinical Skills

Clinical Assessment

Pharmacy is built firmly on the concept of technical rationality.[16] This idea states that practitioners are primarily problem solvers who select technical ways to serve particular purposes. If you are a rigorous practitioner, you solve well-formed problems by applying theory and technique from systematic and scientifically derived knowledge. However, as you become oriented to the "fuzzy" problems of daily practice, you find that the problems you encounter are not well-formed but rather "messy indeterminate situations." It does not take long for novice practitioners to learn that they really don't know how to solve many problems they face in practice. They also learn quickly that defining the actual problem that needs to be solved is difficult and sometimes results in no clear resolution.[17] This book is designed to provide a systematic method to collect and assess the clinical information used to determine the patient's problems and health needs. With repetition and practice, you become proficient at "framing" the patient's problems, achieving concordance with your own professional viewpoint and the patient. (That's why it is called pharmacy practice!)

Drug Information

Today's pharmacists participate in all aspects of patient care. Comprehensive delivery of pharmaceutical care requires that you, as a pharmacist, provide and use accurate and pertinent information to recommend, design, and monitor therapeutic plans. A pharmacist who provides such information readily to patients and the health care team will be recognized for this expertise.

Requests for drug information are frequent and require rapid followup. Time constraints may prohibit referrals to drug information specialists. Furthermore, many organizations do not have such specialists. Therefore, the pharmacist who is directly responsible for the care of a patient must be skilled in drug information retrieval and evaluation.[18–20]

Communication

The pharmacist applies communication skills to interview patients, solicit information from other resources, counsel patients, and advise or consult with other health professionals.

Interaction between the pharmacist and patient must occur to ideally ensure that a relationship is established and maintained based on caring, trust, open communication, cooperation, and mutual decisionmaking. Similarly, the pharmacist must communicate with other health professionals to achieve optimal care for the patient. In this relationship, the pharmacist holds the patient's welfare paramount, maintains an appropriate attitude of caring for the patient's welfare, and uses all of his or her professional knowledge and skills on the patient's behalf. In exchange, the patient agrees to supply personal information and preferences and participate in the therapeutic plan. The pharmacist develops mechanisms to ensure that the patient has access to pharmaceutical care at all times.[5] Many hours may be spent in the process of filling prescriptions or supervising technical support to assist you with the process. This is an important function within the pharmaceutical care concept. Reviewing prescriptions, clarifying their appropri-

ateness, and discussing the patient's care needs in relationship to the medication is central to providing care.

Professional Behavior

Pharmacists are professionally socialized—a process of inculcating a profession's attitudes, values, and behaviors in an individual. The goal is to develop professionalism in all that a pharmacist does. Professionalism is a distinctive competence or an ability to provide a service that is valued by an individual as well as recognized by law and custom collectively.[21] Professional competence requires that the individual possesses skills based on technical and scientific information. This is the basis for expertise. Professional competence also requires that the individuals commit themselves to using their ability for the benefit of those they serve. This is the basis for trust. Finally, professional competence requires a commitment to colleagues to ensure that each individual in the profession meets its standards through self-monitoring and self-discipline.

Knowledge, skill, and beliefs displayed by a professional include

1. maintaining the knowledge and skills of a profession.
2. remaining committed to self-improvement of skills and knowledge.
3. holding a service orientation.
4. displaying pride in the profession.
5. treating the relationship with the patient as covenantal.
6. demonstrating creativity and innovation.
7. demonstrating a conscience and trustworthiness.
8. displaying accountability for the work performed.
9. demonstrating ethically sound decisionmaking.
10. leading.

Caring Behavior

One of your greatest challenges may be to balance patient care with the demanding responsibilities of drug information searching, retrieval, management, and technologies. Yes, caring is knowledge, expertise, and quality delivery of pharmacotherapy and pharmaceuticals. But caring is also interpersonal. Professional caring behaviors have the value of healing, comfort, giving, and social support for those patients who are open to it. The pharmacist must attain the skills listed below to be a professional capable of routinely incorporating these behaviors into practice. For many of your patients, achieving the patient's desired outcomes requires both. Skills and attributes needed by a pharmacist include

- Learning to know and care for self.
- Learning to care for others personally and professionally.

- Seeing others as persons.
- Becoming more accepting of others.
- Seeking help from others.
- Gaining confidence.
- Coping effectively with stress.
- Accepting self.
- Learning to empathize.
- Supporting and helping others.
- Commiting to the future.
- Displaying collegiality instead of competition.
- Treating people as unique individuals.
- Considering the whole picture.
- Being less judgmental.
- Valuing diversity.

In the *ASHP Statement on Pharmaceutical Care*, the following excerpt assists us in understanding that care means the context of pharmaceutical care.[22]

"**Care.** Central to the concept of care is caring, *a personal concern for the well being of another person.* Overall patient care consists of integrated domains of care including (among others) medical care, nursing care and pharmaceutical care. Health professionals in each of these disciplines possess unique expertise and must cooperate in the patient's overall care. At times, they share in the execution of the various types of care (including pharmaceutical care). To pharmaceutical care, however, *the pharmacist contributes unique knowledge and skills to ensure optimal outcomes from the use of medications.* At the heart of any type of patient care, there exists a one-to-one relationship between a caregiver and a patient. *In pharmaceutical care, the irreducible 'unit' of care is one pharmacist in a direct professional relationship with one patient.* In this relationship, the pharmacist provides care directly to the patient and for the benefit of the patient. The health and well being of the patient are paramount. *The pharmacist makes a direct, personal, caring commitment to the individual patient and acts in the patient's best interest.* The pharmacist cooperates directly with other professionals and the patient in designing, implementing, and monitoring a therapeutic plan intended to produce definite therapeutic outcomes that improve a patient's quality of life."

Other text in the statement helps us to better understand the depth and meaning of the term "care." Principal elements within the statement include medication-related, care, outcomes, quality of life, and responsibility.

A specific, purposeful definition for care has been examined extensively by the nursing profession. Jean Watson has developed a framework that has been the primary influence on nurses. This framework is entitled the Carative Factors of Watson and translates fluidly to the practice of pharmacy.[23,24] When caring for a patient,

these factors provide a values basis to the behaviors we choose to adopt. The factors are as follows:

1. Formation of a humanistic-altruistic system of values;
2. Instillation of faith-hope;
3. Cultivation of sensitivity to one's self and to others;
4. Development of a helping-trust relationship;
5. Promotion and acceptance of the expression of positive and negative feelings;
6. Systematic use of the scientific problemsolving method for decisionmaking;
7. Promotion of interpersonal teaching-learning;
8. Provision for a supportive, protective, and (or) corrective mental, physical, sociocultural, and spiritual environment;
9. Assistance with the gratification of human needs; and
10. Allowance of existential-phenomenological forces.

The major assumption underlying these factors is that caring can only be effectively demonstrated and practiced interpersonally. Caring itself consists of carative factors that result in the satisfaction of certain human needs. Effective caring promotes health and individual or family growth. Caring responses accept people not only as they are now but for what they may become. Furthermore, a caring environment offers the development of potential while allowing the person to choose the best action for him- or herself at a given time. Caring is more "healthogenic" than curing. The practice of caring integrates biophysical knowledge with knowledge of human behavior to generate or promote health and to provide ministrations to those who are ill. Therefore, a science of caring is complimentary to the science of curing. The practice of caring must be central to pharmacy.

To be good, caring must be directed at the right things. Pharmacists should concentrate on how we care about patients and the way we express care through professional actions. Models of health are important to understanding the extent to which caring behaviors should be incorporated into the training of pharmacists.[5]

Clinical Reasoning

Clinical reasoning refers to the problemsolving process that you employ with patient problems. Synonyms for the term clinical reasoning include "clinical problemsolving" or "the clinical scientific method." Barrows defines the clinical reasoning process as a dynamic, cyclic, reiterative process in which observation, analysis, synthesis, deduction, induction, hypothesis generation, hypothesis testing, inquiry-strategy design, and skills of examination are interrelated.[25] Important skills that support clinical reasoning include empathy, moral reasoning, and metacognition. A representation of the Clinical Reasoning Process is shown in **Figure 2-3**.

Empathy

At the core of caring behavior in the pharmacist patient relationship is empathy. Empathy is a reflexive understanding of patient and self.[26] In essence, the ability to empathize is to be able to put yourself in someone else's place, sometimes referred to as being able to "walk in someone else's shoes."

Moral Reasoning

Pharmacists who demonstrate the best clinical performance have high moral reasoning skills. A recent work provides an excellent discussion on the application of moral reasoning by pharmacists.[27] Moral reasoning skills are the processes an individual goes through to arrive at decisions. Kohlberg's stages of moral development (**Box 2-2**) describes moral reasoning in the context of development. Moral reasoning is a significant determinant of how pharmacists behave; pharmacists with higher moral reasoning skills demonstrate better clinical performance. Research has demonstrated that a person in the health professions who has more advanced moral reasoning skills will likely not be a poor clinical performer for patients. The idea of being inadequate as a caring professional is morally unacceptable. These individuals work at being competent and effective as a standard of practice behavior.[28,29]

Metacognition

Knowing intuitively is to have a direct understanding without reasoning. Metacognition refers to deliberation and reflection during problemsolving. It is the hallmark of an expert clinical reasoner.

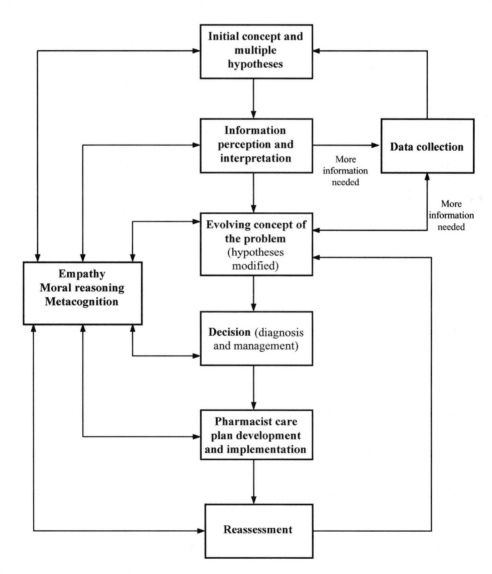

Figure 2-3. *Clinical Reasoning Process for Pharmacists (Adapted from Jones MA. Clinical reasoning in manual therapy. Phys Ther. 1992; 72:875–84.)*

Box 2-2. Kohlberg's Stages of Moral Development Complemented by Case Example

The following six stages of moral development are illustrated with a case example that might be observed in a routine pharmacy practice situation.

Stage 1: The morality of obedience – Do what you are told

Pharmacy example: John the pharmacist is instructed by his regional pharmacy manager to not counsel patients unless they ask today because it will slow down the prescription turnaround time. The pharmacist obeys.

Stage 2: The morality of instrumental egoism and simple exchange – Let's make a deal.

Pharmacy example: John likes to counsel and works out a shift in responsibilities for dispensing to the other pharmacist, Marsha, in order to do it.

Stage 3: The morality of interpersonal concordance – Be considerate, nice, and kind, and you'll make friends.

Pharmacy example: Marsha, the pharmacist who accepted the dispensing role, did it to have a good working relationship with John. She finds counseling rewarding.

Stage 4: The morality of law and duty to the social order – Everyone in society is obliged to and protected by the law.

Pharmacy example: John and Marsha begin to discuss the fact that they feel they are not meeting their responsibilities to their patients by the way they handled this.

Stage 5: The morality of consensus-building procedures. You are obligated by the arrangements that are agreed to by due process procedures.

Pharmacy example: They contact the regional manager to discuss their viewpoints and to seek support for patient counseling. They discuss the obligations in the profession and the oath they took. He does not change his position.

Stage 6: The morality of non-arbitrary social cooperation – Morality is defined by how rational and impartial people would ideally organize cooperation.

Pharmacy example: Marsha and John restructure the work of the technicians. Even though the tasks they have delegated to the technicians are not all legally supported in the state, they are safe based on their two years' employment experience. Both counsel patients.

Modified from: Rest JR and Narvaez D. Moral development in the professions: psychology and applied ethics. Hillsdale, NJ: Lawrence Erlbaum Associates; 1994.

Scope of Practice

Standards of practice represent a consensus of professional judgment, expert opinion, and documented evidence that become society's specific expectations of what a professional should perform. They represent the behaviors for which a professional is accountable. These standards help us by providing guidance and direction to pharmacy practitioners and to other audiences that affect pharmacy practice. Professional organizations often write standards of practice to help practitioners comply with federal and state laws and regulations, to meet accreditation requirements, and to improve pharmacy practice and patient care. They are usually written to establish reasonable goals that can be attained while still being progressive and challenging. They generally do not represent minimum levels of practice but rather what the profession has tacitly or formally agreed represents expectations to achieve.

Standards evolve to meet several needs. A primary reason is to meet a collective need among practitioners for authoritative advice. Another reason is to document the stability often based on sufficient experience that a standard is reasonable. Standards of practice develop because they are relevant to the practice of a significant portion of a profession's members.[30]

The scope of practice is the breadth of responsibilities to the boundaries of what a professional is allowed to do under the legally recognized authority granted. Scope of practice is defined by the practice act of the health professional, and it is interpreted in the context of the standards of practice for that profession. Each pharmacist has the same scope of practice based on the licensure status of the pharmacist. However, some have broadened scopes of practice through collaborative practice agreements with other providers.

Development of Expertise

Pharmacists want to be able to solve problems encountered in clinical practice, and patients want to be treated by health professionals who are highly competent and have a high level of expertise. What elements contribute to development of expertise? Agreement exists that certain factors, identified across professions, distinguish experts from novices. Experts perform complex tasks in their areas of expertise more accurately than novices and solve problems with greater ease. They have superior memory for information related to their area of expertise. Experts are better at perceiving patterns among the cues in their data gathering than are novices and they hold knowledge in a highly specific area, making it readily retrievable when needed.[6]

Experts are believed to have knowledge that is not the same as the knowledge taught in professional schools. The wise actions that professionals use involve practical knowledge. Practitioners add to a practical knowledge base not merely through experience but through a process of reflection. Professionals learn from experience by using reflective inquiry to think about what they are doing, what worked, and what did not work as they are doing it.

A representation model of expertise presented here incorporates elements of knowledge, skills, clinical reasoning, skill acquisition, and reflection similar to Sternberg's model of developing expertise (see **Figure 2-4**). Practical aspects to expertise development are discussed at greater length in a later chapter. The ultimate goal of a pharmacist should be to become expert as a patient-centered practitioner in all roles throughout one's professional career.[31]

Pharmaceutical Care Plan Development and Implementation

Care plan development and implementation are the "start with the end in mind" part of your work. The care plan is the application of your philosophy of practice, knowledge and skills, and clinical reasoning, integrated in a way that best serves the patient's need from the patient's point-of-view. The plan identifies 1) the patient's problems and illnesses, 2) the goals and outcomes expected, 3) care approaches to be implemented, 4) ways they are to be implemented, and 5) ways the patient will be monitored to determine if the needs are being met.

To achieve this, personal integrity in the relationship with the patient is essential. What you believe in must be matched by what you do. We know that empathy is important to being able to put oneself in another's situation. We must also understand that it is right to act on his or her behalf to do whatever we can to improve the person's situation. To achieve this, you may find that you need to involve as many caretakers as possible, when possible. Counsel to build the support structure around the patient while you provide pharmaceutical care.

The Patient–Pharmacist Relationship

Patients sometimes seek pharmacists for help, and sometimes are in highly dependent situations where a pharmacist is part of the health system the patient has entered. Independent of how the pharmacist comes to care for the patient, the patient-centered pharmacist will remain committed to following through with medication management.

The Therapeutic Relationship

There is healing power in the relationship between a health care provider and the patient. The greater emphasis on advanced diagnostic techniques and technologies has deemphasized the value of the therapeutic relationship, long known to the profession of medicine. Pharmacists can and do use their relationship to enhance the patients' therapeutic response to treatments and care. As we develop our relationships with patients, we should be cognizant of our power. An organized approach to the

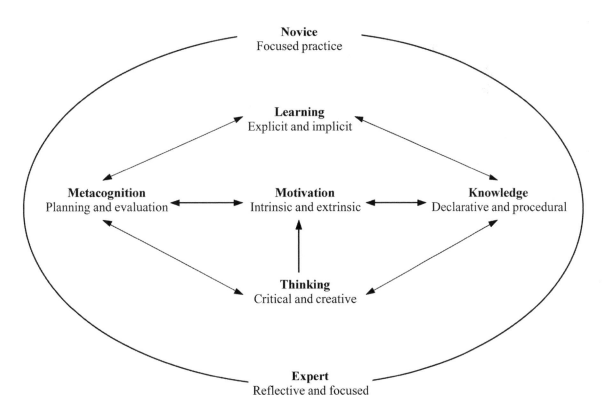

Figure 2-4. *Model of Developing Expertise (Adapted from Sternberg R. Abilities are forms of developing expertise. Educ Researcher. 1998; 28:11–20.)*

therapeutic aspects of the pharmacist–patient relationship should be integrated with the drug therapy evaluation to achieve optimal potential for patient healing. As we progress, we will incorporate learning about the therapeutic strategies that are commonly incorporated when a health care provider uses the therapeutic relationship to enhance patient healing.[32] Pharmacists must develop habits of thinking and acting that fully and accurately recognize the concerns of patients and that demonstrate the empathic commitment of pharmacists to patients.[33,34]

Role as Patient Advocate

Your role as a patient advocate is substantive in today's pharmacist practice. You will increasingly be expected to provide advice, expertise, and direct care related to promoting wellness, improving medication access, and performing social service functions. This role is complementary to your role in the therapeutic relationship. These functions are the extrinsic actions that you take to advance the care necessary for the patient, while the therapeutic relationship is of intrinsic value to the patient.

SUMMARY

As a pharmacist, you must adapt to the changing needs of patients and society. You must develop your own professional identify that includes a sound philosophy of practice as well as a solid set of skills, knowledge, behaviors, and adeptness at clinical reasoning. A patient-centered approach requires you to recognize and accept the patient's desires and expectations. To achieve patient-centered care, you must master the clinical practice skills of clinical assessment, drug information, communication, professional behavior, caring behavior, clinical reasoning including empathy, moral reasoning, and metacognition. As you gain expertise, you will recognize the value of your relationship with the patient, and you will develop advocacy skills to improve the patient's outcomes.

INTRODUCTION TO FOUR PHARMACISTS' CASES

We will follow the lives of four patients and four pharmacists throughout this book as they work together in a pharmacy practice setting related to the patients' care needs. Let's meet the pharmacists (see page 27).

CASE-SPECIFIC QUESTIONS

Instructions: Complete the answer to each of the following questions.

1. Pharmacist 1—Nasir Jabr, PharmD, RPh. What model of health most likely describes the one to which Mr. Jabr relates? What characteristics are likely to influence how he views the health needs of the patients he serves? Which of the 10 carative factors of Watson are less likely to be understood and employed by Jabr?
2. Pharmacist 2—Christine Johnston, PharmD, RPh. What model of health most likely describes the one to which Mrs. Johnston relates? What characteristics are likely to influence how she views the health needs of the patients she serves? Which of the 10 carative factors of Watson are less likely to be understood and employed by Johnston?
3. Pharmacist 3—Luisa Rodriguez, PharmD, RPh. What model of health most likely describes the one to which Rodriguez relates? What characteristics are likely to influence how she views the health needs of the patients she serves? Which of the 10 carative factors of Watson are less likely to be understood and employed by Rodriguez?
4. Pharmacist 4—Michael Jones, MS, RPh. What model of health most likely describes the one to which Jones relates? What characteristics are likely to influence how he views the health needs of the patients he serves? Which of the 10 carative factors of Watson are less likely to be understood and employed by Jones?

GENERAL ASSESSMENT QUESTIONS

1. Distinguish among disease-centered, pharmaceutical-centered, and patient-centered pharmacy practice.
2. Describe the care aspect of pharmaceutical care, as perceived by a patient.
3. What distinguishes a generalist practice from a specialist practice?
4. Describe the characteristics of a pharmacist that separate the novice from the expert.

REFERENCES

1. Albom M. Tuesdays with Morrie: an old man, a young man, and life's greatest lesson. New York: Double Day; 1997.
2. Bezold C, Halperin JA, Ashbaugh RR et al. Pharmacy for the 21st century—planning for an uncertain future; 1984.
3. Allen M. The health dimension in nursing practice, notes on primary care. *J Adv Nurs.* 1981; 6:153–5.
4. Hepler CD, Strand LM. Opportunities and responsibilities in pharmaceutical care. *Am J Hosp Pharm.* 1990; 47:533–43.
5. Galt KA. The need to define care in pharmaceutical

Pharmacist 1—*Nasir Jabr, PharmD, RPh*

Mr. Nasir Jabr is a 37-year-old man who has traveled far in his life journey. He immigrated from Jordan through Canada and is first generation in the United States. Mr. Jabr has worked extremely hard to obtain his education and find a meaningful career in the health professions. Raised in a family of six children, Jabr is the oldest and hopes to have his brothers and sisters join him in the United States. His family is highly educated. They are Muslims, and he is a devout follower of the Islamic faith. Mr. Jabr is generous to his neighbors and remains active in his community as a soccer coach and teacher of religious classes. He resides in Detroit, Michigan, where he has lived for 3 years. Mr. Jabr works for a community pharmacy chain. His own health beliefs are broad, and he emphasizes nutritional approaches to health. When Jabr injured his back during a soccer match several years ago, he consulted a chiropractor.

Pharmacist 2—*Christine Johnston, PharmD, RPh*

Mrs. Christine Johnston is a 35-year-old Caucasian woman of German descent who moved to the San Antonio, Texas, area to complete a pharmacy residency when she was 22 years old. She stayed in Texas because she really enjoyed her ambulatory care clinic experience and was offered a position as an ambulatory care pharmacist after her residency.

Mrs. Johnston is married to a man who works full time at a law firm. They have two children—a 10-year-old daughter and a 7-year-old son. She is an active professional in the local health-system pharmacists' organization. She mentors pharmacy students and offers a clerkship experience. Conservative in her views about health, Johnston's own beliefs separate the spiritual nature of healing from those of the biomedical approach. She does not integrate these ideas for herself and does not connect spirituality to a healing process.

Pharmacist 3—*Luisa Rodriguez, PharmD, RPh*

Ms. Luisa Rodriguez is a second-generation Mexican American woman who resides in Bellevue, Nebraska, just 8 miles south of Omaha. She is a single woman who is 42 years old. She enjoys her work as a hospital pharmacist with a split centralized/decentralized service model in a major hospital with a pediatrics and intensive care unit service.

Ms. Rodriguez lives near her parents and grandparents in the community. Her grandparents are traditional in their beliefs about health and spiritual healing. She is well aware of the cultural differences among her family members, herself, and the patients she generally serves. Ms. Rodriguez has never been sick enough to be dependent upon the health care system. Her mother and grandmother have always integrated their health needs into the traditional family approach and used remedies for comfort. Ms. Rodriguez understands the ways of her family as well as her own scientific discipline and evidence-based approach to her pharmacy practice.

Pharmacist 4—*Michael Jones, MS, RPh*

Mr. Michael Jones has been a practicing pharmacist for 20 years. He has been a community pharmacist with long-term care experience but is presently a hospital pharmacist at a health system in Atlanta, Georgia. He is a 45-year-old white male who was born and raised in Boston, Massachusetts. His family goes back greater than 10 generations in Boston. Extensive clinical care programs were not widespread where he trained 25 years ago. His relocation to Atlanta and his accumulated experiences motivated him professionally to complete a specialized training program in anticoagulation management. He has trained several other pharmacists over the years and is responsible for the pharmacy staff development program in this particular area at the hospital.

Raised as a Jehovah's Witness, Jones is an active follower of this faith and upholds many of the beliefs and practices. He occasionally finds conflicts between the medical treatment choices he is involved in and his own faith. He is married and has one 3-year-old child.

care: an examination across research, practice and education. *Am J Pharm Educ.* 2000; 64:223–33.

6. Kohn LT, Corrigan JM, Donaldson MS. To err is human—building a safer health system. Committee on quality of health care in America, Institute of Medicine. Washington, DC: National Academy Press; 2000.

7. National Wholesale Druggists' Association. Industry profile and healthcare factbook. Reston, VA: 1998.

8. Rupp MT, DeYoung M, Schondelmeyer SW. Prescribing problems and pharmacist interventions in community practice. *Medical Care.* 1992 Oct 30; (10): 926–40.

9. Cabral JD. Poor physician penmanship. *JAMA.* 1997; 278:116–7.

10. Bates DW, Leape LL, Cullen DJ et al. Effect of computerized physician order entry and a team intervention on prevention of serious medication errors. *JAMA.* 1998 Oct 21; 280(15):1311–6.

11. Kroner BA. Anticoagulation clinic in the VA Pittsburgh healthcare system. *Pharm Pract Manag Q.* 1998 Oct; 18(3):17–33.

12. Fuller TS, Christensen DB, Williams DH. Satisfaction with prescriptive authority protocols. *J Am Pharm Assoc (Wash).* 1996 (Dec); NS 36(12):739–45.

13. Covey S. The seven habits of highly effective people. New York: Simon and Schuster; 1995.

14. Zellmer WA. The habits of successful pharmacists. *Am J Health-Syst Pharm.* 2000; 57:1794–6.

15. Tunzi M. Can the patient decide? Evaluating patient capacity in practice. *Am Fam Physician.* 2001; 64:299–306.

16. Shils E. The order of learning in the United States from 1865 to 1920: the ascendancy of the universities. *Minerva.* 1978; 16(2):159–95.

17. Schon DA. Educating the reflective practitioner. San Francisco, CA: Jossey-Bass Inc.; 1990.

18. Galt KA. The ASHP clinical skills program drug information series, module 1: analyzing and recording a drug information request. Bethesda, MD: American Society of Health-System Pharmacists, Inc.; 1997.

19. Smith GH, Horton LL, Ferrill MJ. The ASHP clinical skills program drug information series, module 2: evaluating drug literature. Bethesda, MD: American Society of Health-System Pharmacists; 1995.

20. Sackett DL, Richardson WS, Rosenberg W et al. Evidence-based medicine—how to practice and teach EBM. New York: Churchill Livingstone, Inc.; 1997.

21. Starr P. The social transformation of American medicine. Basic Books, M.Y.; 1982.

22. American Society of Hospital Pharmacists. ASHP statement on pharmaceutical care. *Am J Hosp Pharm.* 1993; 50:1720–3.

23. Watson J. Nursing: the philosophy and science of caring. Boston, MA: Little and Brown; 1979.

24. Gramling L, Nugent K. Teaching caring within the context of health. *Nurse Educator.* 1998; 23:47–51.

25. Barrows HS, Pickell GC. Developing clinical problem solving skills—a guide to more effective diagnosis and treatment. Norton Medical Books; 1991.

26. More ES. "Empathy as a hermeneutic practice." *Theoretical-Medicine.* 1996; 17(3):243–54.

27. Latif DA. The link between moral reasoning scores, social desirability, and patient care performance scores: empirical evidence from the retail pharmacy setting. *Journal of Business Ethics.* 2000:25:255–69.

28. Sheehan TJ, Husted SD, Candee D et al. Moral judgment as a predictor of clinical performance. *Evaluation and the Health Professions.* 1980; 8:379–400.

29. Baldwin DC, Adamson E, Self DJ et al. Moral reasoning and malpractice: a study of orthopedic surgeons. *American Journal of Orthopedics.* 1996; 25(7):481–84.

30. American Society of Health-System Pharmacists. Introduction. In: Deffenbaugh JH, ed. Best practices for health-system pharmacy 2000–2001 edition. Bethesda, MD: 2001; xiii–iv.

31. Adapted from Holyoak KJ. Symbolic connectionism: toward third-generation theories of expertise. In: Ericsson KA, Smith J, eds. Toward a general theory of expertise. New York: Cambridge University Press; 1991.

32. Jensen GM, Gwyer J, Hack LM et al. Expertise in physical therapy practice. Woburn, MA: Butterworth-Heinemann; 1999.

33. Novack DH. Therapeutic aspects of the clinical encounter. *Journal of General Internal Medicine.* 1987; 2:346–55.

34. Miller SZ, Schmidt HJ. The habit of humanism: a framework for making humanistic care a reflexive clinical skill. *Academic Medicine.* 1999; 74(7):800–3.

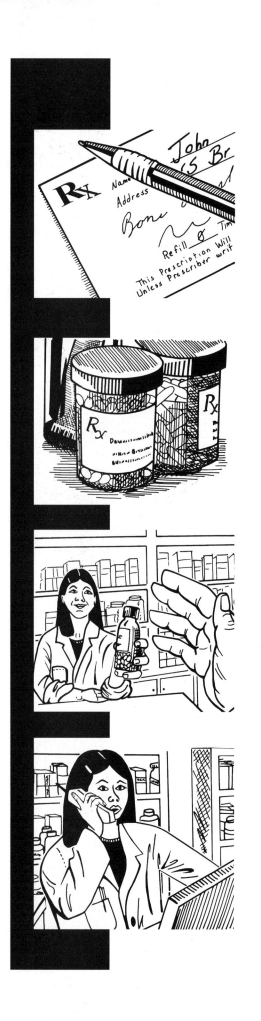

CHAPTER 3

Comprehensive Pharmaceutical Care

"Be compassionate, and take responsibility for each other. If we only learned those lessons, this world would be so much better a place."[1]

Chapter Outline:

Objectives / Be able to describe:

1. patient-centered care as a model for practice;
2. the social context in which pharmacy is practiced;
3. the organizational context in which pharmacy is practiced;
4. the practice settings of pharmacists;
5. the key roles pharmacists occupy in relationship to patient-centered care;
6. pharmaceuticals as treatments; and
7. basic fiscal aspects of pharmacy practice.

Purpose: The purpose of this chapter is to form a framework about comprehensive pharmaceutical care as a patient-centered practice and the varying influences that pharmacists have on the roles.

THE PATIENT-CENTERED CLINICAL METHOD

In the 1970s, the term "patient-centered medicine" was introduced. This concept was developed further into the patient-centered model and method by Levenstein in his own medical practice and refined at the University of Western Ontario.[2–4] The patient-centered model defines what health practitioners should do when they are helping their patients. Because the model is explicit about the behavior of an effective care provider, it provides a vocabulary and focus for teaching and learning. The model also provides a framework of caring as a description of specific behaviors that need to be learned as well as guidelines about when and how to use them. The model transfers to pharmacy practice easily. It applies to the majority of "ordinary" interactions between pharmacists and their patients when patients are seeking the pharmacist's help for consultation or care. It is supportive of a patient-centered philosophy of practice, regardless of the patient type being served. **Figure 3-1** illustrates the interaction model among the patient, pharmacist, and other factors of influence in the patient-centered clinical method.

The following six steps to patient-centered practice support the relationships in this model (see **Box 3-1**):

Component 1. *Exploring both the disease and the illness experience.* This first component involves the pharmacist's understanding of two conceptualizations of ill health: disease and illness.[2–4] *Disease* is a construct by which the health care provider labels a patient's problems in terms of abnormalities with a diagnosis. *Illness* refers to patients' personal experiences of ill health. The diagnostic label explains what each individual has in common with others with the same diagnosis, even though the illness of each person is unique.

Effective patient care requires attending as much to patients' personal experiences of illnesses as to their diseases. A patient-centered method recognizes the identified disease as well as four principal dimensions of patients' illness experiences:

1. Their ideas about what is wrong with them;

2. Their feelings, especially fears about being ill;

3. The impact of their problems on functioning; and

4. Their expectations about what should be done.

A therapeutic understanding of patients' illness experiences requires skill in interviewing to enable the pharmacist to comprehend the illness from the patient's point of view. The pharmacist must be alert for any cues to the patient's ideas, expectations, feelings, or effects on function. Patients may prompt a pharmacist if they miss cues. Sometimes, a crucial comment is made only at the end of a personal interaction. These exiting remarks may indicate that the patient has finally summoned up enough courage to raise a fearful or embarrassing issue before it is too late.

Component 2. *Understanding the whole person.* The second component is an integrated understanding of the whole person. As you interact with the patient, you begin to know the whole person and, in doing so, come to understand the patient's disease and experience of illness in the context of his or her life and health beliefs. This

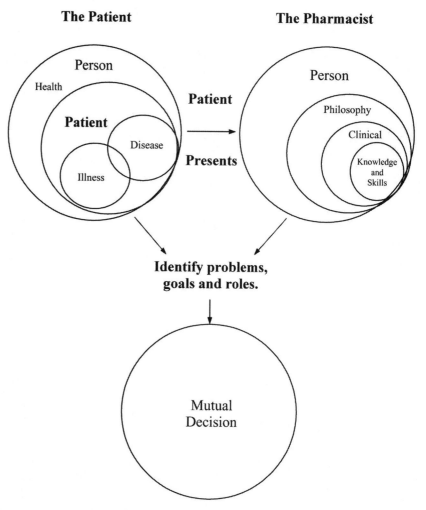

Figure 3-1. *The Patient-Centered Clinical Method Adapted to Pharmacy Practice Health Context*

knowledge of the person may include aspects of his or her life seemingly unrelated to pharmaceutical needs.

An understanding of the whole person can enhance the pharmacist's interactions with the patient at specific times—for example, when medication refills are picked up much later than expected for a chronic condition or the patient seems angry while you are counseling about optimal medication adherence. You will need to determine the reasons why the patient behaves or reacts in these ways. By understanding the patient's circumstances, you enhance your opportunity to assist him or her in achieving the desired behaviors needed to improve health.

Finally, understanding the whole person can deepen your empathic response, especially to those who are suffering or dependent upon your care. Your ethical obligation is to overlook nothing when determining a patient's drug-related problems. A thorough and systematic process will help to ensure that your assessment fulfills this obligation.

Component 3. *Finding common ground.* When a patient has been prescribed treatment, we as pharmacists initially assume that it is consistent with an effective management plan. However, oftentimes patients have not adequately participated in the initial plan determination with their providers and arrive to you with unmet needs. Developing an effective management plan requires that the pharmacist and patient reach agreement in three key areas: 1) the nature of the problems and priorities, 2) the goals of treatment, and 3) the roles of the pharmacist and the patient. Frequently, health care providers and patients have widely divergent views in these areas. Finding a satisfactory resolution requires pharmacists to incorporate patients' ideas, feelings, expectations, and function into treatment planning and care.

Component 4. *Incorporating prevention and health promotion.* The process of finding common ground with patients about opportunities for disease prevention and health promotion is an important component of pharmacist–patient interactions.

With such a supportive process, pharmacists and patients together monitor areas related to medication use, disease, and illness in patients' lives that need strengthening in the interests of long-term emotional and physical health. Pharmacists also monitor recognized problems and screen for unrecognized problems. Finally, pharmacists implement health promotion and screening in practice with an emphasis on expert use and advice of patients' medications. This is done both independently with the patient and collaboratively with other health professionals.

Component 5. *Enhancing the patient–pharmacist relationship.* The fifth component of the patient-centered method is conscious attention to enhancing the patient–pharmacist relationship. At every visit, pharmacists strive to build an effective long-term relationship with

each patient as a foundation for their work together and to use the relationship for its potential to heal and comfort. Pharmacists use self-awareness, unconditional positive regard, empathy, and genuineness to communicate with patients without always having to interpret or intervene. But the approach should be from an empathetic frame. Optimally, you should use your professional caring relationship for a healing purpose with patients. This relationship can provide healing by creating positive emotional support independent of drug treatment. However, this approach combined with treatment will improve the patient's ability to successfully adhere to drug therapy.

Box 3-1. The Patient-Centered Clinical Method Adapted to Pharmacy

The six interactive components of the patient-centered process:

1. Exploring both the disease and the illness experience
   a. Health professionals' differential diagnosis – determining the patients' Problems
   b. Patients' dimensions of illness (ideas, feelings, expectations, and effects on function)
2. Understanding the whole person
   a. The "person" (life history and personal and developmental issues)
   b. The context (the family and anyone else involved in or affected by the patient's illness; the physical environment; the patient's concept of health)
3. Finding common ground regarding management
   a. Problems and priorities
   b. Goals of treatment
   c. Roles of pharmacist and patient in management
4. Incorporating prevention and health promotion
   a. Health enhancement
   b. Risk reduction
   c. Medication problem prevention
   d. Early detection of disease, medication-related problems, and illness
   e. Ameliorating effects of disease, medication-related problems, and illness
5. Enhancing the patient–pharmacist relationship
   a. Characteristics of the therapeutic relationship
   b. Sharing power with the patient
   c. Caring and healing relationship
   d. Self-awareness
   e. Transference and countertransference
6. Being realistic
   a. Time
   b. Resources
   c. Team building

Component 6. *Being realistic.* Pharmacists frequently have competing demands for their time and energy. They must learn to manage their time efficiently for the maximum benefit of their patients. Pharmacists must develop skills of priority setting, resource allocation, and teamwork. Because pharmacists are often the providers with first entry into the health care system, they have an opportunity to steward the patient to needed resources. Pharmacists must also be able to determine reasonable outcomes for their patients. It is important to have the knowledge and expertise to achieve ideal outcomes; however, the patient's specific characteristics, circumstances, and overall health status contribute to what is actually achievable.

Pharmacists have a key role in the care of a patient. The pharmacist must answer, "What role do I occupy with this patient at this time?" Roles include

- The pharmacist as information expert and advisor. In this role, the patient is seeking information to further supplement his or her decisionmaking needs.
- The pharmacist as a primary care provider. In this role, the pharmacist determines the patient's problems and possible treatment options with that patient. This role is illustrated in over-the-counter selections and counseling and in instances where the pharmacist receives delegated authority to manage a patient's drug therapy.
- The pharmacist as one who is carrying out the treatment plan on behalf of the primary provider. This role can include therapeutic drug monitoring as well as compounding and dispensing.

Understanding these roles provides us with a clear guide to our tasks while fulfilling our responsibilities to patients. Each role has specific features of practice that guide our actions by defining what is important. In each patient case, role definition helps us chart a course to effective action.

Although the six interactive components of the patient-centered clinical method have been presented as separate and discrete, they are in fact intricately interwoven. The skilled clinician moves effortlessly back and forth, following the patients' cues, among the six components.

PRIORITIZING PATIENT CARE

Depending on your practice, you may or may not be able to gather a comprehensive database on every patient. A clinical pharmacist in an inpatient dialysis service may see 10–20 patients each day. For the experienced clinician, the resources to efficiently develop a comprehensive database are likely available, so all patients will probably be evaluated. However, a lone pharmacist pro-

viding clinical services to 80 patients in a small community hospital would have to evaluate and prioritize patients to determine which have the greatest need or who would benefit most from direct care. In this setting, the pharmacist may create a modified database for every patient. Similarly, a community pharmacy that provides comprehensive drug therapy monitoring and education within delegated authority protocols will establish these databases on patients. However, a pharmacy providing extensive dispensing and compounding services combined with basic counseling services may need to create only a modified record to provide this service and care. Patients require a wide range of care surrounding their pharmaceutical issues. Whenever a pharmacist evaluates a patient's drug-related needs to determine the level of care, pharmaceutical care as a concept is maintained. The pharmacist's professional expertise is put to its best use when this practice is applied in a patient-centered fashion with an adequate database to best serve the patient.

What types of patients may benefit most from your in-depth evaluation? Depending on your practice site, the following factors have been used to organize patient care delivery and determine priorities:

Patients Who Seek Your Care. These patients are a first priority. The therapeutic process begins when a patient decides to seek care.

Age. Geriatric patients tend to take more medication and have more medication-related problems. Pediatric patients need a substantially greater emphasis on individualized dosing of their medications.

Critical Care. These patients have complex medication regimens that require extensive monitoring as well as complex biotechnology considerations in both preparation and administration.

Consultations. Patients requiring the services of pharmacy consult teams (e.g., nutrition or kinetics) or patients referred by a physician should be monitored by a pharmacist to follow up the consultation.

Drug Use Review or Adverse Drug Reactions. You also may prioritize patients by targeting the medication they are receiving. For example, aminoglycosides or warfarins are often associated with dosing problems, adverse drug reactions, and patient education needs (e.g., warfarin).

Particular Disease States. Patients with renal failure, for example, deserve special attention because of the reduced dosages required for many medications and because some medications and other substances can exacerbate renal failure.

Multiple Prescription Medications or Complex Regimens. Some pharmacists working in ambulatory care settings target patients who take five or more prescribed medications because they often have difficulty managing their regimens.

Nonadherence. Patients who do not adhere to care plan regimens are often the ones who are referred to pharmacists for care. Pharmacists are optimally linked in professional communication networks, communities, and with the health care industry to help patients with medication assistance programs and referral to other professionals, services, and community initiatives. The in-depth interviewing abilities, communication skills, expertise in drug regimen design, and ready access to pharmacists greatly enhance a patient's opportunity to benefit from therapeutic regimens and professional care.

PHARMACEUTICALS AND CARE

Use of Drug Therapies for Prevention and Treatment

Pharmacists are regarded as experts on all forms of drugs. Discussion has occurred both in and outside the profession about the separation of functions among prescribing, counseling, and monitoring of drugs *for* patients and the compounding and dispensing of pharmaceuticals *to* patients. As systems of drug delivery continue to change, we see examples of such separation. However, the role and responsibilities of a pharmacist remain integrally linked with the patient and the pharmaceuticals both selected and used.

Prescription drugs have a status that requires the interaction between patient and pharmacist to ultimately deliver the pharmaceutical. The care associated with these products is interdependent between the pharmacist and patient. Over-the-counter products qualify as self care. As such, the pharmacist's involvement with the patient occurs because the patient desires an interaction with the pharmacist at some level (i.e., information expert, primary care provider, or advisor assisting the patient with carrying out another primary care provider's plan).

Use of Care as Prevention and Treatment

The use of care is another way of describing treatment of the whole patient—mind, body, and spirit as well as disease and illness. Caring is believed to bring comfort and healing, independent of the drug therapies you bring as a pharmacist. The healing relationship is founded in authenticity—a relationship in which the life experiences of both the pharmacist and patient are acknowledged and respected. The healing that occurs in a therapeutic relationship has been described as secondary to the use of therapeutic strategies by health professionals. Some strategies include displays of empathy, suggestion, touch, attending to adherence, and use of family, social supports, or community agencies. These strategies will be discussed further during a more in-depth review of the skills.[5]

Determining the Role of Pharmaceutical Care

To provide effective pharmaceutical care, pharmacists need to view their responsibilities to patients in the context of the medication-use system that is operating around the patient. The patient, pharmacist, treatments, and other providers should be considered within this system. Providers may be physicians, both generalists and specialists, physician assistants, nurse practitioners, parish nurses, physical therapists, occupational therapists, dentists, or others (particularly when varied religions and cultures are involved). These providers may practice care using alternative treatments (e.g., ayurveda, naturopathy, Chinese medicine and acupuncture, homeopathy, chiropractic, and biofeedback). Finally, the patients' self-care practice may be prominent.

All outcomes research related to pharmacists is a measurement of a treatment or model of practice, not specific behaviors of pharmacists which are considered "therapeutic" or "healthogenic." Pharmacists can assist patients with a determination of whether the health practices they follow are helpful, hurtful, or have relatively little impact on outcomes. Outcome success should be defined as responding well to the treatment preferences of the patient. Given the current emphasis on health promotion and the importance of comfort to the process of healing, comfort is an indispensable element of holistic, culturally congruent human care.[6] The role of the pharmacist and pharmaceutical care will have value and context in relationship to this larger picture.

THE PROFESSIONAL WORK ENVIRONMENT

The professional service implied by the setting in which you encounter the patient provides an implicit contract. The setting creates certain expectations in the patient's mind. It can either promote or hinder the pharmacists' use of therapeutic strategies with patients. It also implies a specific set of goals for the pharmacist. For example, a community chain pharmacy practice setting usually encountered by a patient may or may not provide a place for a lengthy evaluation of complex or chronic medical or psychosocial complaints. It may or may not provide a private area that offers privacy, minimizing the importance of this role to the patient. You should determine the tacit or implied service that your patient expects from you. It may be different than you think. Any difference in assumed contract between the patient and you leads to problems in both communication and satisfaction of the patients' and pharmacists' expectations.

Workforce Realities

You and your patients have experiences directly influenced by your practice setting, practice resources that support you, and the opportunity for your ongoing training and development. Practice settings may include hospital, outpatient or community, clinic, long-term care, home care, or physician office-based practices. The practice setting itself goes a long way toward determining the strategies needed to develop, implement, and sustain the services.

The day-to-day challenges of implementing pharmaceutical care are both numerous and imposing. First and foremost, pharmaceutical care must be in your organization's philosophy for you to expect to perform duties at that level. But several other barriers may also be present. Barriers you can overcome include your own philosophy, competency, and commitment to patient-centered care. Other barriers you can influence, but may not control, include your administrator's attitude, knowledge and/or commitment to pharmaceutical care, and the characteristics of your practice area.

In all settings today, excessive workload is a major barrier as is the financial obstacle to employing adequate numbers of pharmacists and support staff. And in all settings, pharmaceutical product volume is a challenge for the limited human resources dedicated to pharmacy. Organizational downsizing is happening concurrently with an increasing portion of the population that needs pharmaceutical care. This problem is further exacerbated by the projected pharmacist shortage over the next 10 years, particularly in the hospital setting.

The outpatient practice setting has an obvious potential conflict of interest. The pharmacy itself depends upon the prescription volume to profit. If pharmacists decrease time spent dispensing prescriptions to provide more comprehensive patient care, there may be an economic disincentive. Another barrier in community practice can be lack of privacy to assess and counsel patients. The environment is often not designed to optimally support this form of patient care.

Home care practice encounters similar barriers to community practice. Payment for pharmacist services is indirectly linked to product dispensing. Moreover, pharmacists in the home care setting generally do not make home visits and are sometimes a distance from their patients.

Hospital setting barriers often include proximity. The pharmacist has an opportunity to work directly with patients if he or she works in a decentralized practice. This form of practice places the pharmacist on the patient care unit, participating in direct activities with the patient and other health care providers. In contrast, centralized services trade off direct patient care contact opportunities for product dispensing efficiencies. Pharmacists work together in one central location, often a substantial distance from the patient care area, making systematic care programs more difficult to implement. The patient has far fewer opportunities to interact directly with the patient.

Payment for Services

The vast majority of pay for pharmacists' services now is done through product reimbursement. Increasingly, however, we see pricing methods and fees for pharmaceutical care services. A mixture of payment methods is likely for a successful health care organization. These methods include direct payment from patients, payment for services incident to a physician's care billed through Medicare, or reimbursement from third-party payors such as private insurance. Demonstration projects concerning pharmacist's reimbursements for pharmaceutical care services have been developed, and the early signs indicate that they are successful.[7,8] This form of payment is expected to increase.

When pharmaceutical care is implemented, pharmacists are shown to reduce excess and inappropriate medication use. This reduction in drug costs has been proven to reduce hospitalizations, adverse events, length of stay, and general burden on patients. Drug costs have been increasing at double digit rates for several years, and they show no signs of decreasing.[9] As pharmacists shift the emphasis from dispensing to decreased pharmaceutical use, it is cheaper for health care payors to reimburse for the professional pharmaceutical care services of a pharmacist.

SUMMARY

A systemic approach to a patient-centered practice provides a clear guide to tasks necessary to fulfilling your patient care responsibility. Role definition in each patient's case helps you to chart a course for effective action. You will need to prioritize patient care needs in all employment settings. It is effective to determine these general priorities so you may handle the most important situations first. Workforce realities pose daily challenges that you must get around to effectively serve your patients. Maintaining a patient-centered approach will provide the context to overcoming these day-to-day problems and setting specific challenges.

INTRODUCTION TO FOUR PHARMACISTS' PRACTICE SETTINGS

Throughout this book, we follow the lives of four patients and four pharmacists as they work together in a pharmacy practice setting related to the patients' care needs. (There are no case-specific questions.) Let's learn about the settings:

Setting 1: Outpatient—general patient-oriented pharmacy practice

Werbert's Pharmacies, a national chain of drug stores, advertises itself as a full-line pharmacy. In addition to traditional pharmaceuticals, the pharmacy also offers a comprehensive nutritional supplement selection, natural products, and durable medical equipment. Nasir Jabr, PharmD, RPh, works at Werbert's; it averages 270–290 prescriptions a day and is staffed with two technicians and another pharmacist overlapping for six hours of the day. Nasir started a counseling program for smoking cessation and a medication refill telephone reminder system for chronic medication users. On request, the pharmacists all agree that they will do semi-private counseling of patients. Appointments are made with the pharmacist for smoking cessation. Nasir is learning about reimbursement for professional charges and will implement some form of payment soon for these services. His store management is lukewarm on the idea of expanding much further on these programs.

Setting 2: Outpatient—collaborative drug therapy practice with delegated authority

Christine Johnston, PharmD, RPh, works for a large organized health care system in San Antonio, Texas. Seven ambulatory care pharmacists hold various clinics to manage patients with chronic conditions who need extensive drug therapy monitoring and adjustment to their regimens. Management is dedicated to this form of patient care and believes the pharmacist is the right person to do it. All of the pharmacists complete an internal privileging process for doing this work. Johnston sees patients by appointment upon formal referral from the physicians who delegate authority to her to perform some practice functions. For specific conditions, Johnston orders laboratory tests, performs physical assessment, and develops a comprehensive pharmaceutical care plan, including the prescribing of medications for this purpose.

Setting 3: Inpatient—general patient-oriented pharmacy practice

Luisa Rodriguez, PharmD, RPh, is a pharmacist at the general tertiary care hospital in Omaha, Nebraska. The hospital pharmacy director has worked several years to build adequate staff to achieve decentralized pharmacy services Monday through Friday from 7 a.m. to 6 p.m. A small drug information support service is available for in-depth questions related to patient care. Rodriguez has access to mainframe drug information sources and carries a personal digital assistant with a few handbooks and key references. It is paid for by the department of pharmacy. She maintains an active practice of 60 to 90 patients a day, with a preference for the pediatric population. She is responsible for medication management, including order review and entry, dispensing, compounding, and distribution. She has a technician assigned to her for working together throughout the day.

Setting 4: Inpatient—collaborative drug therapy practice with delegated authority

Michael Jones, MS, RPh, works at a large hospital in Atlanta, Georgia. Forty-five pharmacists are on staff, all of whom are expected to carry out systematic clinical programs, such as drug usage evaluations and target drug programs. Every clinical program undergoes a privileging process for determination of delegating authority under protocol. Michael is responsible for one such program, anticoagulation, that has gone through this process.

GENERAL ASSESSMENT QUESTIONS

1. Why do some organizations waver in their support of pharmacists in the provision of patient-centered pharmaceutical care?

2. What can the physical layout of a pharmacy or health care facility suggest to a patient?

3. What barriers to the delivery of patient-centered pharmaceutical care can you identify? List them. What strategies might be considered to overcome them?

4. If your workload is too demanding for you to see all patients, what criteria should you consider when making a choice?

ASSIGNMENT

Directions: Spend 5 minutes total examining each of these four questions. Write down a few key thoughts of your own for each question. Discuss each question with someone sitting beside you for a total of 5 minutes.

1. Is care lacking in what pharmacists do?

2. If care skills were applied, would patient outcomes improve?

3. Can caring skills be taught?

4. Is there a need to train care pharmacists / pharmacy students in caring skills?

REFERENCES

1. Albom M. Tuesdays with Morrie: an old man, a young man, and life's greatest lesson. New York: Double Day; 1997.

2. Levenstein JH. The patient-centered general practice consultation. *South Africa Family Practice*. 1984; 5:276–82.

3. Levenstein JH, McCracken EC, McWhikkey IR et al. The patient-centered clinical method: I. A model for the doctor-patient interaction in family medicine. *Family Practice.* 1986; 3(1):24–30.

4. Levenstein JH, Brown JB, Weston WW et al. Patient-centered clinical interviewing. In: Stewart M, Roter D, eds. Communicating with medical patients. Newbury Park: Sage; 1989.

5. Novack DH. Therapeutic aspects of the clinical encounter. *J Gen Intern Med.* 1987; 2:346–55.

6. Malinowski A, Stamler LL. "Comfort: exploration of the concept in nursing." *Journal of Advanced Nursing.* 2002; Sep 39(6):599–606.

7. Hagel HP, Rovers JP. Managing the patient-centered pharmacy. Washington DC: American Pharmaceutical Association; 2002.

8. Farris KB, Kumbera P, Halterman T et al. Outcomes-based pharmacist reimbursement: reimbursing pharmacists for cognitive services. *J Managed Care Pharm.* 2002; (8)5:383–93.

9. Mehl B, Santell J. Projecting future drug expenditures—2001. *Am J Health Syst Pharm.* 2001; 58:125–33.

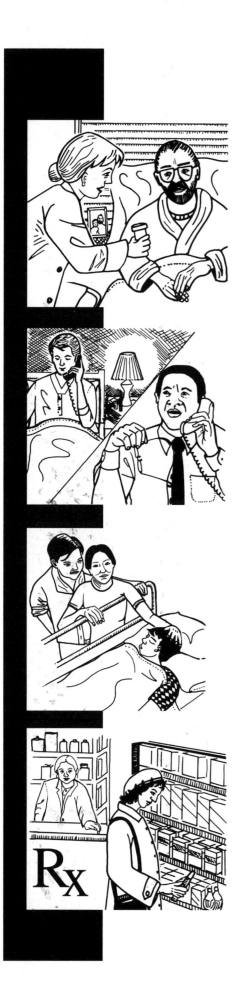

CHAPTER 4

Overview of Pharmaceutical Care Plan Development and Implementation

"There are many ways of caring, and many ways in which patients need caring. We need to know just what it is a patient most needs and what is, in our relationship to that person, in us to give."

Daniel Callahan
The Lost Art of Caring

Chapter Outline:

Objectives / To be able to understand:

1. the interpersonal nature of developing a pharmaceutical care plan with a patient;

2. the components of a pharmaceutical care plan;

3. the importance of determining the patient's care needs;

4. the role of gathering relevant evidence to support development of a pharmaceutical care plan for a patient;

5. the role of applying clinical reasoning to prepare a pharmaceutical care plan for a patient;

6. the importance of applying clinical reasoning in the context of the patient's values, preferences, and beliefs;

7. the design of a pharmaceutical care plan;

8. the implementation of a pharmaceutical care plan;

9. the assessment of a patient's response to care; and

10. the redesign of a patient's care plan in response to progress and outcomes.

Purpose: The purpose of this chapter is to present the pharmaceutical care process that you should follow to provide care.

The provision of pharmaceutical care is a *process*, not a specific task, governed by your cognitive and behavioral actions. This chapter provides an overview of this process as a step-wise approach. Each time you provide care, you apply this process, either in depth or in an abbreviated format. Think of it as a cycle that is repeated whenever you are involved in any step of care. If you become aware of new or modified information, you should update your patient database and evaluate how it influences the modification and implementation of the pharmaceutical care plan (i.e., your care provision). A flow chart representing this pharmaceutical care process is shown in **Figure 4-1**. In the rest of the chapter, you will receive an overview of each step in the process.

DETERMINING THE PATIENT'S CARE NEEDS

Your success in determining the patient's needs is directly dependent upon your ability to gather relevant information from, about, and for use with the patient. Your information is compiled from various sources and *integrated in your mind* to form a patient database. The whole of it is represented by the Pharmacist's Patient Database Model (**Table 4-1**). These bits of information

are also recorded into standard documents to establish a written (or electronic) patient database.

Gathering Background Information

Key sources of information that you can use to form this database include 1) the patient encounter, 2) the medical chart or patient profile, 3) other health professionals caring for the patient, and 4) family members and caregivers who are not health professionals.

You will also gather evidence from drug information sources and clinical literature. Finally, you may choose to seek expert opinions to complement your own clinical experience. The skill of gathering information from various sources reflects different types of expertise. Information may be gathered from the patient, caregivers, and other health care providers and experts. It may involve patient or professional communication, listening skills, direct observation skills, empathy, and a pre-existing knowledge of clinical presentation of conditions and diseases as well as drugs and therapies. Skills required to compile material from drug information and clinical literature include knowledge of available resources, searching strategy, literature evaluation proficiency, and discerning relevance. The greater your skill is in gathering information from various sources, the greater your expertise is in the care of the individual patient.

Sources of Information for patient database:

Patient encounter
- *Patient interview.*
- *Physical assessment of patient*

Patient's medical chart or profile.

Review laboratory test results.

Other health care professionals caring for the patient.

Family members and caregivers who are not health care professionals.

Patient database

Pharmaceutical care plan:

Determine the patient's care needs
(Hypotheses developed through inquiry
and questioning strategies during the patient
encounter)
- *Gather information*
  - *Background information (see sources)*
  - *Evidence from drug information sources and clinical literature*
  - *Obtain expert opinions*

- *Apply clinical reasoning*
  - *Develop the problem list*
  - *Determine therapeutic options*

Design the care plan
- *Specify goals, design the regimen, determine the care behaviors and monitoring plan*

Implement the patient care plan
- *Recommend, initiate and document care provision*

Assess the patient's response to care
- *Evaluate and document the patient progress and outcomes*

Redesign the patient care plan based upon patient progress and outcomes
- *Document changes, progress and outcomes as needed*

Figure 4-1. Pharmaceutical Care Process

The Patient Encounter

The patient encounter is your first opportunity to form a relationship with the patient. This encounter is critical to the future direction of your relationship. Psychologist Carl Rogers identified what he termed the *therapeutic core qualities* of a clinician—*respect* (also described as unconditional positive regard), *genuineness* (congruence), and *empathy*.[1] In the first encounter, the patient must immediately detect these qualities in you. Through your demonstration of these qualities, the patient will give you the privilege of observing his or her problems or concerns and grant you access to all aspects of who he or she is, including physical access through visual inspection, touch, smells, and sounds. If this relationship is not established, you will not succeed in assessing the patient's needs and ultimately developing an effective care plan.

The encounter may be broken into two main sections: the interview and the physical assessment. The interview is your opportunity to gather key information directly from the patient for a comprehensive and accurate database to initiate the pharmaceutical care process. Physical assessment begins immediately upon seeing and hearing the patient. You observe such things as skin color and tone, behaviors, attitude, alertness, and physical comfort level. Data are available immediately that you begin to reason with clinically, such as 1) the patient's concerns, comments, and responses to your initial questions; 2) the patient's appearance, age, sex, dress, and posture; 3) the patient's movements and speech characteristics (e.g., animation, clarity, and the rise and fall of the voice); and 4) the appearance and manner of the people who accompany the patient (spouse, friend, parent, guardian).[2]

To assess a patient's condition and monitor response to treatment and care, you may need to perform specific physical assessment functions. It is taught in medicine that 90% of a diagnosis is based on history alone. The physical examination is often used to confirm what has already been decided by doing the interview.[2] This observation counters a commonly held belief by pharmacists that having no access to the other provider's medical charts precludes the delivery of good pharmaceutical care. Medicine has taught us that most of the care needs are in the patient's story. However, drug therapy monitoring results in the most improved outcomes for patients when you track the desired responses from drug therapy treatment and adjust the care approach to achieve them. Some monitoring parameters require basic physical assessment skills. Chapter 5 will discuss the patient encounter in detail.

Table 4-1. Pharmacist's Patient Database Model

Demographic	Behavioral/Lifestyle	Administrative
Name	*Health beliefs*	*Physicians/prescribers*
Address	*Concepts of Illness*	*Other health providers sought by patient*
Date of birth	*Diet*	*Pharmacist(s)/pharmacy(ies)*
Gender	*Exercise/recreation*	*Room/bed numbers (hospital/long-term*
Religion and religious affiliation	*Tobacco/alcohol/caffeine/ substance use*	*care)*
Occupation	*Sexual history/orientation*	*Consent forms*
	Personality type	*Patient identification number*
Social/Economic	*Daily activities*	
Social history		**Drug Therapy**
Family members	**Medical**	*Prescribed medications*
Significant relationships with others	*Family history*	*Nonprescription medications*
Living arrangement	*Genetic history*	*Medications prior to admission (if*
Ethnic background	*Acute/chronic medical problems*	*hospitalized/long-term care)*
Cultural influences	*Current symptoms*	*Home remedies/folk remedies/herbal*
Primary language/secondary language	*Vital signs/other bedside monitoring*	*products/other types of health products*
Financial/insurance	*information*	*Medication regimen*
	Allergies/intolerances	*Adherence with therapy regimen*
	Past medical history	*Medication allergies/intolerances*
	Laboratory information	*Concerns or questions on therapy*
	Diagnostic/surgical procedures	*Assessment of understanding of therapy*
		Pertinent health beliefs

Modified from Mason NA and Shimp LA. The pharmacist's patient information needs. In: Mason NA and Shimp LA. Building a pharmacist's patient database, module 2. Bethesda, MD: American Society of Hospital Pharmacists, Inc. 1993:7.

The Medical Chart

The medical chart documents the health information of a specific patient. This information is used as a resource by health care providers for treatment planning and care provision. Use the medical chart as a primary source of information for the pharmaceutical care process, when the chart is available to you. The chart is the primary vehicle for communicating among health care professionals involved in a particular patient's care. It is also a legal document of the patient's health information. Medical charts have educational value to health professional students in training who are learning about patient care. The charts are used as research data sources for projects or studies that use a chart review technique to provide data relevant to answering a specific question. They also may be audited as a primary source of data when assessment or evaluation of programs and services occurs or when answers to important questions of safety and effectiveness of patient care practices are sought.

All patient care settings and services maintain some form of the patient medical chart. Charts are maintained in hospitals, clinics, home health care services, extended care facilities, and other practice settings. Historically, they have remained within the physical premises of these settings and services rather than with the patient. Charts are composed of paper materials, can be fully electronic in format, or, commonly, are a combination of both paper and electronic records. The organization of charts vary; however, certain elements exist in each. Chapter 6 will concentrate on the medical chart—its organization and use.

Charts are found in several locations within the practice setting. Typical locations in the hospital are at the end of the patient's bed, in a holder on the room door, in a wall or cabinet by the patient, or by the centrally located patient care (sometimes called nursing) station. Electronic charts are usually accessible through computer screens in locations such as the patient room, hall area just outside the room, or centrally in the patient care station. In clinic settings, charts are usually placed on the door or in the examination room just prior to the patient's visit. In home care practices, charts are maintained and carried by the health professional involved in care delivery. Charts not being used are archived or stored in central locations in hospitals, clinics, home care services, or extended care facilities.

The chart is a private patient document that contains personal health information. The Health Information Privacy and Accountability Act, passed in 2002, provides additional assurances that individuals who do not have a reason to access the patient chart do *not*. In the context of HIPAA, the patient's chart refers to the actual medical chart, pharmacy profile and records, and any official medical documents.

Pharmacists in the hospital setting usually maintain an electronic record of patient medication orders that provide the source of information for active medication orders while a patient is hospitalized. This electronic record is used to generate a document commonly called the medication administration record (MAR). This record is printed and placed in the patient's active medical chart and used by nurses, physicians, pharmacists, and other health professionals to document the time of drug administration and details of the drug regimen to the patient. Similarly, MARs are also prepared for extended care facility patients.

The Patient's Profile

Pharmacists in the community setting maintain records about patient care, often referred to as the patient's profile or pharmacy profile. At a minimum, these patient records contain demographic information similar to the medical chart, a medication list, a listing of conditions or diseases, and general comments related to patient counseling or drug therapy management for the patient. These items are common to most outpatient computerized pharmacy systems that support dispensing activities. In general, the comment areas in computer systems are limited in length, making it difficult to track the care delivery process. Software programs that adequately track pharmacists' dispensing and basic counseling activity are evolving to include documentation features. Most pharmacists maintain two separate systems: one for managing the dispensing process and one for clinical care documentation and monitoring. As software systems and workflow processes improve, integrated software systems that track all aspects of the pharmacists' services to a patient are emerging in the community practice setting. Chapter 6 will cover the patient's profile in detail.

Other Health Professionals Caring for the Patient

Both past and present health care providers are excellent sources of information. However, their evaluations and interpretations of patient data are a product of their experience, cultural background, attitudes, and opinions. The information obtained from health care providers can be written in both medical charts and archived records or else communicated verbally. The primary provider who has cared for a patient over time is the best source of information about that person's past medical history. In addition, the primary provider's assessments of the patient's personality type and interests in various modes of therapy may help you. As you develop your pharmaceutical care practice, you become a primary care provider for some patients whose needs are ongoing medication management.

Health care professionals can be sources of information on numerous topics. For example, dietitians can provide information on nutritional measures instituted by a patient, and social workers may provide insight into the patient's emotional response and financial status. A valuable resource for the institutional pharmacist is the patient's community pharmacist. Dispensing records kept by the community pharmacist often help to determine what medications are being taken, and refill frequencies can provide a good approximation of compliance. Collaborative care is now recognized as an important approach to improving the patient's care.[3] The public has identified the training of health professionals for collaborative care as a priority. Communicating with the various health providers involved with your patient becomes increasingly important as you focus on the pharmaceutical care process. This approach supports the provision of pharmaceutical care and fulfills your responsibilities to the patient.

Family Members and Caregivers Who Are Not Health Professionals

Caregivers are nonhealth professionals who assist with a patient's health care needs. A caregiver is often a family member such as the parent of a young child, the adult child of an elderly person, or the spouse of an ailing person. However, caregivers can be unrelated to the patient such as neighbors, friends, or paid companions.

Caregivers are sources of primarily subjective information. In some cases, they may clarify or elaborate on the information patients report or they may become the spokespersons for patients who cannot speak for themselves. Caregivers are often in a better position to assess therapeutic success or failure than are health care providers because of their regular contact with the patient. For example, a caregiver may be able to describe the improvement in a patient who recently began an antidepressant or confirm the limitations of a person with uncontrolled angina. The caregiver also may be the first person to recognize medication side effects.

The caregiver is often a reliable source of information regarding social drug use and can confirm or deny patient reports on amounts and frequencies of substance use. Objective information that a caregiver may provide could include home blood glucose test results or blood pressure measurements, the patient's medical history, medication use and needs, adherence behaviors, and frequency of self-treatment with over-the-counter products, remedies, and alternative therapies.

Friends, coworkers, good Samaritans, or law enforcement officers may provide information relevant to a specific situation, such as an accident or injury, particularly when patients cannot speak for themselves. When questioning individuals about a patient, you must be aware of the potential to breach privacy. You must approach it in a manner that is consistent with HIPAA rules and regulations. Privacy can be breached if the wording of your question conveys confidential information (unless the patient decides to share it). For example, an appropriate way to inquire about possible illicit substance use of an adolescent would be to ask, "Tell me about your niece's use of illicit street drugs." In contrast, a breach of privacy would occur if you said, "In addition to marijuana, which your niece told us she smoked, do you know what other illicit street drugs she may have used?" Sometimes friends and coworkers may be needed as sources of information and/or participants in a patient's treatment. Information concerning work attendance and performance may be important in assessing a patient's possible overuse of alcohol. Friends and coworkers also may be asked to participate in intervention therapy for alcoholic patients.

Drug Information—Published Evidence

When you are directly responsible for patient care, you must be skilled in obtaining medical-based information and evidence efficiently and effectively. You must be able to formulate a search strategy by retrieving pertinent literature and selecting appropriate drug information. To develop this strategy, you must identify available drug information sources, critically evaluate the information, and select what is immediately and most useful to your patient care needs. Your skills must be so accomplished that you are able to define a framework for your need that reflects the urgency, scope, and depth of information to serve the patient.

Drug information is commonly found in tertiary textbooks (or electronic media versions), secondary resources (bibliographic search systems), or primary literature (published studies in journals). Information is also accessed through resources such as drug or poison information centers and through the assistance of medical librarians, pharmaceutical manufacturers' medical information departments, professional associations or organizations, and government agencies that disseminate evidence and information. You must take ownership of the skills required to comfortably select and draw upon these resources as the needs arise. Chapter 7 will focus on the application of drug information skills to patient care.

Application of Clinical Reasoning

Clinical reasoning is a major component of expert clinical problem solving. It is a dynamic, cyclic, reiterative process in which observation, analysis, synthesis, deduction, induction, hypothesis generation and testing, inquiry-strategy design, and the skills of examination are all interrelated.[2] Expert clinical performance evolves from clinical reasoning, combined with accurate knowledge of background information and evidence, to solve a problem effectively. The use of clinical reasoning skills continues throughout each step in the pharmaceutical care process.

Your ability to use clinical reasoning skills is critical to preparing a patient's care plan incorporating both the individual's health care needs and his or her values. These skills help you determine the best approach that is specific to the patient's needs. With each patient, your approach will vary with each patient based upon the values and specific concerns for that person, not on scientific evidence.

Expert Opinions

Oftentimes, you are unable to find the exact information you need to proceed with care planning decisions. There are two reasons for this problem: 1) you do not have access to the resources you need to find the information or evidence and 2) the information or evidence is not known in the published literature. Clinical knowledge is often tacit, gained through the cumulative experiences with patients. Some information resides with experts who have confidence from prior experience about what you might find valuable in your particular patient's case. Experts from other disciplines can be of great assistance in many cases too. Pharmacists who work in specialized care areas have expertise in comprehensive management of their patients. Areas such as burn units, transplant units, cancer, eye, neurology, pediatrics, intensive care, geriatric units, rehabilitation, and others often have pharmacists who concentrate in the special needs of these patients. If you have exhausted all resources and require expedient information, you should consult these resources for advice.

Developing the Problem List

From the clinical reasoning you apply to the patient-specific information learned through the encounter, available drug information and evidence, and other sources, you will generate a list of problems you identify and concerns of the patient. The problem list must be accurate and consistent with the patients' needs. This list is the format used to determine the therapeutic options for consideration, set patient care goals, and design the care plan. It is documented in the medical chart, patients' profile, or existing documentation system to track the provision of care.

Determining the Therapeutic Options

As you gather information, you develop possible approaches to assist the patient with managing problems. Your options may include recommending a new therapy or modifying an existing therapy. The therapeutic choice may be the use of over-the-counter treatments or prescription medications. You may also recommend supportive care approaches that optimize the patient's existing therapies (e.g., dietary modifications, exercise, or when to use medications to optimize effectiveness). Your accurate knowledge of the possible therapeutic choices to be considered is essential to delivering expert clinical care. In some situations, the most appropriate option is to refer the patient to another health professional for the problem. This interprofessional approach will optimize the patient's outcome by ensuring that competent and appropriate care takes place. It is your advocacy role on behalf of the patient and your professional responsibility.

Once you have determined your therapeutic options, you need to determine the patient care goals, reasonable outcomes to expect, and implementation of the therapeutic options. These steps are involved in designing the patient's care plan.

DESIGNING THE PATIENT CARE PLAN

Specifying Goals

Through your interpersonal care approach, optimal care goals will be established between you and the patient. This is a critical step in decisionmaking, requiring your application of clinical reasoning skills to integrate your knowledge about the patient, the identified problems, potential therapeutic options, and relevant evidence-based information with the patients' values, preferences, and beliefs. You should prioritize the goals that require more immediate attention and assess the patients' interest in achieving them. Remember that the patient's care plan drives the patient's care process. As a result, it needs to be modified in response to how the patient reacts to the treatment approaches implemented. This process has the same core elements independent of care setting. However, the care plan process changes rapidly in the acute care setting and is more prolonged in the ambulatory or home care setting.

Designing the Pharmacotherapeutic Regimen

Meeting *some* goals may only require a minor adjustment to a patient's existing medications. In the outpatient setting, it may warrant a discussion of the optional approaches with the patient and an agreement with the primary prescriber. Other goals may require that you recommend all aspects of drug treatment. Sometimes these goals can be met with you and the patient developing a self-care approach with nonprescription medications and supportive care. Other times, you will be recommending the therapeutic approach desired to another provider.

In the inpatient setting, you are more likely to discuss the approaches with the physician to seek agreement. You may also have been delegated the authority to modify the treatment regimen by the medical staff without prior approval required. You may establish a practice that involves receiving delegated authority from a physician to direct a complete pharmaco-therapeutic plan for a patient in the outpatient setting. Designing the therapeutic regimen takes place in all settings; however, the degree of flexibility you have to implement is dependent upon the formal arrangements with the patient's physician or the medical staff of your employment setting.

Designing the Monitoring Plan

Your monitoring plan is the tool that allows you and your patient to track your patient's progress and the outcomes associated with that care. You should determine if you have achieved the goals that the patient desires through the plan. You should also determine what parameters can be measured (either quantitatively or qualitatively) as indicators that a given goal has or has not been achieved. The monitoring plan should provide you and the patient with feedback, signaling if a redesign of the care plan is warranted. At a minimum, the monitoring plan should include specifying drug therapy monitoring parameters, identifying desired endpoints, determining the frequency or schedule for monitoring, and educating the patient about how to participate in the plan. The monitoring plan will also be influenced by the needs of other professionals caring for the patient and policies of the health care setting itself.

Determining the Amount of Support Necessary

Patients should be included in the decision processes and educated about how to achieve the care goals. Patient needs vary about how much supportive behavior and assistance is necessary. It may not be possible for the patient to independently participate in all aspects of care, requiring a support system to be designed into the care plan. Examples include periodic phone call reminders from you about the patient's drug therapy monitoring responsibility and education of the caregiver about specific responsibilities needed to successfully implement the care plan. The support system for achieving the health goals should be designed along with the pharmacotherapeutic regimen. The design of the care plan will be emphasized in Chapter 9.

IMPLEMENTING THE PATIENT CARE PLAN

Recommending the Regimen, Care, and Monitoring Plan

To implement your care plan, you must communicate your recommendations to the appropriate person. If you are suggesting that a prescriber change his or her ap-proach to treatment, you must select the appropriate information to convey and the optimal communication style and technique to convey it. Key elements of the recommendation include reviewing the patients' health care needs that you are addressing and identifying as the pharmacotherapeutic goal(s), the treatment recom-mendation(s), and your suggestions for monitoring. These same guidelines govern recommendations to the patient or a caregiver. You may have to negotiate the final treatment and monitoring plan when another health care professional or caregiver is involved. However, it is important to know this from the outset so that a success-ful approach can be implemented.

Oral Communication

Oral communication can take place face to face or over the telephone. These responses are more personal than written communication. An oral medium also allows for immediate clarification if someone does not understand a particular issue. Moreover, oral communication provides an open forum to facilitate discussion about a recommendation. Face-to-face interactions allow both people to interpret and evaluate important nonverbal cues. These cues include a nod of one's head, a smile, a crossing of arms, and a raised eyebrow. A limitation of telephone communication is that you do not have the opportunity to process nonverbal cues from the requester. Verbal communication also promotes pharmacy as a profession, especially when talking to another member of the health care team or to a patient. This communication gives recognition to the role of a pharmacist as a problemsolver and contributor to direct patient care.

Oral communication is not without its limitations. Misinterpretation of information is dangerous and more likely to occur with this method. If loud noise or activity is present in the background, the requester may be distracted from listening to the response and, therefore, not understand it. Additionally, oral consultations are time consuming. The depth of your response also may be limited due to time constraints imposed by your other work responsibilities.

Characteristics of an Effective Oral Response

The level of information and the terminology in your response should be appropriate for the person to whom you are communicating. If the request is initiated by a physician, your communication should include profes-sional terminology and scientific evidence. Your goal is to provide expert guidance necessary for the physician to modify the patient's care plan in the physician's area of responsibility. This communication will influence the physician's decision to make the recommended change by reviewing your evidence and feedback to determine that the change is optimal for the patient's care and health care goals. Your recommendation should improve the patient's care plan from this present state. A summary of skills to optimize the physician–pharmacist encounter are described in **Box 4-1**.

Box 4-1. Optimal Skills for the Physician–Pharmacist Encounter

Skill Category	Criteria
Environment	• Pick a location that ensures privacy between you and the physician when you communicate.
	• Do not communicate in front of the patient. This may cause the physician to feel you are being confrontational. It may cause discomfort – reducing your potential for success.
Preparation	• Prepare your communication to: 1. state your recommendation first. 2. provide a brief summary of the background and evidence that supports the recommendation. 3. anticipate the questions the physician may have. 4. prepare your recommendation to emphasize patient centeredness.
Greeting	• Introduce yourself; identify who the patient is; indicate you are contacting the physician to make a recommendation.
Body of Communication	• State recommendation. • Provide a summary of the background and evidence that supports it. • Answer any questions the physician poses.
Closure	• Confirm the physician's agreement with the recommendation. • Thank the physician for supporting the change.
Documentation	• Record the key elements of the encounter in the appropriate patient records.
Assessment of Barriers	• If the physician rejects your recommendation: 1. solicit the physician's reasons. 2. acknowledge the legitimacy of these. 3. reconsider your recommendation.
General Guidelines	• The physician may be aware of other information that is not familiar to you; accept and consider this additional information.

A response to a patient should include lay language. When dealing with a patient, you should know the advice that the patient has received from the primary provider so you do not offer confusing information and recommendations. You also must consider the impact of your response on a patient. Be sure that you are providing useful and pertinent information. The decision about what and how much information to impart depends on your relationship with the patient, the amount of background information you have about that patient, and the role of other involved providers. You may need to be selective about what you communicate.

Initiating Care

Through the process, you monitor all aspects of what has been agreed upon and take responsibility for the patient's safety and care. A key to effective care is communication. You should provide the direct care you are responsible for, communicate all relevant information to other providers proactively, and pay attention to and monitor the patient's progress as needed.

Documenting Care Provision

Care provision should be recorded in the medical chart, patient profile, or existing documentation system. Documentation is the primary method of sharing how you have approached the patient's care, what care you have provided, and information useful for other health professionals. All basic care and services provided to patients should also be documented for legal reasons. For example, a well-documented allergy history can be useful in determining if an untoward event is drug related. If it is a standard of practice in your facility to conduct medication histories and identify agents that patients bring to the hospital, documentation of this information could be regarded as a minimum standard of practice. You also must document any therapeutic preferences expressed by patients. This documentation can provide a rationale for therapeutic decisions and decrease overall liability. If a situation arises that may have legal implications, you should take care in what you document in a written note. The note should express the care provided and observations made in an objective and patient-centered manner. The note is not a forum to record opinion or conjecture about confidential issues in the care of the patient. Written responses may also be a letter or a memorandum, a pharmacy newsletter, or a communication from your department's Pharmacy and Therapeutics Committee.

You should find out your institution's policy governing use of the patient chart. Because of sensitive and legal issues, some institutions restrict who can write in the chart. However, with an increased emphasis on documentation of patient care, pharmacists should expect to record their recommendations. *How* and *where* the pharmacist documents care varies by the local health setting.

Written Communication

Documentation provides specific information and becomes a formal record for both you and the patient and for the health setting or facility where care is provided. Although it may seem that oral communication is less time consuming, writing sometimes can be more expedient. Written communication also allows you to explain as much information in as much depth as desired, including the use of tables, graphs, and charts to display data visually. One limitation of the written method is that it usually is not as immediate as oral communication. However, it is an essential method for documentation of care.

Although no rules are absolute for selecting the method of response, certain situations are better suited to a written format. Written notes in the patient chart allow you to evaluate the existing literature on a topic and to synthesize a patient-specific response. If the content of your documentation is complex or requires a lengthy answer, the best way to communicate it may be in writing. Written responses also are useful because they provide documentation about what types of services you provide in your practice setting.

Methods of Written Response

After you decide that a written note is warranted, the amount of information you provide depends on the purpose of your note. Two methods can be used: medical chart entry or a letter/memorandum. Chart entries are appropriate when

- An official consultation requests your services.
- The patient's physician requests it.
- You need to communicate information to the health care team.
- You have delivered care directly to the patient and need to document the care provision and plan for followup.

You may record your medical chart entry on a consultation document, form, or progress note. In certain circumstances, a letter or memorandum may be appropriate.

An official consultation is a written request for expert services. When you are asked to conduct an official consultation, you usually write on the report or findings section of a consultation form. A formal consultation requires an expert evaluation of a patient for a specific purpose. It must include a comprehensive discussion of findings and recommendations. Furthermore, the level and depth of expertise applied to these requests must be documented. Conversely, a brief communication in the Progress Notes section of a chart is not comprehensive. Its primary purpose is to provide key facts for determining any necessary changes in the patient's care plan. You should prioritize your information to determine its importance. Your background information, including literature summary, should be clearly separate from your conclusions and recommendations. If attachments are needed, refer to them in the body of your consultation and label them accordingly.

Suppose that you are the pharmacist who provides decentralized services to the general medicine inpatient floor of a hospital. At 2:00 p.m., a clerk on the patient care unit pages you to provide a written consultation on behalf of a physician. This physician needs to know the likelihood that a patient's full body rash is drug related. In this case, you should evaluate the urgency of this request, determine an information-gathering strategy, conduct an evaluation, and formulate a response. Ultimately, you should write your response and recommendations on the consultation form that was originally generated by the physician. This form should then be placed in the chart.

A physician may orally request a consultation and ask that you "leave a note in the chart." At the beginning of the medical chart note, you should indicate that the note is provided at the physician's request.

A chart entry is the only way of ensuring that your information is communicated to everyone who needs it. This entry becomes essential when the patient is transferred among different providers or levels of care. For example, when a patient is preparing for discharge, your information may be needed by outpatient or home care providers. Therefore, it should be part of the documentation supporting the discharge plan.

A chart note is useful when you want to provide a brief reply to a question. However, information placed in the medical chart becomes the patient's legal document. Because some issues are sensitive, chart information should include only what is essential to deliver appropriate patient care. Although you may have expertise in a particular area, the note you write in the chart could result in litigation.

For example, a female patient on the obstetrics/gynecology (OB/GYN) floor asks whether phenytoin can cause fetal malformation. The pharmacist researches the literature and discovers that phenytoin is indeed a possible culprit; however, he is unable to interview the patient or reach the physician who monitored her pregnancy and knew her medication-use history. Although this pharmacist could write about phenytoin-induced fetal malformation in the chart, he should discuss the information in person with the physician. He also should describe his limited knowledge of the patient's case to the physician and record it in a written response.

If your recommendations conflict with other providers, you must understand your role and obligations in patient care. Limit the extent of your chart entry to reflect what you are asked. Before submitting a chart note, you also may contact the provider to work out an appropriate conclusion. Include a notation in your entry that the expert was consulted and then summarize the comments pertinent to your recommendation. You can include a brief explanation about the differences in your conclusions.

If your recommendations conflict with an organizational policy, you should identify the issue and determine if you can modify it to conform. If you cannot conform, evaluate the purpose of the policy and determine if your recommendations are a reasonable exception. Include these explanations in your entry to substantiate your recommendations and to protect yourself as a practitioner. In these situations, a countersignature from a physician or supervisor may ensure all professionals that appropriate orders or activities can be performed. The endorsement by suitable authorities also strengthens the credibility of controversial or highly judgmental recommendations.

You should document your oral response to a request in the patient care plan of the pharmacy department. Consequently, all pharmacists who provide care to the patient will know about your recommendations. Moreover, the data are recorded in the workload statistics of the department. However, not all oral responses need chart documentation. If you believe that it is essential for proper patient care or the physician has requested it, you should do so.

If you decide that documentation should appear in the patient's medical chart, your entry should be placed in the Progress Notes section. The documentation must include

- Date and time the note is entered.
- Purpose of the note.
- Person who requested services or consultation.
- The content summarizing your findings, assessment, and recommendations. It is usually prepared in S.O.A.P. note format.
- Your contact information for additional followup.

SOAP Note

The most common method for documenting information about the patient encounter is the "S.O.A.P." note.

This acronym describes both the type and order of information that should be included in the note. The "S" represents subjective information or information told to you by the patient or others. Subjective information is reported to you.

Objective information, represented by "O," is the information that you directly observe. This includes your physical and mental assessment of the patient and measurable data (e.g., blood pressure, temperature or heart rate, and laboratory data).

Assessment information, represented by "A," is the clinical opinion of the patient's problems and an evaluation of how the patient is progressing based upon the subjective and objective information. Outcomes evaluation of a patient's response to a prior plan is expressed here. This section also incorporates relevant published evidence or guidelines to be applied in a patient's case.

The Plan, represented by "P," summarizes the care approach you will use with the patient. The plan includes a prioritization of the patient's problems, care steps intended for each problem, monitoring indicators and timeframe for evaluation, and the future period for followup. A forward thinking approach to the plan is helpful to you and others. A comprehensive care plan involves patient and provider education and documents communication to other health care providers when relevant.

When a written response is provided in the medical chart, you also should document it in the pharmacist's care plan. Documentation in the pharmacist's care plan varies, depending on what is used by your organization. Remember to be concise. If your written response to an information request is a letter or memorandum, it may or may not be appropriate to refer to it in the patient's medical chart. You must decide whether it can add to the quality of a patient's care and/or provide the minimum documentation to ensure that other providers are properly informed. Again, you should document the fact that you provided a letter or memorandum response to a particular request in the pharmacist's care plan.

Case Study

Suppose that a clinic physician asks your advice about how to adjust allopurinol in Mrs. Caines, a 67-year-old white female with a history of gout. Her only other medication is indomethacin for acute gout flares. Her creatinine clearance, estimated at 30 ml/min, has remained stable for at least 1 month. Her serum uric acid concentration is 9.8 mg/dl, and her serum creatinine is 2.4 mg/dl. Moreover, Mrs. Caines was hospitalized for an elective surgical procedure. As in the previous case study, you should look up information on allopurinol used for the treatment of gout and then continue to develop recommendations.

In this case, you should give your recommendation orally and follow up with written documentation in the pharmacist's care plan. If the physician wants you to document a response in the patient's medical chart, you should prepare a brief progress note that identifies the patient, confirms the creatinine clearance estimate and stable but impaired renal function, and states the information you are using to recommend a dose adjustment. Then, you should sign and date the note. You also should document on the pharmacist's care plan that this recommendation was recorded in the patient's medical chart.

A letter is the usual format for communicating information to someone outside of your employment setting. Letters can be sent to health care professionals, patients, administrators, government agencies, and media professionals. Conversely, a memorandum usually communicates a response to someone in your employment setting. It is a brief, formal communication and usually does not exceed two pages. A memorandum is used to

- Document a communication for several people who need a common understanding of content.
- Provide information for later reference.
- Disseminate important information rapidly.
- Communicate important changes in policy.
- Communicate expectations about a behavior.
- Communicate information about a patient or patient care that is not appropriate for the medical record.

The implementation of the care plan will be detailed in Chapter 10.

Assessing the Patient's Response to Care

Evaluating the Results/Outcomes from Implementation of the Plan

Whenever you have incorporated a monitoring plan in the delivery of care, this evaluation should take place. Your evaluation of progress should be documented in the appropriate patient care records. Not all care situations require this followup, as in the example of a patient who seeks information for self-treatment in a community setting. However, the offer to be available to a patient for further followup may be just what was needed to have that patient return for assistance in the future.

Redesigning the Patient Care Plan Based Upon Patient Progress and Outcomes

You should take action to change the patient care approach if the desired goals are not being met. The pharmaceutical care process is iterative. New patient information about progress and outcomes should be used, and clinical reasoning skills can be applied to redesign the care plan with a greater potential for success. All changes to the plan as a result of outcomes assessment should be documented in the patient profile

or medical chart. The redesign of the care plan will be detailed in Chapter 11.

Summary

Your success in determining the patient's needs is directly dependent upon your ability to gather relevant information from, about, and for use with the patient. You formulate your own patient database from the patient encounter, the medical chart or patient profile, other health care professionals caring for the patient, and family members and caregivers who are not health professionals. A systemic use of clinical skills is applied to develop a problem list, determine therapeutic options, design a care plan, implement the care plan, and document and communicate about the care provided. You will assess the patient's response and redesign the care plan based upon the patient's progress and outcomes.

Cases

See pages 54–57 for cases.

Case-Specific Questions

Case 1: Lauren Smith
1. In Chapter 1, we discussed three types of patients you generally will encounter. What type of patient does Lauren Smith seem to be?
2. To what extent do you think Nasir Jabr's professional services will be used by Lauren?
3. What impact will the interaction between Nasir Jabr and Lauren Smith have on her likelihood of returning to the pharmacy? Seeking counsel from Nasir Jabr?

Case 2: Eduardo Montanez
1. What background sources of information are accessible to Christine Johnston to learn about Mr. Montanez before his next clinic visit?
2. What is likely to be the primary method of documenting care provided to Mr. Montanez?
3. Who should Christine Johnston be sure to communicate with each time she has a care visit with Mr. Montanez?

Case 3: Huong Tran
1. What are the cultural and language considerations that have affected Dr. Rodriguez's ability to establish a productive relationship with Huong and his parents?
2. What are some actions she can take to minimize the negative impact of these considerations on caring for

Huong? What should she do in order to prepare for caring for Huong?

Case 4: Mr. Robinson

1. What did Michael Jones do well in relationship to managing Mr. Robinson's case?

2. Do you think that Nurse Charlotte did the right thing in response to Mr. Robinson's request?

GENERAL ASSESSMENT QUESTIONS

1. What are the therapeutic core qualities of a clinician? Why are they so important to patient care?

2. When do you obtain expert opinions in the delivery of patient care?

3. Describe the reasons why you document care provision in writing.

4. What is the purpose of a S.O.A.P. note?

5. What circumstances warrant redesigning a patient's care plan?

ASSIGNMENT

See page 51 for reference tables.

1. For each of the four cases, determine the sources of information that were used by the pharmacist in the case presented.

2. For each of the four cases, determine which of the steps were involved in the care plan development and implementation.

REFERENCES

1. Coulehan JL, Marian RB. The medical interview: a primer for students of the art—edition 3. Philadelphia, PA: F. A. Davis Company; 1997.

2. Barrows HS, Pickell GC. Developing clinical problem solving skills—A guide to more effective diagnosis and treatment. New York, NY: Norton Medical Books; 1991.

3. Committee on the Health Professions Education Summit. Board on Health Care Service. Institute of Medicine. Health professions education: a bridge to quality. Greiner AC, Knebel E, eds. Washington, DC: The National Academies Press; 2004.

Assignment Question 1

Sources of Information	Case 1: Lauren Smith	Case 2: Eduardo Montanez	Case 3: Huong Tran	Case 4: Samuel Robinson
Patient interview				
Physical assessment of patient				
Patient's medical chart or profile				
Laboratory test results				
Other health care professionals caring for the patient				
Family members and caregivers who are not health care professionals				

Assignment Question 2

Care Plan Development and Implementation	Case 1: Lauren Smith	Case 2: Eduardo Montanez	Case 3: Huong Tran	Case 4: Samuel Robinson
Determine the patient's care needs				
Apply clinical reasoning				
Design the care plan				
Implement the care plan				
Assess the patient's response to care				
Redesign the care plan based upon patient progress and outcomes				

Case 1: *Lauren Smith visits Werbert's Pharmacy and meets Nasir Jabr, PharmD, RPh.*

Lauren decides to visit Werbert's Pharmacy because she is having some uncomfortable symptoms (i.e., itching and burning when she urinates). She decides that her discomfort is too great and wants to seek some relief. She hopes that there is an over-the-counter product that she can use. This pharmacy is the one she most frequents, once every few months.

Lauren first browses through the Analgesic/Pain Management section of the store. Advil® has worked for her in the past, so she picks up another bottle of 200-mg strength tablets, 100 count. Then she reconsiders, because she thinks that she might have a vaginal infection. Lauren uses Internet access at home to look at consumer-oriented health sources. Consequently, she decides to purchase Vagisil Gel® prescription checkout area, so she takes these products there to pay for them. Nasir Jabr is the pharmacist on duty and offers to assist her.

As he is completing the checkout process, **Nasir Jabr asks**: "Can I assist you with any information or help?"

Lauren: "No thank you. I think I have what I need for today."

(Dr. Jabr quickly evaluates her overall appearance, facial expressions, general appearance of health, and attitude. These observations, along with her strong individualist approach to communication, suggest that she will not be responsive to further offers.)

Nasir Jabr: "Our phone number is listed on my business card. Do not hesitate to contact me if you decide you would like assistance. I would be most pleased to answer any questions or conduct a preliminary clinical evaluation about your concerns. Call me if you decide you would like further assistance."

Lauren: "Thank you very much. I appreciate your concern. I'll consider this." (She was surprised and impressed by his professional approach and politeness toward her.)

Case 2: *Eduardo Montanez attends his outpatient primary care clinic appointment and is referred to Christine Johnston, PharmD, for followup.*

Mr. Montanez was taken to his primary care physician, Dr. Mattis, at Heart of Texas Health System Clinics, by his daughter-in-law Maria. Dr. Mattis spoke with him and his daughter-in-law in some detail about his health status and health practices. Dr. Mattis concluded that a more individualized drug therapy management approach would likely benefit Mr. Montanez. He obtained agreement from both Mr. Montanez and Maria to visit Christine Johnston, PharmD, ambulatory clinical pharmacist who assists patients with chronic condition drug therapy management. Dr. Mattis gets Christine Johnston from her work area to facilitate introductions.

Christine Johnston: "Bueños dias, Señor Montanez and Maria." Mr. Montanez smiles and Maria responds: Buenos dias, Senora Johnston."

Christine Johnston: "It is my great pleasure to have the opportunity to work with you, Mr. Montanez. I speak very little Spanish. However, I am able to provide information in writing that has been translated from English to Spanish. I can also arrange for a translator when you come to visit. Would you prefer that I do this?"

Mr. Montanez (looks slightly confused): "Translator? Won't Maria come?" (Mr. Montanez speaks with limited confidence.)

Maria: "Yes, Señora Johnston. Please let me serve as a translator for my father-in-law. He has some beliefs about his health and problems that I could help to explain. He is very comfortable coming here. This would be best."

Christine Johnston: "Very well. I appreciate the support and care you are providing Maria and will look forward to both of you visiting. When you return to visit, Mr. Montanez, will you please bring all of your medications and treatments with you?"

Maria: "Oh, I take care of all of that for him. I will make sure to do this."

Christine Johnston: "Good. I enjoyed meeting you both and look forward to your visit."

She turns to leave the room thinking Mr. Montanez seems to understand most of what she is saying. She makes a mental note to speak directly to him and not allow Maria to distract her from this approach. (She also notes the very close caregiving relationship Maria has with her father-in-law.)

Case 3: *Huong Tran is admitted through the Emergency Room to Midcity Hospital and meets Luisa Rodriguez, PharmD.*

Dr. Mooris, the Emergency Room physician, evaluates Huong's respiratory status. He hears severe wheezing through the stethoscope. Huong is trying to take deep breaths, but he is unable to because of severe restriction of his airways.

Dr. Mooris: "Huong, do you have asthma?"

(Huong nods his head yes, as it is too difficult for him to answer. Huong's parents came with him. They appear frightened. Unable to speak English, they depend on Huong to tell them what they need to know. They try to treat Huong's respiratory condition with herbal remedies and an acupuncturist.)

Dr. Mooris: "I want you to inhale this medication by spraying it directly in front of your mouth and breathing deeply."

(Huong appears to have difficulty manipulating his handheld inhaler. Luisa Rodriguez, PharmD, was delivering another medication to the Emergency Room and noticed Huong struggling with self-administration of the albuterol.)

She approached Dr. Mooris and asked: "Dr. Mooris, I noticed this child is having a difficult time using this device. Would it be alright if I showed him how to use it?"

Dr. Mooris: "That would be terrific. Huong, this is Luisa Rodriguez; she is a pharmacist. She will help you to use this medicine correctly. Please do what she says. It will make you feel much better in just a few minutes."

(Ms. Rodriguez works with Huong while Dr. Mooris completes Huong's hospital admission process. Once Huong is stabilized, the pharmacist informs him and his family that she will be working with him while he is in the hospital. Huong's parents look worried and frightened, and she feels badly that she cannot speak with them to alleviate their fears and concerns.)

Case 4: *Mr. Robinson meets Michael Jones, MS, RPh, while hospitalized for an exacerbation of congestive heart failure.*

Mr. Robinson rings the bed alarm from his semi-private room on the 3rd floor on the internal medicine ward.

Nurse Charlotte (over speaker): "What is it, Mr. Robinson?"

Mr. Robinson (over speaker): "Yes, nurse. I think I am supposed to take my blood thinner this morning. It is almost noon, and I am sure I didn't get it."

Nurse Charlotte (over speaker): "Thanks Mr. Robinson. I'll check and see what is happening with your medication and get right back to you."

(Michael Jones, decentralized pharmacist, was just getting to his patient care rounds when the nurse stops him in the hallway.)

Nurse Charlotte: "Michael, Mr. Robinson in Room 347 believes he should receive his warfarin and thinks that it is late. I did not give him any because I saw that you were consulted by Dr. Rangert to manage his anticoagulation."

Michael Jones: "Thank you Charlotte. I will go and speak with him right away. I have not met him yet."

(Michael goes to see Mr. Robinson. He knocks on the room door.)

Mr. Robinson: "Hello . . . come on in . . . it's okay, I'm dressed."

Michael Jones: "Hello Mr. Robinson. My name is Michael Jones, and I am a pharmacist. Dr. Rangert, your physician in the hospital, asked me to see you and take care of your warfarin and other blood thinner medication while you are in the hospital."

Mr. Robinson: "It's nice to meet you, Michael. I didn't know there were pharmacists in the hospital. I guess I shouldn't be surprised . . . I just never really thought about it."

Michael Jones: "Yes Mr. Robinson. There are several pharmacists on duty, and we staff the hospital 24 hours a day. Most of our work is behind the scenes, ensuring that your medication is being dosed correctly, preparing it for your use, and watching how you respond to the medicine you are taking. We make recommendations to adjust medications as we see areas for improvement."

Mr. Robinson: "Great. Well . . . I think you guys are late with my warfarin."

Michael Jones: "That is why I am here. I will be evaluating some information about your response to warfarin and deciding the correct dose for you while you are here. This will take me another 15 minutes or so. I will get back to you to let you know what I recommend."

Mr. Robinson: "Thank you. I just don't want anyone to make any mistakes. My wife used to watch everyone for me . . . she really took care of me . . . but now I have to do this on my own. She taught me well though!"

Michael Jones: "She certainly did. And you are doing a good job. I will communicate with you shortly. Thank you Mr. Robinson."

(Michael leaves the room.)

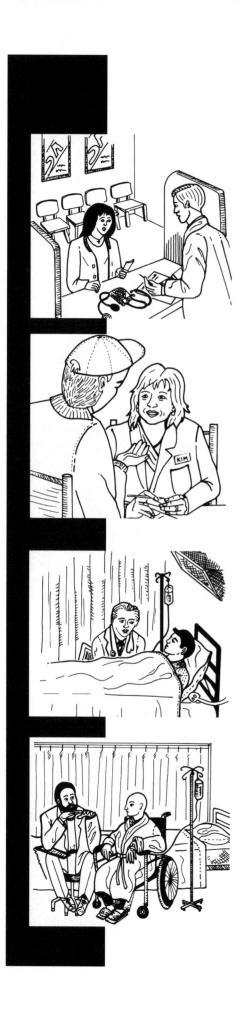

CHAPTER 5

The Patient– Pharmacist Encounter: A Primary Source of Information

"If you think the cost of education is high, think about ignorance."

Derek Bok
President
Harvard University

Chapter Outline:

Objectives / To be able to understand:

1. why various types of patient encounters take place;
2. the purpose, structure, and processes of the patient encounter;
3. unique aspects of the patient encounter to consider with special populations;
4. how to conduct a patient interview;
5. how to design a questioning strategy and use questioning skills to elicit information;
6. how to use different communication techniques to optimize the patient's experience;
7. how to respond to a patient's questions during an interview;
8. the use of physical assessment for problem identification and drug therapy monitoring;
9. the value and use of the mental status assessment in the patient encounter;
10. the value and use of the review of systems in the patient encounter;
11. how to conclude the patient encounter; and
12. the importance of documenting your findings from the patient encounter.

Purpose: The purpose of this chapter is to describe the structure and process of the pharmacist–patient encounter.

"I walked into the patient's room and instantly realized how fragile this patient was. She lay in the hospital bed looking thin and nearly as flat as the mattress itself. She couldn't be more than 5 feet tall and weighed no more than 100 pounds. But it was her slow, methodical, labored breathing...her pale, faded thin skin...her thin white hair, her sunken cheeks, and her colorless lips that told me her condition. She was poorly nourished and dehydrated. I didn't need her chart to identify this."

Kim Galt

THE PATIENT ENCOUNTER

Patient encounters occur in order to gather information, determine the care a patient needs, and provide care. You will have patient encounters in almost all employment settings. In the hospital setting, the encounter may occur initially to gather an admission history, compile specific information in response to you being asked to consult, solve a problem you or another professional has identified, or prepare a patient for discharge. Other reasons may include gathering information to participate in an interprofessional care planning session, counseling a patient about a mediation for self-use, or responding to a request from a patient to discuss an issue with a pharmacist. In the community setting, patient encounters routinely occur when a prescription is presented for filling and when a patient receives the dispensed medications. Encounters occur when you are resolving a conflict or problem on a prescription, or when a patient requests advice or guidance on self-treatment. In some community settings, pharmacists provide comprehensive care evaluations, drug therapy monitoring, and drug therapy management. In this role, you will have patient encounters that require complete privacy. You will conduct physical examinations and assessments important to drug therapy management.

No matter what the circumstances and setting, therapeutic care is the purpose of your encounter with the patient. With each patient, you have the opportunity to form a *therapeutic relationship*.[1] The patient encounter consists of the patient interview and physical assessment; the scientific tools used to investigate the patient's problems, determine treatment options that are acceptable to the patient, and monitor treatment response. When you first see the patient, you will pose questions that encourage a conversation intended to have the patient describe his or her concerns. As you continue to listen to the patient, you will form an initial impression or concept of this patient's problems. Then you will formulate an inquiry strategy to focus on the emerging areas of need. Inquiry involves conversation, observation, and physical assessment to generate data. You will use your clinical reasoning skills to analyze this infor-

mation and eventually synthesize your concept of the patient's needs with a degree of confidence that draws you to the next step—development of the care plan. **Figure 5-1** and **Box 5-1** provide guidance about the content collected and approaches used to communicate during a patient encounter. You should refer to them as you progress through the chapter.

The Interview

Interviews and good patient–pharmacist communication are essential to pharmacy practice. A primary source of information to determine the patient's needs in all practice settings is the patient interview. Interviewing is a basic skill that can be broken down into its component parts and be learned. Coulehan and Block describe the fundamental skill of the interview as "understanding exactly."[2]

Preparing for the Interview

The environment surrounding an interview implies what is expected of you to the patient and what you can provide to the patient. This environment is referred to as the patient care setting. In general, patients expect certain services from you based upon the practice setting. Patients who are interviewed by you in the community pharmacy, at a minimum, expect their questions to be answered, to be given a recommendation for care or referral, and possibly to receive a prescription or over-the-counter treatment. Patients who are interviewed in the hospital, outpatient clinic, and home care or nursing home setting may be unclear about what to expect from you at your first interaction. It is not customary for the patient to work with a pharmacist in this setting. You may have to assist the patient with this understanding.

Most often, interviews in community pharmacy are initiated by the patient, making it impossible to prepare ahead of time for the unplanned interaction. But if you have ready access to the patient pharmacy profile and are prepared with skillful questions, you can efficiently and effectively turn the interaction into a meaningful interview, consistent with the patient's expectations.

Ideally, the environment should be private and relatively quiet to enhance communication between you and the patient. A sense of privacy can be created by drawing curtains between beds in a hospital or nursing home or sitting away from other people in a waiting area. This same sense of privacy can be created in a community pharmacy by having an area slightly separate for interviewing and counseling. If you are involved in using physical assessment skills that involve directly touching the patient, manipulating clothing to assess or view an area, or some other act that is perceived as personal or intimate, a private area that blocks the view of others is necessary. If such an area is not available, you will be limited to fewer methods of drug therapy monitoring and outcomes assessment.

PATIENT'S HISTORY FORM – PHARMACIST'S RECOMMENDATIONS/PLAN

Demographic and Administrative Information:	Room No.		ID No.		
Date:	Gender:		Primary Language:		
Name:	DOB:		Height:		Weight:
Street Address:	BP:		Temp:		Pulse:
City, State, Zip	Race/Ethnicity:			Religion:	
Home Phone #:	MD/Phone No.				
Work Phone #:	Pharmacist/Phone No.				
Occupation:	Insurance:				
Family Members/Care Givers:					

Problem List:	Pharmacist's Recommendations/Plan:
1.	
2.	
3.	
4.	
5.	
6.	
7.	
8.	
9.	
10.	

Pharmacist's Name: _____   Date: _____   Phone/Pager #: _____

Chief Complaint/History of Present Illness:

Past Medical History/Surgery/Genetics:

Family and Social History (significant relationship/co-habitants):

Physical Examination/Review of Systems:

ADL:

Lifestyle/Diet/Exercise:

Acute and Chronic Medical Problems/Associated Symptoms:	
1.	6.
2.	7.
3.	8.
4.	9.
5.	10.

Describe Patient's Health Beliefs and Values:

Figure 5-1. Sample Patient's History Form—Pharmacist's Recommendations/Plan (cont'd)

Does Patient Receive Assistance in Medication Administration? Describe:

Allergies/Intolerances: ( ) No Known Drug Allergies

Allergen:	Reaction:	Treatment:
Allergen:	Reaction:	Treatment:
Allergen:	Reaction:	Treatment:

Social Drug Use: Alcohol: Caffeine: Tobacco: Other:

Current Drug Therapy (prescription and over the counter, vitamins, remedies, alternative treatment):

Drug Name Strength/Route	Problem Number	Usual Schedule	Describe PRN Use	Does Med Work?	Side Effects or Concerns	Compliance Issues
1.						
2.						
3.						
4.						
5.						
6.						
7.						
8.						
9.						
10.						
11.						
12.						
13.						
14.						
15.						

Past Drug Therapy:

Time Line: Circle administration times and record appropriate medications and meals below:

Patient's Actual Use:

6 7 8 9 10 11 12 1 2 3 4 5 6 7 8 9 10 11 12 1 2 3 4 5
am   noon   pm   midnight   am

Prescribed Schedule:

6 7 8 9 10 11 12 1 2 3 4 5 6 7 8 9 10 11 12 1 2 3 4 5
am   noon   pm   midnight   am

Costs of Meds/Month: $ Insurance: ( ) Yes   ( ) No

                           Co-pay: Medicaid: Annual Income:

Completed by: _____   **Date:** _____

Figure 5-1. Sample Patient's History Form—Pharmacist's Recommendations/Plan

Box 5-1. Optimal Skills for the Patient–Pharmacist Encounter

Interview Category
* *Specific Skills*

Environmental preparation
* Assure adequate patient privacy.
* Appropriate level of privacy for the clinical care occurring in the encounter. A completely private area is required for physical assessment.
* Is away from physical barriers (glass windows, high countertops).
* Area is relatively quiet.

Interview preparation
* Reviews background sources of information, i.e., medical chart or pharmacy profile.

Greeting
* Introduces self; explains purpose; assures confidentiality.
* Establishes rapport; demonstrates respect, genuineness, empathy, competence.
* Determine patient's willingness to participate.

Assessment of patient communication barriers
* Primary language and interpretation is known. If you are unable to communicate effectively, seek another person known to the patient for assistance or an interpreter.
* Assesses visual impairment. Alternatives to assist the patient's vision are available and used when needed (magnifying glass, large print patient education, supplementary written instructions to medication labels).
* Assess hearing impairment. Communicates by looking directly at the patient and not covering mouth during speaking.
* Assess physical limitations. Determine if patient has inadequate strength or dexterity to open medication containers or handle small medical devices. Does patient require a wheel chair, walker or cane? Is patient limited in gait and distance her or she can walk?
* Assess if others present during the encounter is desired by the patient.
* Determine the need for an interpreter.

Establishment of therapeutic relationship
* Responsiveness to patient's questions.
* Display intent to advocate for the patient's needs.

Assessment of patient expectations
* Communicates in a way that demonstrates you understand the patient's expectations.

Closure
* Reviews findings of importance.
* Generates problem list and priorities.
* Reaches agreed upon action plan with patient.

Documentation
* Writes summary of care in S.O.A.P. format for medical chart and pharmacy care plan or pharmacy profile.

General Category
* *Specific Skills*

General
* Communication conveys care for the other person.
* Communication conveys an open and non-judgmental attitude.

Non-verbal communication
* Maintains eye contact with the patient (exception: cultural considerations)
* Keeps arms open, not folded across body.

Listening skills
* Is attentive to the patient.
* Responds to the patient's comments and requests.

Speaking skills
* Present information at a level of understanding that matches the patient's abilities and needs.

Questioning strategies
* *Communication style*: Responses show respect for the interviewee's attitudes and feelings.
* *Closed-ended questions*: Uses closed-ended questions to obtain precise, narrow focused information.
* *Open-ended questions*: Uses open-ended questions when obtaining as much information as the interviewee is willing to provide.
* *Probing questions*: Probing questions are assertive, not aggressive.
* *Indirect questions*: Chooses indirect questions when the goal is to encourage the interviewee to elaborate on a particular matter.

Quality of questions in interview
* Questions are appropriate for the care needs of the patient.
* Questions are productive, i.e., yield useful information needed to optimize patient care.

Verbal caring behaviors
* Verbally responds to an expressed concern.
* Explains procedure/touch of patient prior to initiation.
* Verbally validates patient's physical status.
* Verbally validates patient's emotional status.
* Shares personal observations or feelings (self-disclosing) in response to patient's expression of concern.
* Verbally reassures patient during care.
* Discusses topics of patient's concern other than current health problems.

Non-verbal caring behaviors
* Sits down at bedside.
* Touches patient exclusive of procedure.
* Sustains eye contact during patient interaction.
* Enters patient room without solicitation.
* Provides physical comfort measures.

Communication at eye level improves comfort for patients. Therefore, you should sit across from the patient to enhance interaction. Physical barriers, such as glass windows or relatively high counter tops separating you and the patient, should be eliminated. Communication barriers can also result from language (e.g., the patient is not able to speak or understand your language), sensory impairments (e.g., dementia), or affective disorders (e.g., depression). And always, you should determine the patient's willingness to participate in this process. Patients will participate when they are ready.

An alternative plan can be developed, if required.

You may be able to gather information in advance of an actual interview. A brief review of the medical chart or the patient's pharmacy profile may improve your efficiency in your interview strategy through familiarizing yourself with the known history of this patient, alerting you to areas of inquiry and providing you with insight into what you may need to know prior to the interview (e.g., unfamiliar medication in patient's current regimen).

Developing an Organized Interview Approach

During an interview, you must gather a considerable amount of information by using a written history or interview document or by adhering to a structured or ordered sequence of questions. Figure 5-1 provides you with a history-taking form that is complementary to Table 1-2, the pharmacist's database model. Use of such tools will help to improve your efficiency of documentation and prompt you to not miss important aspects of questioning. However, the structure itself is only part of the interview process. When patients have concerns, you always start with insufficient information. The process of inquiry is inductive, and it requires you to solicit information that reveals insight into the patient's needs. In essence, you hypothesize the patient's problems as you conduct the inquiry and formulate a questioning strategy to further support or refute your hypotheses.[3] Your ability to define and revise the definition of the patient's problem is a skill that develops with increasing expertise. Some problems remain ill-defined, challenging you as a clinician to develop a plan for care. Equally challenging is knowing what the optimal plan choices are for managing a particular problem. Some treatment choices have greater uncertainty of the outcomes that are achievable than others. The process of inquiry is the feedback loop that makes the pharmaceutical care process cyclic, allowing you to redesign your care plan as is needed based upon these outcomes.

Opening the Interview

Start with a broad-based question or statement that elicits the patient's concerns right away. When the patient initiates the interview, you might consider examples such as "I understand you want to speak with me about medications" or "What might I assist you with today?" However, if you have initiated the interview, it is best to begin with questions that fit a patient's expectations of a pharmacist. For example, after introductions and statement of your purpose for interviewing the patient, you might consider "Do you have any concerns or questions about your medications?"

Interacting with the Patient

Greet the person initially, introduce yourself, and briefly explain the purpose of the interview. You also may want to assure the patient that the information shared is confidential. In many instances, you may offer the patient a document to sign that is a consent allowing you access to the medical information and health data you need to properly care for him or her. This is a requirement induced by the HIPAA legislation approval in 2002. Work to establish rapport at the outset by establishing the therapeutic core qualities with the patient through demonstration of respect, genuineness, and empathy as well as competence.[2] Rapport is also enhanced by a clean, neat, professional appearance and, where customary, a white coat and nametag. Use proper names and titles, such as Mr., Mrs., Miss, or Ms.; when referring to colleagues, use their titles (e.g., Dr.).

If a patient's family member is present, either include that person in the conversation, if appropriate, or ask that person to return after the interview. The patient may feel uncomfortable discussing certain topics in the presence of another person; in that case, politely ask the individual to leave. In other situations, the patient may prefer to have a family member present. For example, a patient's spouse may be able to confirm or expand on the information being provided by the patient. One important caveat is to avoid shifting your attention away from the patient when another person is speaking. While you may record information from both sources, it is usually best to direct your questions primarily to the patient. For example, when the patient is a child who is old enough to speak with you, you should keep focused on the child even when the parent speaks.

As your conversation with the patient unfolds, you should stay alert to the patient characteristics that may influence the interview. How a person reacts and performs in the role of patient or caregiver will be influenced largely by social, familial, cultural, spiritual or religious and socioeconomic background, age, gender, and sensory or communication impairments. Refer to Chapter 1 about the patient for a review. The specific influences of each are discussed here in the context of the interview.

Patient Characteristics

Social Background

Social distance is a term used to describe the social, cultural, and economic differences between a patient and health care provider.[4] The greater the social difference, the more difficult it is to establish an open and trusting relationship, and the more likely it is that misinterpretations will occur. Work and lifestyle considerations should be brought out in order to understand the influences they may have on problem identification and care planning. Refer to Chapter 1 for a more detailed discussion.

Cultural Background

Language barriers exist if the patient does not speak or understand your language. Translation by a family member may allow for communication, but it also may alter either the questions asked or the patient's responses. Studies of reporting styles have demonstrated differences among various cultural groups. Different ethnic groups are apt to respond to and describe pain differently; some are more vocal, while others more stoic. An important consequence of these differences is the interpretation by health professionals. You need to consider your own cultural competency when interacting with patients. To achieve cultural competence in your practice, consider these guidelines offered by Ann Zweber:[5]

1. Examine your own cultural background.
2. Learn about the cultures you serve.
3. Demonstrate sincere interest in your client's culture. Ask open-ended questions.
4. Recognize cultural differences.
5. Don't generalize or stereotype. Determine individual perceptions, beliefs, preferences, and needs.
6. Make the pharmacy environment welcoming and attractive based on clients' cultural backgrounds.
7. Negotiate and educate to develop therapeutic plans that are compatible with cultural beliefs.
8. Use culturally sensitive educational approaches and materials.
9. Learn some phrases of the predominant non-English speaking population in your community.
10. Be aware of culturally based resources in your community. Have materials available for referral if needed.
11. For language barriers, use a trained interpreter if possible. If not, a family member may be helpful.
12. Pictograms may help convey some messages.

Spirituality

Spirituality is an important source of meaning for many patients. Your understanding of the patient's spiritual history is a critical element to understanding the ways in which you will be perceived by the patient. Spiritual tradition may dictate that perception. Again, it is the patient's values and beliefs that must determine how you approach your communication with the patient. If you are a devout Catholic, communicating about birth control may be a substantial challenge for you. But you must place the values of the patient first. You must find an acceptable way to serve the patient. It might include, for example, finding an alternative pharmacist who feels capable of working with these patients and their needs. But the spiritual basis of a person's belief system might be more subtle. For example, an individual's concepts of death may determine their choices in life. It is possible that a patient chooses nonadherence to a regimen because he or she believes that medication use is prolonging life in a way that is inconsistent with personal beliefs. These understandings of the person further explain why we see conflict or discord between a patient and one's family members. Family members may want something different (i.e., they may want to not lose this loved one, no matter what the "price" of treatment). This difference is often observed in what are termed "code" situations in hospitals. A code situation means an urgent, lifesaving call to have a trained interprofessional team rapidly respond to manage it. A code is commonly called when a patient stops breathing or develops a life-threatening cardiac arrhythmia.

Alternative approaches to healing and health may involve shamanism, faith healers, and medicine healing. Shamanism is the practice of a native healer. This person acts as a spiritual advisor, medical care provider, and counselor. Shamans exist in cultures worldwide. Similarly, faith healers are a common health provider in many areas of the world, including South Africa, Australia, and in the Pennsylvanian Dutch communities across the United States. Shamans and faith healers commonly use prayer in their modes of treatment.

Socioeconomic Background

Some evidence shows that the reporting of symptoms and the seeking of medical attention occur less frequently for certain symptoms among patients of lower socioeconomic classes.[6] This difference is referred to as health disparities. Health disparities are differences in the incidence, prevalence, mortality, and burden of diseases and other adverse health conditions that exist among specific groups in the United States. It is the outcome of racial and ethnic differences in rates of access, utilization, and prescription health care services. Recent reports indicate differences in the kind and quality of health care both sought and received by different race or ethnic groups. You may elicit more information if you actively inquire about symptoms, such as potential adverse drug effects, rather than assume that the patient will mention significant ones. Patients with limited incomes may have difficulty adhering to their medication regimen because of insufficient funds to purchase medicine. Moreover, patients in lower socioeconomic classes experience higher illiteracy rates and complete fewer years of formal education. This is particularly true for the elderly on fixed incomes. To ascertain literacy and correct usage, ask patients to demonstrate medical use rather than just describe it. You should ask the patient to read the medical label back to you, draw insulin in a syringe, or use an inhaler to show true understanding.

Family Background
During the interview, you may be able to gather information that provides insight into family dynamics and social support. For example, the person's role in the family may influence his or her reaction to a chronic illness. Reluctant to accept this role, the patient's attitude may translate to nonadherence with medications. Family members may also be the care providers needed to support the patient. For example, a grandson may organize his grandmother's medications so that she can continue to live in her own home.

Family history is relevant to the probability that a patient presents with certain conditions due to genetic predisposition. The role of the family history, when interpreted in combination with genetic testing, is emerging as an important component to this future method of diagnostics, treatment, and prevention. An excellent source to assist care providers with comprehensive, reliable family history is the General Primary Care Family History Tool Kit. This tool kit uses three approaches: 1) genetic disease screening; 2) a traditional family medical history; and 3) genogram/pedigree history. Both the American Association of Family Practice and the American Medical Association provide resources. One disadvantage to the family history is the amount of time it takes to construct it. Experienced clinicians report 30–45 minute sessions to accurately complete them. If this information is already available for use in records, it is well worth saving time to not repeat it. Use proper judgment to determine if the value of what you will learn can substantially contribute to your ability to perform care responsibilities.

Gender and Age Considerations
Men tend to report fewer symptoms or problems than women. Elderly people are less likely to report symptoms and problems than younger people. Because of the overlap between common drug side effects and symptoms (e.g., upset stomach, fatigue, drowsiness, dizziness, headache, constipation, and diarrhea), you should actively inquire about symptoms rather than wait for older patients to volunteer information. Pediatric patients may not be able to accurately express the symptoms (e.g., scratching at ear for otitis), and younger pediatric patients will require an adult to describe the patient's history and presentation. The content of the interview changes from small children to teenagers to adult and elderly based upon the needs and concerns present.

Sensory or Communication Impairments
Sensory loss ranks second as a cause of low morale among the elderly, with 1 out of 4 people over the age of 65 affected by some degree of hearing loss.[7] Patients with sensory or communication impairments will require assistive techniques to optimize communication. These impairments include hearing impaired or deaf, visually impaired or blind, and literacy, language, or cultural barriers to communication.

Visually impaired patients are more dependent upon the auditory form of communication. Speaking clearly, not necessarily louder, so that the patient can understand you and confirm it is important. Large print reading materials may also help. A practical tool is the magnifying glass. Some patients may find it an adequate assist device. There are also effective teaching tools/aids for visually impaired individuals. However, the poorer the vision, the less useful the visual aids. Make sure to introduce yourself as the pharmacist so the patient knows who he or she is speaking with. If you intend to touch the patient, let him or her know your intentions and request permission to do so beforehand. Warm your hands briefly so that you do not startle the patient. Make sure to speak to the patient while you are performing any physical contact to keep him or her informed of your intentions.

Take responsibility for enhancing communication with a person who is hard of hearing. Background noise such as conversation, radios, television, or traffic make it more difficult to hear. Hearing impaired patients are more dependent upon visual forms of communication. Having written and pictorial materials available can be good assists. Gestures are helpful. In general, you should be directly in front of the patient for the benefit of the person who uses lip reading as a technique. Get the patient's attention before you speak by a gentle touch on the arm. Medications may affect the patient's ability to pay attention. Speak clearly in short sentences and not too quickly. If the patient asks you to repeat yourself more than once, find a different way to say what you want. Make sure to continue looking at and speaking directly to the patient rather than to others who are present. Patients who are hard of hearing only know what they are capable of hearing. The use of sign language interpreters may be effective if available.[8] Generalizations should be applied cautiously and tentatively since they have the potential to become stereotyping. Be observant of these possible influences during the interview, but then decide on their impact and relevance.

Continuing the Interview

Once you have started the patient talking, use a focused approach to inquiry and design the questioning strategy based upon your hypotheses of the patient's problems or needs. You must look, listen, be aware of odors, and pay attention, while trying to be as objective as possible about what you are observing. Sometimes, knowing exactly what the patient means by the words they are using is difficult. You can easily misinterpret or *translate the patient's words incorrectly*. A way to avoid this mistake is to inquire until you know what it would be like yourself to experience what the patient is telling you. Do not assume anything about the patient.

Questioning Skills

Use different types of questioning to get the patient to tell you what you really need to know. In general, express your questions in a way that elicits more than a "yes" or "no" answer. For example, you will learn more information by asking "How do you remember to take your medicines?" than by asking "Do you use a reminder package to help you remember to take your medicines?" In this example, the first question—known as an open-ended question—encourages the patient to talk, but the second question is closed and can be answered with one word or a short phrase. Closed questions are most useful when gathering precise, narrowly focused information. They can help fill in details after open-ended questions have established a general framework within a topic area. Let's examine a short interview where the pharmacist combines both types of questions:

Pharmacist: "Now, I'd like to discuss the nonprescription medicines you use. Can you tell me what you would take if you got a headache?"

Patient: "I'd most likely use some Tylenol, maybe Advil."

Pharmacist: "Do you ever take any aspirin?"

Patient: "Yes sometimes. My wife swears by Bufferin and sometimes gives me that."

Pharmacist: "How do you manage constipation if it occurs?"

Patient: "I try to manage it by watching what I eat. I've been eating a couple of prunes every morning."

Pharmacist: "What if the prunes don't work? Do you take any laxatives?"

Patient: "If I need something, my wife gives me some of her Nature's Remedy to take. That's something else she swears by—says it keeps her regular as a clock, and it's natural."

Pharmacist: "Tell me about the vitamins and minerals you use."

Patient: "Well, I take a B-complex pill because the lady at the health shop at the mall said most people like me have stress and it would help. She also said the body needs more minerals than what were in regular vitamins, so I'm taking a pill that has calcium, magnesium, and zinc in it."

Pharmacist: "Any others?"

Patient: "No. No one seems to agree about how much vitamin C is a good idea, so I just drink some orange juice every day. I figure that it can't hurt me."

This combination of question types elicits the most complete information. The closed questions were most effectively used to follow up on the open-ended questions.

With direct questions, you attempt to learn information. With indirect questions or reflective statements, you encourage a patient to elaborate or clarify a previous comment. A reflective statement summarizes or simply restates the idea or feelings that were expressed. It demonstrates interest and understanding but does not imply approval. Indirect questions are most useful for eliciting a patient's feelings or concerns.

The following examples illustrate how both direct and indirect questions might be used to gather information on a patient's negative feelings about taking several medications. Direct questions on this topic include "Why are you unhappy about taking all of these medicines?" or "What bothers you about taking these medicines?" Comparable, reflective statements might be "So, you're unhappy about taking all of these medicines" or "What you seem to be saying is that it bothers you to have to take all of these medications." In this situation, the strength of the indirect question is that it is not too instructive to the patient as to how to express concerns or feelings. The direct question, conversely, can limit the patient's response. Depending on the topic, a direct question may evoke defensiveness.

A probe is a direct question designed to elicit specific information about a portion of what was said. There are two main purposes for probes: one is to redirect the patient's attention on something in order to ask about it again, and the other is to clarify a statement or obtain more detailed information. Probing is really a way of eliciting sufficient detail for an assessment. A common example is asking a patient to provide more information about the frequency of medication use. You may ask "How often do you take aspirin?" Then a patient may reply "Oh, just occasionally." This answer is not detailed enough for you to decide if the patient's aspirin use has any therapeutic implications. A suitable probe in this case might be "Which would describe how often you take this medication—a couple of times a week, a couple of times a month, or almost every day?" More than one probing question may be necessary to obtain enough detail for assessment purposes. **Table 5-1** provides an overview of the questioning strategies discussed here.

Listening Skills

Listening is a complex activity that requires openness and sensitivity. In many ways, an opportunity to listen can be lost. One common way is to talk. If you are talking, you are not listening. To maximize your opportunity to gather information, the person you are interviewing should be talking. Some keys to effective listening include

1. Give the person 100% of your attention.
2. Begin listening with an open, neutral mind.
3. Respond either verbally or nonverbally (nod, express interest) to demonstrate that you heard and understand. If your response is verbal, speak at approximately the same energy level.
4. Respond to the person in a way that shows you understand what he or she was saying.
5. Pay attention to the logical content of what the patient says, but also pay attention to how he or she says it. It reveals one's true feelings on the subject.
6. Demonstrate respect for the person's point of view.

Facilitation means to encourage patients to say more but do so without directing the conversation. Facilitation can be done either verbally or nonverbally. The message behind facilitative gestures is that you are interested in what the patient is saying. A common verbal facilitative gesture is to repeat the last words said by the patient (reflection) or to say a short phrase such as "go on," "I see," or "mm-hmm." These gestures encourage the patient to provide greater detail.

Attentive silence is an important facet of skillful interviewing. Silence essentially provides the opportunity for the patient to talk; as long as the patient is sharing relevant information, you are gathering important data. However, the word "attentive" is critical. Although you are not speaking, you must provide nonverbal cues that demonstrate your interest and encourage the patient to continue. In this way, silence is a nonverbal facilitative gesture or technique. Silence may also occur because the patient is confused, resistant, embarrassed, or has strong emotion. If the patient is confused, rephrase your question. If the patient is resistant to answering the question, acknowledge the patient's reluctance and explain the usefulness of the information to the pharmacy assessment. You might say, for example,

"I know that you are reluctant to discuss the frequency of use of your inhaler. However, I think that you are using it more often than what is intended. Knowing how often you use it now will help us determine how to change your medications to control your shortness of breath." A silence from embarrassment should be acknowledged. You might consider saying "I can see this is hard for you to talk about." Finally, if a strong emotion is evoked in the interview, a patient may become silent. If given a moment, most patients will "collect" themselves and continue with the interview.

Responding to Patients' Questions

Patients and others often raise questions during an interview. In fact, you may be seen as more accessible than physicians or as able to offer a "second opinion." However, these questions can create an uncomfortable situation if you do not know how much information has been shared with a patient or if the response would reveal unpleasant information. In general, it is appropriate to refer many questions about care or procedures to either a nurse or physician; questions on prognosis or medical problems should be referred to the patient's physician. You can acknowledge the patient's concerns, encourage him or her to seek the appropriate professional, and also let that professional know about the patient's concerns. Taking responsibility for interdisciplinary communication is an important part of the pharmaceutical care process.

You will often have requests for information as a pharmacist. However, patients also sometimes pose questions as a way of expressing concerns or underlying feelings. Before answering a question, think about what it might imply and then try to elicit the person's true

Table 5-1. Questioning Strategies

Type	Purpose	Usual Response	Example
Open ended	*Encourage patient to talk; elicit additional information*	*Conversational / large quantity of information*	*How do you manage a headache?*
Closed ended	*Gather specific, narrow-focused information*	*"yes"–"no" short phrases*	*Does your headache respond to aspirin?*
Direct	*Learn information*	*Specific information*	*What medication do you take for a headache?*
Indirect	*Elaborate or clarify information*	*Information about feelings or concerns*	*I hear you saying it bothers you that your headaches don't respond to aspirin.*
Probe	*Elicit specific information about a portion of something already said*	*Detailed information*	*What is the most aspirin you've taken at one time for a headache? And you've never felt relief from this?*

concern. For example, if a patient asks "What are the effects of this blood pressure medicine?," you might describe its pharmacologic actions. But if you respond with "The medication has several effects—why do you ask?," the patient has the opportunity to share a concern such as "Well, I read that it might cause memory problems."

Similarly, a question may convey an attitude that you should acknowledge. For example, a recent pharmacy school graduate is asked by an older patient, "How old are you?" This question may convey the attitude that the pharmacist is too young to be giving advice. The pharmacist may respond to the presumed attitude rather than to the factual question by saying "I realize that I may seem young, but I am a licensed pharmacist and am knowledgeable about your medicines." An alternative response may be, "I can help you get the most out of your medicines and stay safe while using them."

Patients and caregivers frequently ask a health professional for advice, and these questions can be taken at face value and answered accordingly. However, people also ask about personal situations where your advice would be inappropriate. For example, a man whose mother is having difficulty managing her medications at home may ask, "Do you think she should be placed in a nursing home?" While you may have an opinion, it is inappropriate to share it; the decision must be made by the family, not the pharmacist. As a reply, "Many factors have to be considered before you decide how best to care for your mother. In terms of her medication management, several options could be tried to improve her medication compliance at home."

Interpreting Nonverbal Communication

Both you and the patient communicate with words and behavior. Communication via behavior is a nonverbal exchange. Just as you carefully select the wording for a question, you must also control your nonverbal messages. Nonverbal messages are expressed by posture, facial expressions, gestures, activities, voice quality, and eye contact. A patient also may form impressions based on your personal appearance (just as you are likely to do in return). The general demeanor that facilitates communication conveys an unhurried calm style and interest. If you are collecting more than a small amount of information, it is appropriate to sit while talking with the patient; standing often implies being "too busy to spend time talking." Likewise, if you do other things while talking (e.g., leafing through a chart or fidgeting), the patient can interpret your behavior as indicating a lack of interest. Attentiveness and interest can be communicated by leaning forward, by maintaining eye contact, and by voice inflection. Open-body posture (arms extended or hanging loosely at the side) suggests to the patient that you are relaxed. Closed-body posture (limbs crossed or held in a defensive position) suggests mistrust or anxiousness. One gesture that will inhibit almost any conversation is looking at a watch.

Facial expressions are an important nonverbal behavior. Your expressions might be misinterpreted and negatively affect a patient's willingness to communicate. If you frown, for example, a patient may interpret this as indicating anger or annoyance. Your expressions may also convey judgmental feelings, such as embarrassment, disapproval, or boredom, about what the patient is saying. Although you may experience these feelings, nonverbal expression of them is likely to inhibit further sharing by the patient.

Making eye contact is generally regarded as a positive way to engage the patient in communication. However, eye contact and its meaning vary by culture. In Asian, Native American, Indochinese, Arab, and Appalachian cultures, directly looking at someone may indicate a sign of disrespect or aggression. In some cultures, it is not acceptable for women or younger people to make direct eye contact.[9]

In summary, Platt and Gordon recommend the following behaviors.[10] Avoid outside interruptions when you are speaking with a patient. Look like you're listening. Look like you are there for a while. Sit down when speaking with the patient. Use touch appropriately. Even when you are not talking, your body language is talking for you.

Special Situations

The Pediatric Patient

Parents or guardians are a usual source of information when a child is evaluated. For the very young, adults may describe the child's health experience as what they observe rather than how the child feels. Coulehan and Block point out that participation in the pediatric interview changes when children reach the age of 5–6 years. These children are able to broadly speak about their concerns but may need an adult to provide accuracy and precision. Adolescents take an active role in their own health care and may need to speak with you in confidence. Local regulations govern confidentiality issues.

The Geriatric Patient

Older patients are more likely to have multiple conditions and complex medication regimens that challenge the patient and you in successfully managing medication use. A larger proportion of the elderly population have low income, decreased mental acuity, impaired memory and access to care, and reliance on caregivers. These patients need you to spend more time initially in assessing their health and medication management needs. You are more likely to encounter adverse drug events, undertreatment of conditions, and overtreatment of conditions in this population. These patients often go to multiple providers for their varying problems and may use multiple pharmacies. Constructing an effective history may require the input of people who know the older patient well enough to fill in the details. You are likely to interact with caretakers to obtain information and make decisions when dealing with elderly patients. You must discern who has the authority to make decisions on behalf of the patient and take care to manage these relationships appropriately.

Working with an Interpreter

It has been argued that every clinical encounter with a patient is actually a cross-cultural event.[10] We might classify this in two ways. Patients may not speak your language nor you theirs, and many patients lack conversational English language skills. Alternatively, you may both speak the same language but use the words for different ideas about the problems that the patient is experiencing. In both situations, translation is needed, and it always involves both language and culture.[11]

The roles of interpreters vary. Interpreters may translate the meaning of words in a neutral way; alternatively, they may advocate or negotiate for the patient by controlling and filtering information between you and the patient. Therefore, it is important to communicate to the interpreter what you want and expect from the encounter, such as the following:

- Tell translators what you need to obtain good and useful information.
- Determine the translation technique that you would like (simultaneous, consequential, or summary)
- Encourage the translator to ask questions when clarification is needed for the translator or patient.
- Tell the translator that you expect the patient to be assured of confidentiality and privacy.
- Determine how the exchange is progressing. Ask the translator to provide you feedback about the patient's comprehension of the exchange.

Translation will take time and may create distance between you and the patient. To make the most of the encounter, communicate to the patient that you are interested in doing your best to understand and also ask that of the patient. Keep eye contact with the patient, rather than the translator, as much as possible. This may best be accomplished by sitting next to the translator, with both of you across from the patient. This way the patient can make contact with both of you, and you keep your eye contact directed toward the patient.[12] Use touch and nonverbal communication techniques to enhance your understanding as cultural considerations permit.

In general, family members, especially children, and friends make poor translators for communication about personal and private matters. However, a family member may be the only available translator. There may be a need for you to provide brief training about the role of a translator and the need to communicate in a neutral and nonfiltered fashion.

Physical Assessment

Physical assessment activities are used to assist patients determine their self-treatment needs (e.g., selecting an OTC product or referring to another provider), monitor drug therapy response, and determine the success of the care plan or recommendations you have made. In this context, physical assessment will provide you with valuable baseline data about your patient. If your patient is being managed for hypertension, taking the patient's blood pressure at the initiation of therapy will provide you with a frame of reference to monitor his or her response to treatment. If your patient is being treated for atrial fibrillation, assessing the patient's pulse for rate and rhythm will provide you with a simple monitoring parameter to determine treatment response.

The skills of physical assessment include observation or inspection, palpation or manipulation, percussion, and auscultation. The skill used most by pharmacists to collect physical data is observation. Physical data collected by pharmacists includes age (as birth date), weight, height, pulse rate and rhythm, respiratory rate, and blood pressure.

Review of Systems Approach

You may use the review of systems (ROS) approach to elicit a more complete assessment of symptoms that a patient may be experiencing as you are interviewing the patient to gather data. The ROS approach asks questions by geographically beginning at the head and working down through the body systems, ending at the toes. This approach is sometimes used when you are not getting adequate and specific information to assist you in further determining the patient's problems or response to treatment.

Mental Status Assessment

Physical assessment includes those assessments related to the mental state. Conducting a mental status examination for a patient who appears to have inconsistencies with memory and substantial medication nonadherence problems may reveal findings that should be used in plan redesign and possible referral to a primary care physician. Coulehan and Block state that you can quickly and nonintrusively assess cognitive function of a patient at the start of the interview without a formal mental status examination.[2] When you first meet a patient, you should assess the level of *alertness* demonstrated. You should also pay attention to the person's *general appearance* and *behavior.* As the patient begins to speak, assess the *verbal output* or *speech*. As the person converses with you, determine if the patient demonstrates a pattern of *thought process that is logical and of appropriate content*. Notice the patient's *mood and affect*. Many patients who have cognitive difficulties will give the impression of being *oriented to time, place, and person*. However, as you continue to talk, the patient's *ability to remember* may become more apparent when specific questions are asked. This approach gives you insight into the patient's mental state without a formal test or measurement. Alternatively, the Mini-Mental Status Examination (MMSE) can be used to rapidly quantify the patient's overall cognitive function.[13] Pharmacists have found it useful as an indicator of cognitive impairment in relationship to medication use (see **Figure 5-2**).

Activities of Daily Living (ADLs) and Instrumental Activities of Daily Living (IADLs) are methods to assess a patient's inability to manage the basic tasks of everyday life. ADLs are in the form of questionnaires and assess such things as eating, bathing, dressing, toileting, and transferring. The IADL assess the functional capabilities, such as using the telephone, traveling, shopping for meals, doing housework, managing money, and taking medicines. The goal of using these instruments is to determine how well and in what areas your patient is able to maintain personal independence in daily life. This tool is commonly used by nurses or occupational and physical therapists—individuals who often manage the long-term adaptation abilities of patients. The IADL is a useful tool for pharmacists' general assessment of a patient's ability to take medications independently of assistance and to determine one's mobility in getting to the pharmacy and obtaining medication. There are many versions of the ADL and IADL, but a representative IADL is included in **Figure 5-3**.[14]

Closing the Encounter

Closing the encounter is an important communication that outlines your understanding of the patient's needs and the responsibilities you have to the patient. In most situations, the closure should include reviewing what your findings of importance are—the problems you have identified and the signs and symptoms that support it. If you are ready at this time, you should also generate the problem list with priorities. From this, you should agree on an action plan and determine your responsibilities and the patient's responsibilities. This should culminate in patient education and answering any last questions from the patient. The appropriate point to end the encounter and how long the encounter should take depend on the nature of the patient's problem, its urgency, and your own constraints.

Documenting the Encounter

Once you have heard the patient's story, you should document it in writing. How do you do this given the breadth of information, symptoms, experiences, and feelings shared with you? What do you write—knowing it will be included in the permanent record? You must select the facts or observations that appear most important from all of the information you can access. As you gain experience, you will almost automatically decide what problems have surfaced. You should record your findings in a way that will facilitate your own work with the patient and enlighten others also caring for the patient who have access to your documentation records. Chapter 4 introduced you to documentation; more detail will be presented throughout the case studies.

SUMMARY

This chapter has provided an introduction to the structure and process of the patient encounter. No matter what the circumstances or setting, therapeutic care is the purpose of your encounter with the patient. The well conducted interview is a primary source of information to determine the patient's needs. You should now be able to properly prepare for the interview, construct an organized approach, open and close the interview properly, and listen, respond, and use questioning strategies appropriately. Your interaction with the patient (and others) should be broad and open based upon the patient's cues. Physical assessment may be an important component to some patient interviews. Once completed, the interview should be documented in retrievable records for you and others involved in the care of the patient if appropriate.

CASES

See pages 74–85 for cases.

The Mini-Mental State Examination

Items			Points

Orientation

1. What is the   Year?   1
Season?   1
Date?   1
Day?   1
Month?   1

2. Where are we?   State?   1
County?   1
Town or city?   1
Hospital?   1
Floor?   1

Registration

3. Name three objects, taking one second to say each. Then ask the patient all three after you have said them. Give one point for each correct answer. Repeat the answers until the patient learns all three.   3

Attention and calculation

4. Serial sevens. Give one point for each correct answer. Stop after five answers. *Alternate*: Spell WORLD backwards.   5

Recall

5. Ask for names of three objects learned in Question 3. Give one point for each correct answer.   3

Language

6. Point to a pencil and a watch. Have the patient name them as you point.   2
7. Have the patient repeat "No ifs, ands, or buts."   1
8. Have the patient follow a three-stage command: "Take the paper in your right hand. Fold the paper in half. Put the paper on the floor."   3
9. Have the patient read and obey the following: "CLOSE YOUR EYES." (Write it in large letters.)   1
10. Have the patient write a sentence of his or her own choice. (The sentence should contain a subject and an object and should make sense. Ignore spelling errors when scoring.)   1
11. Enlarge the design printed below to 1 – 5 cm per side and have the patient copy it. (Give one point if all sides and angles are preserved and if the intersecting sides form a quadrangle.)   1

Figure 5-2. The Mini-Mental State Examination (Reproduced, with permission, from Folstein MF. The Mini-Mental State Examination. In: Crook T, Ferris S, Bartus R, eds. Assessment in geriatric psychopharmacology. New Canaan, CT: Mark Powley; 1983:50–1.)

Instrumental Activities of Daily Living (IADL)

Patient's Name: _____ **Date:**_____

I = Independent   *A = Assistance Required*   *D = Dependent*

Obtained from Patient	Obtained from Informant	Activity	Guidelines for Assessment
I A D	I A D	**Using Telephone**	I = Able to look up numbers, dial, receive and make calls without help A = Unable to use telephone D = Able to answer phone or dial operator in an emergency but needs special phone or help in getting number, dialing
I A D	I A D	**Traveling**	I = Able to drive own car or travel alone on buses, taxis A = Able to travel but needs someone to travel with D = Unable to travel
I A D	I A D	**Shopping**	I = Able to take care of all food/clothes A = Able to shop but needs someone to shop with D = Unable to shop
I A D	I A D	**Preparing Meals**	I = Able to plan and cook full meals A = Able to prepare light foods but unable to cook full meals alone D = Unable to prepare any meals
I A D	I A D	**Housework**	I = Able to do heavy housework, i.e., scrub floors A = Able to do light housework, but needs help with heavy tasks D = Unable to do any housework
I A D	I A D	**Taking Medicine**	I = Able to prepare/take medications in the right dose at the right time A = Able to take medications, but needs reminding or someone to prepare them D = Unable to take medications
I A D	I A D	**Managing Money**	I = Able to manage buying needs, i.e., write checks, pay bills A = Able to manage daily buying needs but needs help managing checkbook, paying bills D = Unable to handle money

Figure 5-3. Instrumental Activities of Daily Living (IADL) (Adapted from Lawton MP, Brody EM. Assessment of older people: self-maintaing and instrumental activities of daily living. Gerontologist. 1969; 9:179–86.)

Case 1: *Lauren Smith calls Nasir Jabr, PharmD, RPh, 2 days later.*

Please read the following telephone interview. You will evaluate this encounter for appropriateness and completeness.

Pharmacy Technician (answers telephone): "Hello, you have reached Werbert's Pharmacy. This is Nancy, Pharmacy Technician, how may I help you?"

Lauren: "This is Lauren Smith. Is Nasir Jabr available?"

Nancy, Pharmacy Technician: "Yes, just a moment, will you hold please?"

Lauren: "Yes."

Nasir Jabr, Pharmacist: "Hello Lauren; it is nice to hear from you. What may I help you with?"

Lauren: "Nasir, you mentioned to me if my symptoms did not go away to give you a call. Well, they haven't."

Nasir Jabr: "Tell me what symptoms you are having."

Lauren: "I am having a burning sensation when I go to the bathroom."

Nasir Jabr: "Do you mean when you urinate?"

Lauren: "Yes. And it has worsened. It hurts so much that I just can't stand it anymore."

Nasir Jabr: "Lauren, it sounds like you have an acute urinary tract infection. I would like to refer you to a physician so that he can confirm this and start antibiotic treatment."

Lauren: "I never have experienced anything like this before. Do you think I should go to the Emergency Room?"

Nasir Jabr: "No, this is a common problem that many women of your age experience. There are several things you can do to reduce your chances of having this problem again. In the meantime, you need to get in to see a physician and start treatment. Do you have a physician that you see?"

Lauren: "No, I really haven't had any problems that I haven't been able to treat on my own. Would you refer me to someone?"

Nasir Jabr: "Dr. Joyce Miller is nearby and has a general family practice. The office phone number is 501-2963. You need to tell the office when you call that you are having this pain and that the pharmacist referred you to the physician."

Lauren: "Good. Thank you Nasir."

Nasir Jabr: "You are welcome. I would also like to know a few additional things. Do you have any other medical problems that you are self-treating?"

Lauren: "No."

Nasir Jabr: "What about birth control? Do you use birth control pills?"

Lauren: "Why do you ask?"

Nasir Jabr: "Women often are more susceptible to urinary tract infections if they are currently on birth control pills."

Lauren: "I didn't know that. Yes, I do."

Nasir Jabr: "Please tell that to Dr. Miller. Do you smoke?"

Lauren: "Well, yes. Why do you ask that?"

Nasir Jabr: "I noticed you bought cigarettes when you were in here last. I also noticed that you bought Advil. Do you use this for any other problems beside the pain that you describe now?"

Lauren: "Well, yes again. I often get headaches and find that this relieves most of my discomfort."

Nasir Jabr: "Lauren. Let Dr. Miller also know this history. Will you please let me know how it goes after you see her?"

Lauren: "Yes, Nasir; I will. Thank you so much for your help."

CASE 1: SPECIFIC QUESTIONS

Evaluate the initial encounter, the main encounter, and the closure to the encounter.

1. What were the correct communication skills demonstrated in this encounter?

2. What improvements in the communication skills would you recommend?

3. What types of information were not accessible to you because of the telephone communication?

Case 2: *Christine Johnston, PharmD, RPh, conducts the initial patient encounter with Mr. Montanez in the clinic.*

Mr. Montanez and his daughter Maria return to Christine Johnson's medication assessment clinic. She maintains an evaluation area in a clinic examination room that she has been set up with assessment tools and patient teaching materials, including the Patient History form (Figure 5-1).

Christine Johnston: "Bueños dias Señor Montanez and Maria. It is very nice to see you. Please have a seat and make yourself comfortable."

Maria: "I have brought everything that you asked of us last time when we met. I wrote down this list of medications my father takes and have also brought his prescription bottles."

Christine Johnston: "This is wonderful Maria. Thank you for bringing all of this. Let me take a few moments to look them over."

[Christine reads the list of medications and finds the following:

Diabinese 1 tablet every day

Tolinase 1 tablet every day

Mevacor 1 tablet every day

Tylox 1 tablet if leg pain

She examines the medication bottles and finds the following on the labels:

Chlorpropamide 125 mgs tab. Take 1 tab po qd for diabetes.

Tolazamide 250 mgs tab. Take 1 tab po qd for diabetes.

Mevacor 20 mgs tab. Take 1 tab with evening meal.

Tylox (325 mg acetaminophen/7.5 mg oxycodone) tab. Take 1 every 4 hours if needed for leg pain.

She thinks about what she is seeing and asks a few questions of Mr. Montanez.]

Christine Johnston (hands Mr. Montanez each medication container as she asks the questions): "Mr. Montanez, can you please tell me what this medication name is and how you take it?"

Mr. Montanez (looks at Maria with an alarmed expression): "I take this one in the morning. This one is (he moves the medication container back and forth like he is trying to focus his vision) well, I think this one is for my diabetes."

(Maria looks a little embarrassed for her father-in-law.)

Christine Johnston: "What about this one Mr. Montanez? Tell me what it is and how you use it."

(Mr. Montanez repeats the same episode. Christine decides not to pursue this further and asks a different line of questions.)

Christine Johnston: "Okay then Mr. Montanez. Thank you very much. Have you ever been told that you have allergies to any medicine?"

Mr. Montanez: "Yes. I was told I am allergic to codeine."

Christine Johnston [pulls out her opioid allergy decision tree developed by the pharmacists at her facility (**Figure 5-4**)]: "Do you have asthma?"

Mr. Montanez: "No."

Christine Johnston: "Why do you think you are allergic to codeine?"

Mr. Montanez: "Because the last time I had some I had an upset stomach and was dizzy. I called the pharmacy, and the pharmacist said I might be allergic to codeine. He told me I might need to switch to some other medicine."

Christine Johnston: "Have you ever had codeine before that?"

Mr. Montanez: "I am not really sure."

Christine Johnston: "When you had that upset stomach and were dizzy, did you develop a rash or itching?"

Mr. Montanez: "No."

Christine Johnston: "How about difficulty breathing soon afterward?"

Mr. Montanez: "No."

Christine Johnston: "Did you have to go into the emergency room or hospital for any reason right after taking it?"

Mr. Montanez: "No, oh no, not at all. I just didn't really feel good in my stomach, and I would get a little dizzy when I stood up. That's all."

Christine Johnston: "Mr. Montanez, do you find that you must use the bathroom to urinate frequently?"

Mr. Montanez: "I usually go every hour or two…I guess that's a lot. But I am thirsty and drink a lot of water too."

Maria interjects: "And beer too!" (she laughs)

continued

Case 2: *Christine Johnston, PharmD, RPh, conducts the initial patient encounter with Mr. Montanez in clinic. (cont'd)*

Christine Johnston: "How many beers a day do you drink sir?"

Mr. Montanez: "Well, usually 1 or 2." (Maria confirms by nodding her head "yes.")

Christine Johnston: "Do you lose the feeling in your hands or feet?"

Mr. Montanez: "Sometimes. Mostly I get pain in my feet and lower legs…it comes and goes."

Christine Johnston: "What do you do when you get this pain?"

Mr. Montanez: "Sometimes I take one of those medicines."

Maria: "I usually give him one of the Tylox tablets."

Christine Johnston: "Do you test your blood sugar at home?"

Maria (interjects): "Yes, I do this for him once a week with a machine."

Christine Johnston: "Did you bring this with you today?"

Maria: "No."

Christine Johnston: "Is there anything else that you do to take care of your health that we haven't discussed?"

Mr. Montanez (joking): "Well, I come here a lot." (everyone laughs)

Christine Johnston: "Okay Mr. Montanez. Thank you so much. I am going to have the nurse check your urine for protein and check your blood sugar too. Let me escort you to the laboratory area."

(Christine walks Mr. Montanez to the outpatient stat lab and returns to discuss the case further with Maria.)

Christine Johnston: "Maria, is there anything else that your father-in-law takes or is given to him for his health?"

Maria: "Well, I probably should not talk to you about this, but I am not sure if this is good for him or not. You see, he is from the old country…and he has beliefs about his health that are different than what goes on here in this clinic. He believes that his diabetes was caused by 'susto.' This is the word for him having a 'fright' or 'scare' many years ago. This is commonly believed by my older relatives. So he has also been told to use some of the plants to get better."

Christine Johnston: "What do you mean 'plants'?"

Maria: "Well, his sister started him using Cactus Flowers, from the Prickly Pear Cactus."

Christine Johnston: "How does he take this?"

Maria: "She says to broil the stems and eat them each day. She says if he feels worse, to eat them three times during the day, if he feels better, to eat one. I tell him not to do this, but he ignores me and tells me I am not helping him. So I buy these at the market and help him with it."

Christine Johnston: "Is there anything else that he uses?"

Maria: "His sister also buys him Yucca root from the store and brings it over. She boils it into a tea and has him drink a few cups each day. She taught me how to do this. We do it some days."

Christine Johnston: "I really appreciate you telling me about this. I will need to check on whether there is any evidence that this is helpful to diabetes; or for that matter, whether this may cause harm."

Maria: "Thank you so much, no matter what you find, it will be difficult for my father-in-law to believe what you tell him about these things. These beliefs are strong and founded in his culture and family."

Christine Johnston: "I understand. Why don't I go get your father now. In the meantime, if he has a worsening of symptoms, including dizziness, thirst, or the frequency of his urination, please call me. What I plan to do is evaluate the information you have provided to me today and have you return in 1 week for a followup plan."

Maria: "Very good. We will do this."

Opioid Allergy Decision Tree

Patient Interview

Do you have asthma?

_____Yes_____No Patients with asthma are more likely to develop difficulty breathing because of opioid-induced histamine release.

> **Recommendation:** **If yes**, consider pretreatment of asthma patients who have previously reacted to opioids with diphenhydramine or prednisone. Continue on with patient interview.
> > **If no**, continue on with patient interview.

Have you ever been told that you are allergic to or should not receive codeine, morphine, or other opioid medication?

_____Yes_____No *Pharmacist: Common brand names to prompt patient with:* Vicodin®, Lorcet®, Percocet®, Tylox®, Roxicet®, Percodan®, Oxycontin®, Darvon 65®, Darvon N®, Darvocet N-100®, Demerol®, Duragesic®, Dilaudid®, Numorphan®, Talwin NX®

> **Recommendation:** **If yes**, continue on with patient interview.
> > **If no,** correct allergy status documentation in the chart. No further interview necessary.

Did you (patient) report any of the following symptoms or did any of your health care providers observe one or more of the following symptoms after taking codeine/morphine or <u>drug(s) identified by patient above?</u> (Check all that apply from both list A and list B.)

List A	List B
____ Upset stomach	____ Drug-related fever
____ Dizziness	____ Severe systemic rash or itching
____ Previous history of taking codeine/morphine	____ Localized hives (late onset urticaria > 72 hours)
	____ Immediate hypotension or hypertension after administration
____ Mild, localized itching	____ Major total body rash (early onset urticaria within 1 – 72 hrs)
____ Difficulty breathing (due to laryngeal edema or bronchospasm)	____ Hospitalization/emergency room visits due to opioid allergy
	____ Documented anaphylaxis to codeine/morphine

Recommendations:

> **If yes to any symptoms in list A, and no to any in List B**, then the risk of anaphylaxis approximates that of the general population. Continue with current agent.

> **If yes to any symptoms in List B,** then risk of anaphylaxis is greater than that of the general population. Opioid agents are listed in three distinct classes below. If allergy is confirmed, switch to an alternative from one of the other two available classes.

> > I. <u>**Most structurally similar to morphine/codeine:**</u> Hydromorphone, hydrocodone, oxymorphone, oxycodone, buprenorphine, butorphanol[*], nalbuphine, pentazocine[**]

> > II. <u>**Less structurally similar to morphine/codeine:**</u> Meperidine, fentanyl, sufentanil, alfentanil

> > III. <u>**Least structurally similar to morphine/codeine:**</u> Methadone[***], propoxyphene

Figure 5-4. *Opioid Allergy Decision Tree: standard method to determine the likelihood of true allergy and cross-sensitivity to opioid derivatives.*

CASE 2: SPECIFIC QUESTIONS

Evaluate the initial encounter, the main encounter, and the closure to the encounter.

1. How was communication affected by the language and cultural differences among Mr. Montanez, Maria, and Christine Johnston in this encounter?

2. How might the information revealed through this visit be affected by the use of a professional interpreter?

3. What possible communication problems emerged about Mr. Montanez through this routine encounter?

Case 3: *Luisa Rodriguez, PharmD, conducts an admission history on Huong Tran in the Emergency Room.*

Luisa grabs a spacer device to help Huong with his Metered Dose Inhaler of albuterol.

Luisa Rodriguez: "Huong, I am attaching this to the inhaler…all you have to do is breathe as soon as you push it down. I would like you to do this now."

[Huong does this, trying to breathe deeply. Luisa has him repeat this each minute three more times. Huong's breathing improves substantially within 5 minutes. Luisa has him wait 5 minutes and repeat the 4 inhalations one minute apart each. Huong's breathing improves further. While Luisa is working with Huong, the Emergency Room nurse was administering Solu-Medrol 40 mgs (1 mg/kg dose) intravenously. Huong's parents became frightened. Luisa tries to reassure them that Huong is receiving the right care, but they do not understand and watch in great fear.

The metered dose inhaler process is repeated again in 20 minutes. By the end of one hour, Huong is breathing normally.]

(Huong speaks to his parents in Vietnamese.)

Huong: "It is okay Mom and Dad. I am better now. These people have done the right things for me."

(His parents are relieved and ask him what will happen next. Huong translates this back to Luisa.)

Luisa Rodriguez: "Well Huong, because you have been here three times in these past 2 weeks, the doctor wants to admit you to the hospital. I need to interview you about any medicines you are on and how you take care of yourself. Then we will provide you with medication and send you home. But, I am concerned that your parents

will not understand everything that we have to discuss. Is there anyone else in your family that speaks English and Vietnamese… an older brother, sister, or a relative of your parents?"

Huong: "No. It is just us. There are other people in the neighborhood. But I pretty much do all of the translating for our family."

Luisa Rodriguez: "We have a translator who speaks Chinese. I wonder if this is close enough to be helpful to your parents. In addition, there is a social worker who may be able to contact a volunteer translator in the community. Dr. Mooris will be back in a minute to explain what will happen to your parents. I will let him know that you are the family translator."

(Huong is transferred to the general pediatric floor in the hospital. Luisa visits him to conduct a medication admission history.)

Luisa Rodriguez: "Hello again Huong, Mr. and Mrs. Tran. I hope you are comfortable here. This is the area of the hospital I usually work in. Huong, tell me what medicines you are supposed to take."

Huong: "I have the inhaler just like the one you had me use in the Emergency Room. But I don't have one of those things that you put on it…that really worked better."

Luisa Rodriguez: "That is called a spacer device. We will get you started with that in the future. How do you get this medicine?"

Huong: "Well the school nurse has been working with a doctor in our neighborhood. She worked it out so that I could see her after school sometimes. She gives me the inhaler from her cabinet."

Case 3: *Luisa Rodriguez, PharmD, conducts an admission history on Huong Tran in the Emergency Room. (cont'd)*

Luisa Rodriguez: "Do you run out of medicine?"

Huong: "Yes. I tell the nurse and she works it out for me to get some more. That is what happened about 2 weeks ago. I ran out and told her about it, but she couldn't find any yet. So I have been having trouble."

Luisa Rodriguez: "What other medicines do you take?"

Huong: "My mother gives me something that she gets from Vietnam. Mom, what is it called?"

(Huong asks his mother in Vietnamese.)

Mrs. Tran: "Bai Guo Ye."

Huong: "I do not know what it is exactly. She takes a powder and mixes a little bit of water with it.

She grinds it up and lets it soak into the water. Then I drink the small amount of liquid."

(Luisa makes a note to herself to look up this substance and find out what it is.)

Luisa Rodriguez: "Does she do anything else for you?"

Huong: "There is a doctor, he uses the needles."

Luisa Rodriguez: "Does he call it acupuncture?"

Huong: "Yes. That is it. And sometimes she takes me there. It's okay; it really doesn't hurt or anything."

Luisa Rodriguez: "Thank you Huong, Mr. and Mrs. Tran. I will be back later to discuss your medicines with you."

CASE 3: SPECIFIC QUESTIONS

Evaluate the initial encounter, the main encounter, and the closure to the encounter.

1. What were the difficulties that Luisa Rodriguez was faced with during this emergency room encounter?

2. What issues in patient care management might Luisa face, even if she is able to arrange for an interpreter that speaks their language?

Case 4: *Michael Jones, PharmD, conducts a patient interview and limited physical examination with Mr. Robinson.*

Please read the face-to-face interview text. You will evaluate this encounter for appropriateness and completeness.

(Michael returns back to Mr. Robinson's room to conduct his initial patient interview. Before entering the room he checks to make sure that he has his pocket notepad and his stethoscope and that his pager is on vibrator mode so it doesn't disrupt Mr. Robinson during the interview. He knocks on Mr. Robinson's door.)

Michael Jones, Pharmacist: "Hello Mr. Robinson. It's me, Michael the pharmacist. May I come in to speak with you?"

Mr. Robinson: "Yes. I've been anxious for your return. Please come in."

Michael Jones: "Mr. Robinson, I'd like to ask you several questions. I need some information from you directly to be able to recommend to Dr. Rangert the best approach for your anticoagulation while you are hospitalized. This means I need to know information about how you are feeling, how your body is responding to this medicine, and about other general aspects of your health. I would also like to respond to any questions you have. Please be assured that whatever you and I discuss will remain private."

continued

Case 4: *Michael Jones, PharmD, conducts a patient interview and limited physical examination with Mr. Robinson. (cont'd)*

(As he is speaking, Michael finds a chair and brings it up alongside Mr. Robinson's bed so that he can face him at eye level. He also partially closes the room door to assure privacy in the conversation. He sits down.)

Mr. Robinson: "Go ahead. I'm not going anywhere."

Michael Jones: "Thank you. I'm going to ask you some general questions, and then I will follow up with specific questions about your blood thinner medicine."

[Michael uses the Patient's History Form (**Figure 5-5**) first to guide his questions and take notes and record relevant information from the interview.]

Michael Jones: "Tell me about yourself. How old are you?"

Mr. Robinson: "I am 76 years old."

Michael Jones: "Where do you live?"

Mr. Robinson: "At my home. It's been mine and my wife's now for over 50 years."

Michael Jones: "Are you still working?"

Mr. Robinson: "Well, not really. I retired several years ago from farming. I have a pension, but I still take fresh vegetables to the market for a little extra when they are in season."

Michael Jones: "Does your wife help you with your medicines?"

Mr. Robinson: "Well she used to. But she died 1 year ago, and I am having a very hard time keeping track of things. I live alone now."

Michael Jones: "I am sorry to hear that. Do you have anyone who helps you with your work around the house?"

Mr. Robinson: "Not really. There are a couple of lady friends of my wife who look in on me now and then. They pick up my medicines or take me to see Joe Daly, the pharmacist at Daly Apothecary in town. He's been the most help to me."

Michael Jones: "What is the main problem that caused you to come to the hospital Mr. Robinson?"

Mr. Robinson: "I was having a real hard time breathing, I just felt like I was gonna suffocate. I called Joe, and he asked me a few questions. He said he'd call me right back. When he did, he said

that he talked to Dr. Friedland in town who said that I should get to the hospital right away."

Michael Jones: "Who is Dr. Friedland?"

Mr. Robinson: "He's the doctor I usually see. He works with Dr. Rangert."

Michael Jones: "What medical problems have you been told you have?"

Mr. Robinson: "I was told I had a congested heart…and bad blood pressure…and that my heart beats in a funny way, so they give me a blood thinner for that problem."

Michael Jones: "Could you tell me what medicines you take?"

Mr. Robinson: "Well I can never remember names. But I know my blood thinner, my heart pills, there are three of them…and my thyroid medicine too. You know I put all of these medicines in a bag and brought them to the hospital. That nurse, you know, Charlotte, she has them."

Michael Jones: "Okay Mr. Robinson. I will get them and be back with a couple more questions. Thanks. That will help us to do better with your medicine. Do you remember the last time you took your blood thinner?"

Mr. Robinson: "I don't miss that one. I took that yesterday morning."

Michael Jones: "Now Mr. Robinson. I'd like to take a closer look at you. Do you mind if I take your pulse and blood pressure?"

Mr. Robinson: "No—that's fine. Go ahead."

(Michael Jones measures his blood pressure. It is 156/102 mm Hg at rest. He then takes his pulse rate of 110 beats/minute-rhythm irregular. While he is doing this, he examines Mr. Robinson's skin and eyes for evidence of bleeding or bruising. There is no evidence of a problem.)

Michael Jones: "Mr. Robinson, your blood pressure is higher than normal and your heart rate, which I am checking by monitoring your pulse, is higher than we like to see it. The rhythm of your heart is also irregular. Have you been told you have atrial fibrillation?"

Mr. Robinson: "Yes…that's it. That's what it's called."

Michael Jones: "Do you drink alcohol sir? Beer or whiskey or anything?"

continued

PATIENT'S HISTORY FORM – PHARMACIST'S RECOMMENDATIONS/PLAN

Demographic and Administrative Information:		Room No.	ID No. 02946372	
Date:		Gender: M	Primary Language: ENGLISH	
Name: SAMUEL ROBINSON		DOB:	Height:	Weight:
Street Address: 1362 MOCKINGDALE LANE		BP:	Temp:	Pulse:
City, State, Zip BILOXI, MISSISSIPPI 78023		Race/Ethnicity: AF-AMER	Religion:	
Home Phone #: (901) 468-4832		MD/Phone No.		
Work Phone #: N/A		Pharmacist/Phone No.		
Occupation: RETIRED		Insurance: MEDICARE		
Family Members/Care Givers: WIFE DECEASED				

Problem List:	Pharmacist's Recommendations/Plan:
1.	
2.	
3.	
4.	
5.	
6.	
7.	
8.	
9.	
10.	

Pharmacist's Name: _____   Date: _____   Phone/Pager #: _____

Chief Complaint/History of Present Illness:

Past Medical History/Surgery/Genetics:

Family and Social History (significant relationship/co-habitants):

Physical Examination/Review of Systems:

ADL:

Lifestyle/Diet/Exercise:

Acute and Chronic Medical Problems/Associated Symptoms:	
1.	6.
2.	7.
3.	8.
4.	9.
5.	10.

Describe Patient's Health Beliefs and Values:

Does Patient Receive Assistance in Medication Administration? Describe:

Figure 5-5. Patient's History Form—Pharmacist's Recommendations/Plan (cont'd)

Allergies/Intolerances: ( ) No Known Drug Allergies		
Allergen:	Reaction:	Treatment:
Allergen:	Reaction:	Treatment:
Allergen:	Reaction:	Treatment:

Social Drug Use: Alcohol: Caffeine: Tobacco: Other:

Current Drug Therapy (prescription and over the counter, vitamins, remedies, alternative treatment):

Drug Name Strength/Route	Problem Number	Usual Schedule	Describe PRN Use	Does Med Work?	Side Effects or Concerns	Compliance Issues
1.						
2.						
3.						
4.						
5.						
6.						
7.						
8.						
9.						
10.						
11.						
12.						
13.						
14.						
15.						

Past Drug Therapy:

Time Line: Circle administration times and record appropriate medications and meals below:

Patient's Actual Use:

6 7 8 9 10 11 12 1 2 3 4 5 6 7 8 9 10 11 12 1 2 3 4 5
am   noon   pm   midnight   am

Prescribed Schedule:

6 7 8 9 10 11 12 1 2 3 4 5 6 7 8 9 10 11 12 1 2 3 4 5
am   noon   pm   midnight   am

Costs of Meds/Month: $ Insurance: (   ) Yes   (   ) No
Co-pay: Medicaid: Annual Income:

Completed by: _____   **Date:** _____

Figure 5-5. Patient's History Form—Pharmacist's Recommendations/Plan

Case 4: *Michael Jones, PharmD, conducts a patient interview and limited physical examination with Mr. Robinson. (cont'd)*

Mr. Robinson: "No sir—don't touch it." (He frowns at Michael with displeasure.)

Michael Jones: "How about smoking?"

Mr. Robinson: "Well yes, I do smoke. I smoke cigarettes."

Michael Jones: "How many cigarettes do you smoke in a day sir?"

Mr. Robinson: "Well—for sure about 20 or so—1 pack a day or so."

(Michael switches to his Anticoagulation Assessment Record, **Figure 5-6**.)

Michael Jones: "Have you had any bleeding of any kind recently Mr. Robinson?"

Mr. Robinson: "What do you mean?"

Michael Jones: "Do you have bleeding of your gums when you brush your teeth?"

Mr. Robinson: "No."

Michael Jones: "Have you noticed any blood in your stool or urine when you use the bathroom?"

Mr. Robinson: "No."

Michael Jones: "Okay then. Do you take any over-the-counter medicine?"

Mr. Robinson: "What is that?"

Michael Jones: "The kind you can buy without a prescription. For example, do you use any acetaminophen? Some people know it as Tylenol®."

Mr. Robinson: "No."

Michael Jones: "How about ibuprofen—some people know that as Advil®?"

Mr. Robinson: "You know…some times when I get a headache, I think I take that Advil® medicine."

Michael Jones: "How about vitamins. Do you take any?"

Mr. Robinson: "Yes. I know that I take a once-a-day vitamin of some kind. And also vitamin E. My wife told me that vitamin E was good for my heart."

Michael Jones: "I have a few things to look at in your medical record, and then I will recommend what to do to both you and your doctor."

Mr. Robinson: "Thank you Michael."

CASE 4: SPECIFIC QUESTIONS

1. Evaluate Michael's initial greeting in the encounter with Mr. Robinson. What did he do to "set the stage" correctly for the interview?

2. What additional questions could Michael Jones have asked to learn more about Mr. Robinson's Advil® use?

3. Is Mr. Robinson someone who should be assessed with the IADL? The MMSE?

GENERAL ASSESSMENT QUESTIONS

1. Describe the optimal environment for conducting a patient interview.

2. What should you communicate to the patient when you first meet him or her?

3. What will you evaluate about the patient when you have your initial interaction?

4. Describe ways to enhance your communication with a visually impaired patient.

5. Describe ways to enhance your communication with a hearing impaired patient.

6. What key points should you communicate with the patient about when you close the patient encounter?

ASSIGNMENT

1. Interview a friend or family member, practicing the communication skills and clinical observation skills presented in this chapter. You may use the Patient's History Form—Pharmacist's Recommendations/ Plan document (Figure 5-1) to keep track of your observations.

2. Conduct a Mini-Mental Status Examination on three different people. Reflect on the variation you observe in the responses from these individuals.

REFERENCES

1. Cipolle RJ, Strand LM, Morley PC. Pharmaceutical care practice. New York, NY: McGraw Hill; 1998.

ANTICOAGULATION ASSESSMENT RECORD   Patient's Name _____   Age _____ Date of Birth _____ Race _____

Home Telephone ( )_____ **Alternate Telephone** ( )_____
Emergency Contact Person _____ **Telephone** ( )_____

Habits (describe pattern of use): Smoking _____ **Alcohol** _____ **Drugs** _____

Indication for Anticoagulation	Check One	INR Goal
Prophylaxis of DVT		2-3
Treatment of Venous Thrombosis		2-3
Treatment of PE		2-3
Prevention of systemic embolism		2-3
Tissue heart valves		2-3
Acute MI		2-3
Valvular heart disease		2-3
Bileaflet mechanical valve/aortic position		2-3
Mechanical prosthetic valve		2.5-3.5
Antiphospholipid syndrome		2.5-3.5
Acute MI (prevent recurrence)		2.5-3.5

Bleeding History/Risk Factors for Bleeding	
Factor	**Check if present**
Hosp. Admission for bleed	
Falls	
Oral bleed	
Vaginal bleed	
Lower GI bleed	
Upper GI Bleed	
Rectal bleed	
Guaiac + - __/__/__ ND	
hemorrhoids	
Seizure	
Urinary bleed	
Hct <30%	
Hematuria	

Conditions Requiring Dose Adjustment	
Condition	**Dose Change**
ETOH Acute	No change
ETOH Chronic	Inc dose
Advanced renal disease	Dec dose
>65 years old	Dec dose
Liver disease	Dec dose
Congestive heart failure	Dec dose
Thyroid disease	Dec dose

Baseline Hematology	
Hemoglobin	
Hematocrit	
Platelets	
WBC's	
Stool Guaiac	

Drug Interactions
Dietary/alternative sources of Vitamin K

Considerations for dosage determination:
Concurrent conditions requiring dosage adjustment
Bleeding history/risk factors for bleeding

Indication for anticoagulation
Target INR
Initial dose recommendation taking into consideration all factors:

Date	Dose	INR	RP Initials	Comments

Date	Dose	INR	RP Initials	Comments

ANTICOAGULATION ASSESSMENT RECORD   (page 2)
Vitamin K Food Intake History (Foods High in Vitamin K)

Food Source	Amount	Consumption Qty	Food Source	Amount	Consumption Qty
Fats and Dressings			Green Scallion - raw	2/3 cup	
Mayonnaise	7 tbsp		Kale - raw	3/4 cup	
Oils: Cannola, Salad, Soybean	7 tbsp		Lettuce - raw bib, red leaf	1-3/4 cup	
Vegetables			Mustard greens - raw	1-1/2 cup	
Broccoli	1/2 cup		Parsley - chopped	1-1/2 cups	
Brussel Sprouts	5 sprouts		Spinach - raw leaf	1-1/2 cups	

Figure 5-6. Anticoagulation Assessment Record   (cont'd)

			Turnip greens - raw	1-1/2 cups
Cabbage	1-1/2 cups		Watercress - raw chopped	3 cups
Collard greens	1/2 cup			
Endive - raw	2 cups			

Concurrent Medications Known to Interact with Warfarin (Prescriptions and OTC—name, dose, frequency):

Drug	Using	Action to be Taken	Drug	Using	Action to be Taken
Acetaminophen - large dose>1week		None	Dicloxacillin		Inc W dose
Alcohol - acute ingestion		Redraw INR in 24 hrs	Diflunisal		DecW dose
Alcohol - chronic ingestion		Inc W dose-stop ETOH	Disulfiram		DecW dose
Allopurinol		?Inc W dose	Fluconazole		DecW dose
Aminoglutethimide		Inc W dose	Griseofulvin		Inc W dose
Aminoglycosides		?DecW dose	Isoniazid		DecW dose
Amiodarone		DecW dose - delayed effect	Ketoconazole		DecW dose
>500 mgs/day ascorbic acid		?Inc W dose	Lovastatin		DecW dose
Azathioprine		?Inc W dose	Metronidazole		DecW dose
Azithromycin		?DecW dose	Miconazole		DecW dose
Barbiturates		Inc W dose	NSAIDS-varies with each agent		Inc/DecW dose
Carbamazepine		Inc W dose	Omeprazole- slight increase in INR		DecW dose
Cephalosporins		?DecW dose	Phenytoin		Inc/Dec W dose
Cholestyramine		Inc W dose/displace time of administration	Quinidine		DecW dose
Chloramphenicol		DecW dose	Simvastatin		DecW dose
Cimetidine		?DecW dose	Sulfinpyrazone		DecW dose
Ciprofloxacin		?DecW dose	Tamoxifen		DecW dose
Clofibrate/Gemfibrozil		DecW dose	Thyroid hormones		DecW dose
Colestipol		Inc W dose/displace time of administration	Tricyclic Antidepressants		?DecW dose
Corticosteroids		Unpredictable	TMP-SMX		DecW dose by 1/3
Cyclophosphamide		Inc W dose	Vitamin E		DecW dose
Cyclosporine		IncW dose	Valproic Acid		DecW dose
Danazol		DecW dose	Zafirleukast		DecW dose

Figure 5-6. Anticoagulation Assessment Record

2. Coulehan JL, Block MR. The medical interview: mastering skills for clinical practice, 3rd ed. Philadelphia, PA: F.A. Davis and Company; 1997.

3. Barrows HS, Pickell GC. Developing clinical problem solving skills—a guide to more effective diagnosis and treatment. New York, NY: Norton Medical Books; 1991.

4. Bernstein L, Bernstein RS. Interviewing: a guide for health professionals, 4th ed. Norwalk, CT: Appleton-Century-Crofts; 1985.

5. Zweber A. Cultural competence in pharmacy practice. *Am J Pharm Educ.* 2002; 66:172–6.

6. Addressing racial and ethnic disparities in health care fact sheet. AHRQ Publication No. 00-P041. Rockville, MD: Agency for Healthcare Research and Quality; February 2000. www.ahrq.gov/research/disparit.htm.

7. Clark M. Culture and aging: an anthropologic study of older Americans. Springfield, IL: Thomas; 1967.

8. McNamee C. Chapter 8—communicating with the hard of hearing. In: Physician–patient communication—reading and recommendation. George Henderson, ed. Springfield, IL: Thomas; 1981.

9. Barkauskas VH, Stoltenberg-Allen K, Baumann LC et al. Health and physical assessment. Mosby-Year Book, Inc.; 1998.

10. Platt FW, Gordon GH. Field guide to the difficult patient interview. Baltimore MD and Philadelphia PA: Lippincott Williams and Wilkins; 1999.

11. Myerscough PR. Talking with patients—a basic clinical skill. New York, NY: Oxford University Press; 1989.

12. Billings JA, Stoeckle JD. The clinical encounter—a guide to the medical interview and case presentation. Use touch and nonverbal communication techniques to enhance your understanding. Mosby-Year Book, Inc.; 1999.

13. Folstein JF, Folstein SE, McHugh PR. Mini-mental state: a practical method for grading the cognitive state of patients for the clinician. *J Psychiatry Res.* 1975; 12:189–98.

14. Lawton MP, Brody EM. Assessment of older people: self-maintaining and instrumental activities of daily living. *Gerontologist.* 1969; 179–86.

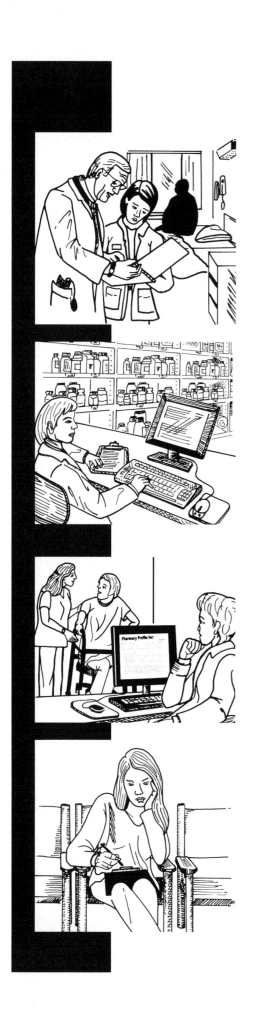

CHAPTER 6

The Patient's Record: A Primary Source of Information

"Let your policy be quality…"
Dad—*A Father's Book of Wisdom*

Chapter Outline:

Objectives / To be able to understand:

1. use of the patient medical chart or patient profile as a key source of information for providing patient care;
2. use of the medical chart or patient profile as a vehicle for documenting the provision of patient care; and
3. how to act legally and ethically to safeguard the confidentiality of patient information.

THE MEDICAL CHART

General Discussion of the Patient Medical Chart

Each patient who receives care within an organized health care institution (e.g., hospital, nursing home, or clinic) has a medical chart. The chart is the repository for all written information concerning that patient's care, condition, and treatment. Health professionals use it to record their assessments, diagnoses, treatment plans, and other pertinent information. In it, you will find laboratory values, test results, and descriptions of procedures you need to assess. The chart is the primary mode of communication between you and other health care professionals providing treatment to a patient. Use it to obtain the data you need to make good drug therapy decisions and then communicate those decisions to the rest of the health care team.

Uses of the Chart

A patient's medical chart is most commonly used by health professionals during patient care. However, the chart may be used by several individuals for multiple purposes:

The Clinician Who Writes in the Medical Record. Preparing a medical record aids in organizing and remembering information about patients, developing clinical skills, reflecting on the diagnosis and management, and planning continuing care.

Health Care Professionals within the Hospital. The chart serves as the primary mode of communication of patient information among health care professionals who collaborate in the patient's care. Medical professionals such as physicians, pharmacists, and nurses use the medical chart daily. Physical and occupational therapists, dieticians, respiratory therapists, and other allied health professionals also consistently refer to patient charts. When your care notes are available, you potentially enhance the quality of care these professionals can provide. With the increasing use of e-mail, fax machines, and computerized medical records, your notes are readily available to other clinicians who are collaborating in the patient's care.

Patients. Patients may access the chart to help them understand and review their treatment, allowing them to be more active in their self-care. They may also secure chart information to provide to outpatient health care providers or other professionals, such as insurance agents. Doctors' offices often request a copy of a patient's chart when seeing a patient for the first time, especially if the patient has an extensive medical history.

Administrative Personnel. Hospital administrators, risk managers, medical records personnel, and ward clerks all need to access the chart. Your supervisors may use the record to evaluate and guide your clinical development. Insofar as the record is an accurate account of what you observed, concluded, and did for the patient, it is one measure of your clinical performance. Similarly, record audits have been used to evaluate the quality of care, though their usefulness has been limited by discrepancies between what is recorded and what is actually done. The medical record contains data for assessing disability, mental competency, and eligibility for insurance billing, while also being used in utilization review and lawsuits.

Research Use. Patient medical charts can provide data for clinical research. Personnel researching drugs and medical devices use the chart to document information relevant to patient care. The information may be collected retrospectively, concurrently, or prospectively from patient charts. Pharmacy schools may have a research requirement as part of their degree program, and pharmacy residency programs usually have a research project requirement. Medical charts are a common source of data for such projects.

Public Health. Health agencies and registries use data from patient charts to compute health statistics. The Centers for Disease Control (CDC), the Public Health Department, and the Food and Drug Administration (FDA) are a few of the many administrative offices that collect data from patient charts for statistical analysis. For example, the CDC might gather data from patient charts to study the long-term complications of diabetes.

Legal Use. Lawyers and other legal personnel may wish to review a patient's medical chart for legal purposes. The patient's medical chart then may be used as evidence against the health care professional to prove that harm was done, or it may be used as evidence in defense of the professional that proper care was provided. Malpractice suits may be filed against health care professionals for various reasons. Patients (or their families) may sue because of poor judgment of standard of care, medication or treatment errors, or negligence.

Educational Use. The education of future health care professionals is another use of the patient medical chart. Students of the health professions receive valuable instruction from "real life" patient charts. During didactic training, patient case presentations excerpted from charts help students to integrate "book learning" and the "real world." Students get additional, hands-on training during hospital clerkships and rotations where they have direct contact with patients and see the medical chart system in action. In both cases, the students become familiar with the chart's contents, organization, and patient care uses.

Audit Use. Patient medical charts are used in audits of patient care. Within an institution, the Quality Assurance or Continuous Quality Management Department professionals may review patient charts to monitor hospital health care practices and to determine if standards for care are being met. Plans to improve patient care can be developed from the information. For example, patient charts may be audited to assess the appropriateness of blood product use or to determine the necessity of a specific surgical procedure. Or drug-use evaluation studies may be conducted by gathering information from patient charts on the appropriateness of medication use within a hospital. Hospital Medical Records Departments also routinely review patient charts for accuracy and completeness. The review commonly includes the following:

- Is there a signed consent form for every surgical or diagnostic procedure performed?
- Is there patient identification on every page of the chart?
- Have physicians signed or countersigned every order written?

These audits increase the accuracy of information and ensure that legal requirements are met. From outside the health care setting, third-party payors employ auditors to review patient charts; payment or reimbursement is based on the results of these audits. Medicare/Medicaid, Blue Cross/Blue Shield, indemnity carriers, and managed care organizations routinely audit patient charts for this purpose.

Program Evaluation. Hospital administrators are interested in patient information that helps them plan for the hospital's future. Statistics gained from medical charts aid administrators in budgeting and financial planning, expansion or reduction of hospital services, and personnel management.

Inpatient and Outpatient Medical Charts

Inpatient and outpatient charts exist for the same purposes and are similar in content. This chapter discusses "the chart" in a comprehensive way. Discussion about different aspects of the chart will identify the inpatient or outpatient setting when appropriate.

Chart Organization

The Problem-Oriented Medical Record (POMR) represents a useful attempt to systematize the recording and processing of clinical information. Many aspects of this approach have been widely adopted. Rational, orderly clinical action is facilitated by the POMR requirement of defining a list of clinical problems, identifying the database relevant to each problem, and providing an assessment and a plan for each. All charts are generally organized in this way so that information retrieval can be both efficient and consistent. A typical organization scheme is as follows:

- Admitting or Initial Clinic Visit Data
- Physician Orders

- Graphic Charts
- Nursing Notes
- Laboratory (lab) Data
- Diagnostic Procedures/Consults
- Operating Room (OR) or Outpatient Procedures
- History and Physical
- Progress Notes
- Medical Administration Record (MAR) or Medication List
- Miscellaneous

Charts are located in common centralized areas in hospitals, clinics, nursing homes, medical offices, home health agencies, and pharmacies when they are not actively being used. However, when a patient is actively receiving care, the chart is retrieved from the storage area and may be found in several places as previously discussed.

In any practice setting, the chart follows the patient. For example, if a patient goes to surgery or is having a procedure performed in the endoscopy department of the hospital, the chart is with that patient so it is available for reference and documentation. When the patient returns to the hospital room, the chart is returned to its permanent location. If a chart is not in its assigned location, it may be found with physicians, medical residents, or medical students while they are on rounds. Sometimes, other members of the health care team (e.g., nurses, pharmacists, or physical therapists) may have it. Or you may find a medical chart in the transcription or dictation rooms. Often, physicians, medical residents, or medical students take the charts of all their patients to a quiet place to work. When patients have been hospitalized for an extended period or have received chronic care in an office or clinic for several years, the amount of paper generated becomes too great to fit into the chart binder. Then, charts may be "thinned" (i.e., information rarely used from the start of the hospitalization or from earlier clinic visits is filed in a separate location). Early physician orders, MARs, and graphic sheets are often thinned. Summary type reports, such as dictated consultations and diagnostic procedures, usually are kept in the binder.

The future goal of most health-related industries is to become "paperless," by storing, exchanging, and using all information electronically. Increasingly, components of the medical record are electronic. For example, the MAR produced by a pharmacy is available on computer and printed in most health facilities. However, as facilities gradually invest in computer-based information technology infrastructures, these printed documents will be accessed "on-line" throughout the patient care facilities. Presently the U.S. Department of Veterans Affairs has most of its inpatient facilities supported with an information technology infrastructure that supports the complete electronic medical record. The information presented here will hold true whether the chart is totally paper based, totally electronic, or integrated. You should expect to encounter the different methods of chart information access, retrieval, and documentation and adapt in your practice setting, as required.

Chart Content

We turn now to a more detailed look at what is contained in each section of the medical chart. Considerable overlap and duplication exist among sections. Understanding both the routine contents of each section and the logic of this overlap and duplication will help you search efficiently for specific information. We discuss the Patient Profile commonly used in community and outpatient pharmacy settings later on in this chapter. We shall describe highlights of each section of the chart. **Figure 6-1** shows common locations for specific types of clinical information in the typical medical chart.

Inpatient Admitting or Initial Outpatient Visit Data

In most cases, admitting data is the first section of the patient medical chart. This information is usually gathered by the admitting department when the patient enters the health care institution. Information is collected on standardized forms to ensure consistent, accurate, and complete data collection. The data usually are divided into four groups: biographical, financial/insurance, admission-related, and consent forms.

Biographical Data
Biographical data serve to identify the patient. Typical information collected may include the patient's name, address, date of birth, sex, marital status, religious affiliation, emergency contact, occupation, employer, and social security number. Most demographic information you need about a patient appears in this section.

Financial/Insurance Data
Financial and insurance data are collected so that the hospital's billing department can receive payment from the appropriate source(s). The guarantor, or party who guarantees payment, often is the patient, patient's spouse, or parent/guardian. The patient's financial status, or ability to pay, is noted as well as insurance information (i.e., insurance companies and policy numbers) and other methods of payment (e.g., self, Medicare, or worker's compensation).

Inpatient Admission-Related Data
Admission-related data apply only to the current admission. Common categories of admission-related data are name of admitting physician, date and time of admission, admitting diagnosis for problem, room or bed number, and admission or account number.

In the initial outpatient visit data, the name of the primary care practitioner, date and time of visit, and initial problem list are generally identified.

Consent Forms
Consent forms are statements that must be read, understood, and signed by the patient or his or her guardian. The types of consent forms that you can expect to find in a patient's medical chart include forms for medical

Patient Data	Admission Form	Consent Form	Admit Summary	Admission Orders	Progress Notes/Transfer	Progress Notes/General	Flow Sheet	Rehab Form	Consultant Report	Procedure Req. Form	Clin Path Lab Rpt.	Patient Interview	Med Admin Record
Demographic information	X												
Chief Complaint			X				X						
Past Medical History			X										
Problem List			X										
Medication History on Admission			X										
Social History			X									X	
Allergies			X									X	
Physical Examination			X		X	X	X						
Laboratory Tests											X		
Pulmonary Function Tests							X	X		X			
Arterial Blood Gasses											X		
Emergency Room Txt Plan			X										
General Medicine Progress						X							
Medications Used in Hosp.													X
Patient's Medication Use Behavior												X	
Consent to be Taped/Info Shown to Others Publicly		X											

Figure 6-1. Sections of medical chart where specific information is usually found.

treatment, tests, procedures, investigational treatments or drugs, release of information, and photographs, videotapes, or films of the patient. Many of these forms are often presented to the patient at the time of the initial admission or visit. Others are presented when decisions must be made to take a particular course of action.

Patient confidentiality and privacy are specific concerns in patient care. Pharmacists must also ensure the privacy of the patient's health information in a manner that complies with the Kennedy-Kassebaum Health Insurance Portability and Accountability Act of 1996 (HIPAA).

Physician Orders

Physician orders are directives for patient treatment written either directly by a physician or by another health care professional and then countersigned by a physician. In office or clinic charts, the physician's orders are usually summarized in the progress note that describes the visit. The orders themselves are usually written on order sheets for services (e.g., laboratory or X-ray services) or prescriptions (e.g., medications, devices, other treatments).

Physician orders in hospitals are usually written on a standardized form specific to each hospital. The form usually is in three parts and preprinted with the hospital's name or logo and space for the date, time, and patient's allergies. The patient's addressograph is stamped prominently on the form. Often, there is space for the patient's height and weight; preprinted statements specific to hospital policy may be present. Clinicians in the outpatient setting write prescriptions that are usually given to the patient or transmitted to the pharmacy requested by the patient.

Computerized practitioner order entry (CPOE) may be taking place in your practice setting. This is a paperless method for clinicians to order tests and procedures, labs, or treatments using computer access. If CPOE is active in your setting, then it is highly likely the entire patient medical record is computerized. The practitioner orders may be reviewed online by viewing the patient's electronic medical record.

Written or Transcribed Orders

Orders may be written directly on the chart by a physician or transcribed to the chart by another health care professional after discussion with the physician. Transcription usually occurs when a physician gives orders to a registered nurse, pharmacist, or other professional over the telephone or from some place remote from the patient chart. The order is then written in the chart by the health care professional who signs the physician's name and his or her own name, separated from the physician's name with a slash (/) mark. A physician must countersign or initial the order within a specified time that is identified by institutional policy.

Electronic Transmission of Orders

Orders also may be transmitted from a physician's office to the hospital nursing unit, nursing home, or outpatient or clinic pharmacy using facsimile (fax) technology. Orders can be faxed prior to a patient's hospital or nursing home admission to be ready for the patient on arrival. Fax technology also is used within the hospital to speed order processing; nursing units may fax orders to the pharmacy or other departments. This process usually gets the order to its destination faster than if a courier or other transport system is used.

Pre-Printed Routine or Standard Orders

Some facilities or practices solve the poor handwriting issue and also standardize and streamline the order-writing process by pre-printing routine or standard orders. Individual physician or physician groups often write the same set of orders for every patient they admit or after a specific test or procedure is performed. To avoid writing the same order repeatedly, routine orders are typed and duplicated ahead of time. Orders that may vary, such as site of treatment, length of therapy, or drug dose, may be typed with blanks to be filled in later. Using this format, a physician can implement a set of routine orders on the order sheet by filling in the blanks, dating and signing it, and inserting it in the patient's chart. Chemotherapy, pre- and postpartum procedures, pre- and postsurgical procedures, and other complex orders readily lend themselves to this format.

Clarification of Orders

What do you do when you cannot read a word or even an entire order or prescription? Sometimes, you may be able to decipher the order if it is taken in context of other orders and the patient's condition. Usually, it is not that easy. The pharmacist is generally responsible for contacting the physician who wrote the order to ask for clarification. If the handwriting makes it difficult to determine the physician's name, a nurse, ward clerk, or other pharmacist may be familiar with the physician's handwriting and "translate" the name for you. Sometimes, the physician may have discussed the order with another pharmacist who can tell you what is ordered. However, it is a poor safety practice to have an order translated secondhand. Pharmacists should always contact the prescriber when any aspect of an order is unclear.

Graphic Charts

Graphic charts, sometimes called flowsheets, are standardized forms that simplify data collection and retrieval. They are quantitative records of repetitive monitoring activities and are usually arranged so that trends and patterns are easy to visualize. Information suitable for graphic charts includes the patient's vital signs, intake and output data, and activities of daily living. Other patient parameters that are frequently assessed or administered, such as blood glucose values, insulin doses, intravenous (IV) fluids and blood products, or neurologic checks, often are documented on graphic charts. The charts are printed with the word "data" and various time intervals so that the person documenting the data, usually a nurse or nurse's aide, needs only enter the information. The frequency of data collection and documentation depends on the parameters and the patient's clinical status.

Nursing Notes

The Nursing Notes section sometimes is a subsection under Progress Notes. If not, hospitals, clinics, and offices may use an integrated approach where Nursing Notes are eliminated and all health professionals make entries in the Progress Notes section. The kinds of information you may find routinely in the Nursing Notes section are described here.

- *Physical functioning.* Physical functioning is usually reported in narrative notes made by the nurse or clinician who has observed it. Vital signs are examples of data recorded about physical functioning.
- *Behavior/mental status.* Behavior and mental status descriptions are identified.
- *Clinical signs and symptoms.* A clinical description of observed signs or reported symptoms is included.
- Nursing interventions. Nursing interventions include P.R.N. medications administered, risk assessments, and pain assessments or interventions. Sometimes checklists rather than a narration are used to assess progress.
- *Documentation of care.* These entries record implementation of patient care directives by the nursing staff (i.e., physical restriction, tests, procedures, blood samples, and routine treatments).
- *Patient education.* Patient education may be documented on specialized custom forms or as a narrative in the progress notes or profile.
- *Additional types of educational activities that may be recorded.* This includes the patient's attendance in education classes, viewing of videotapes, and demonstration of self-care skills, such as Hickman catheter care or administration of insulin.
- *Consults.* Consults from various health care professionals, such as physicians, pharmacists, enterostomy nurses, or physical therapists, can be found in this section.
- *Nursing care plans.* Nursing staff plans describe what nursing intends to do in the care of the patient.
- *Nursing admission data.* A nursing admission database is established by nurses who interview patients.
- *Discharge plans.* Discharge planning entries are made in the Nursing Notes section of a chart.

In summary, the Nursing Notes section reflects the diversity of functions performed by the nursing staff.

The categorization scheme offered gives some order to this information. As you can see from the examples, these notes and sections are not categorized easily and may overlap with other sections of the patient medical chart.

Laboratory Data

Lab test results are found in this section. The format of the lab report is tailored to each institution or outpatient contract laboratory, although the same basic information is found regardless of the format. The lab results are separated into several categories:

- Hematology
- Urinalysis
- Type and screen
- Chemistry
- Microbiology
- Arterial blood gases

When appropriate, the normal range is given for each test. Most lab reports highlight abnormal values in some fashion, perhaps with an asterisk (*). An "H" next to values higher than the normal range and an "L" next to values lower than the normal range are commonly found on laboratory reports. Hematologic test results include measurements of red blood cell, white blood cell, and coagulation parameters. The urinalysis section divides test results into macroscopic and microscopic categories. A section on type and screen lists the results for ABO & RH testing and antibody screening.

The chemistry–renal function category lists the BUN, creatinine, sodium, potassium, chloride, carbon dioxide, and other tests of renal function. In the chemistry–metabolic category, you will find glucose, calcium, magnesium, phosphorus, total protein, albumin, cholesterol, and triglyceride measurements. The cardiac and liver chemistries are reported next, followed by cardiac enzymes and therapeutic drug concentrations.

The microbiology section reports information on blood and other body fluids and tissue cultures. Gram stain (if performed) and culture results are given. Antibiotic susceptibility and minimum inhibitory concentration (MIC) information is usually presented. Other microbiologic results, such as spinal or joint fluid examinations, also are found here.

The final section under Lab Data is arterial blood gases. Here, information about the patient's oxygen source (i.e., room air, ventilator, and FiO_2) and blood gas results are given.

The lab reports include all lab tests performed during a patient's admission or clinic visit. In the hospital, an updated cumulative report must be printed and placed in the chart daily, usually during the night. The report from the previous day can then be discarded. After discharge, a final cumulative summary is compiled and becomes a permanent part of the medical chart.

Sometimes, test results are not available when the updated reports are printed. This problem often occurs for tests sent to an off-site laboratory or in outpatient clinics or pharmacies. In these cases, the updated report may list the time and date of sample collection, but a notation of "pending," "in lab," "sent out," or some other similar term appears instead of a result. Once results are known, the next updated report is corrected.

Therapeutic Drug Monitoring Test Results

Several drug therapies are used by pharmacists and other health professionals to monitor for both effectiveness or toxicity by including the collection and interpretation of serum, whole blood, saliva, or sometimes urine drug concentration samples. Examples of such drugs include phenytoin, aminoglycosides, or digoxin. Other drug therapies are monitored for effectiveness and/or toxicity by using clinical laboratory tests that are proxy indicators for effectiveness and/or toxicity. One example is the monitoring of the International Normalized Ratio (INR) as a reflection of warfarin sodium. These test results are usually reported by identifying the monitored substance, the concentration of the substance reflecting the time that the sample was collected, and the desired or target ranges of the substance.

Home Test Kits and Monitoring Devices Results

Many patients use home test kits to monitor their progress in controlling their condition [e.g., blood sugar for diabetes, total cholesterol for dyslipidemia, or blood pressure cuff (sphygmomanometer) for essential hypertension]. Others use tests to determine the status of a condition (e.g., pregnancy testing or ovulation prediction tests). These results are usually brought in by patients or their family members to share how they are doing with clinicians. Clinicians will often regard this data as "subjective" when reported by the patient and will often verify the accuracy of them through clinical laboratory testing. As testing accuracy improves and community quality laboratory standards have been set, more clinicians accept the data generated by these methods. They offer the pharmacist a unique opportunity to incorporate monitoring tools into practice in a variety of settings.

Diagnostic Procedures/Consults

The diagnostic procedure reports are presented in a standardized format as a typed narrative, either a diagram or graph. Examples of the common diagnostic procedures included in this section are X-rays, electrocardiograms (ECGs), electroencephalograms (EEGs), computed axial tomography (CT) scans, magnetic resonance imaging (MRI), arteriograms, and invasive hemodynamic monitoring.

Operating Room Procedures

This section contains information presented in a typed narrative or graphic/diagrammatic format. Some hospitals may combine the Diagnostic Procedures/Consults section with the OR Procedures. Included in this section is documentation of surgical procedures, biopsies, and other invasive procedures. The same documentation is required for outpatient or office-based procedures.

History and Physical

Information about the patient's past and present medical history and physical examination findings appears in the eighth section of the medical chart. This information is presented in a standardized format and may be handwritten or dictated.

When a patient is admitted, the physician often writes a note about his or her initial findings and impressions in addition to the patient's medical history in the Progress Notes section. Then, when more information is available or when the physician has more time, a complete history and physical note are dictated. The History and Physical section documents subjective and objective information about the patient. Subjective information is open to individual interpretation (e.g., assessments of pain, comfort, and orientation). Objective information is based on replicable or quantifiable data. This type of information usually is measurable and has a numerical value (e.g., body temperature, serum drug concentrations, and urine output). Both subjective and objective information is obtained from multiple sources: the patient, the patient's family members, caregivers such as nurses and physicians, and other health care professionals such as pharmacists, dieticians, and physical therapists. The contents of the History and Physical section usually appear in the following order:

Chief Complaint

The patient's chief complaint is exactly what brought the patient to the hospital. Often, the physician will document the patient's own words to describe his or her medical problem. Chief complaints may include "My chest feels like there's an elephant standing on it," "I've been coughing up blood for 3 days now," or "I slipped and fell."

History of Present Illness

The history of the present illness chronologically outlines the events of the patient's current medical problem(s) and gives details about the characteristics of the chief complaint. If a patient's chief complaint is "My chest feels like there's an elephant standing on it," the history of present illness may say "The patient had been mowing the lawn about 9:00 this morning when, suddenly, he experienced sharp pain in the chest. He sat down to rest and took three nitroglycerin tablets with no relief. After 6 hrs of constant chest pain, the patient's wife convinced him to go to the emergency room."

Past Medical History

The past medical history describes the patient's more remote history such as past surgeries, diseases, and medical conditions. Also included are patient allergies and resulting reactions, family history, and social history (e.g., smoking and alcohol habits, prescription and over-the-counter medication use, recreational drug use, occupation, and marital history). The health history may be obtained from the patient, the patient's family, other caregivers (e.g., private nurse or nursing home personnel), the present or previous physician(s), and/or charts of the patient's previous hospitalization(s).

Review of Systems

The review of systems is an attempt by the examining health professional to elicit information from the patient. The patient is systematically questioned about each organ system and its functional status. The organ systems are grouped and presented in the review of systems in a top-to-bottom order: head, eyes, ears, nose, and throat (HEENT); respiratory system; breasts; cardiovascular (CV) system; gastrointestinal (GI) system; skin, bones, joints and muscles; endocrine system; and nervous system. Questions that a clinician may ask a patient about his or her respiratory system include the following:

- Do you have any trouble breathing?
- Do you get short of breath when climbing stairs?
- Do you wake up short of breath at night?
- Do you cough up blood?

If the answers are negative, the clinician may note that "patient denies shortness of breath, exertional shortness of breath, paroxysmal nocturnal dyspnea (PND), or hemoptysis."

Other questions that health care professionals may ask include

- Do you suffer from dizziness or lightheadedness? (cardiovascular system assessment)
- Do you have trouble urinating or pain when urinating? (genitourinary system assessment)
- Do you have trouble with diarrhea or constipation? (gastrointestinal system assessment)

Physical Examination

The physical examination can be considered physical evidence that supports and verifies the information discovered in the review of systems. This examination report describes what the health care professional saw, heard, felt, and sometimes smelled while examining the patient. Documentation of the examination may start with a short statement describing the patient's general status and a summary of the vital signs. Then, the results of the physical examination are again presented by organ system in a head-to-toe order: HEENT; neck, thorax or chest, and lungs; breasts; CV system; abdomen; extremities; lymph nodes; bones, joints and muscles; genitals; rectum; and neurological system. Statements that you may read in a physical examination report include "pupils reactive to light," "abdomen soft, nontender, no masses or organomegaly," "fingers cyanotic with clubbing," and "regular cardiac rhythm without murmur or gallop." It is not always possible or convenient to examine every organ system. In these situations, the physician may note "deferred." Short statements may explain why a particular organ system was not examined. Examples include "unable to assess" or "patient refused."

Admission Tests

When available, results of admission tests follow the physical examination. Lab data and report of diagnostic procedures are documented. Occasionally, a patient may have had relevant lab tests or diagnostic procedures as an outpatient before being admitted to the hospital. If the information is pertinent, that data may be presented here as well.

Assessment and Plan

A description of the clinician's assessment or impression of the patient's condition is the clinician's working diagnosis. The clinician compiles all of the data presented in the History and Physical and integrates them to determine known and/or possible explanations for the patient's medical problem(s). The clinician usually concludes the History and Physical with an initial plan of therapy based on the aforementioned impressions. The plan may include medications, surgical procedures, or diagnostic tests. These plans are not final; they may change during the patient's hospitalization. Standards for good records also structure what information is collected and thus promote self-teaching and self-critique of clinical work. For instance, the standard format for a writeup helps you remember what data to collect (e.g., do a family history and a stool guaiac). The format for the assessment and plan should help you ask the following sorts of questions: What problems have been identified? What is the significance of each finding? What other information has been collected (or should have been collected) that bears on this finding? What do I make of each problem? What do I intend to do to clarify my diagnosis? What treatment will I undertake for each problem? How has the patient been educated?

Progress Notes

The Progress Notes provide a running commentary on the patient's condition and treatments throughout the entire hospital stay. Progress Notes document the patient's response to treatment from admission to discharge. Events of the hospitalization and the patient's physical condition are described. These notes are a chronological log of how the patient is feeling and what is happening on a day-by-day, or even hour-by-hour, basis.

Various health care professionals write entries in the Progress Notes section. Each person who cares for the patient documents what he or she did to or for the patient; when, where, and why; and how the patient reacted or responded. As discussed previously, some institutions ask nurses to record their notes in a separate Nursing Notes section, while others integrate all health professionals' entries into a single Progress Notes section. The following are characteristics of correctly written progress notes:

- Date note is written is documented.
- Time of note is documented.
- Note is entitled, "Pharmacist Consultation" or "Pharmacist Progress Note." Each discipline identifies itself on the notes prepared for the chart (e.g., Cardiology Consult for cardiologists note).
- Note is handwritten, dictated, or typed. Note is neat, legible, professional in appearance, and written in black or blue ink.
- Note is well organized using the S.O.A.P. format.
- Content is written in either outline or narrative format.
- Note is signed with a cursive signature with the name printed clearly below it.
- Errors are documented with a cross out; "error" is written above the line with the writer's initials.

Progress notes are filed in forward or reverse chronological order, depending on the preference of the institution.

Progress note entries may take one of two formats: outline or narrative. A standardized outline approach in common use is the SOAP format where the entry is divided into four sections: subjective data (S), objective data (O), assessment (A) or impression, and therapeutic plan (P) or recommendation.

To review, subjective data are open to individual interpretation, while objective data are easily duplicated or quantified. As in the Historical and Physical section, the assessment portion of SOAP note describes the writer's interpretation of the aforementioned subjective and objective data and subsequent impressions. Finally, the writer outlines a therapeutic plan just as in the History and Physical section.

Sometimes an author may combine the subjective and objective data (S/O) and the assessment and plan portions (A/P). If no data are available for one section, the note writer may choose not to mention that section. Sometimes the data to be documented are not easily adapted to a SOAP format. This situation is especially true if there are a lot of subjective data to record with little or no objective data available.

Medication Administration Record (MAR)

Most facilities produce a typed form, the MAR, which documents all of the medications that are active on a patient (see **Figures 6-2 A and B**). This record usually includes the start date, stop date, name, strength, route, and frequency of administration. It is also common to see the recommended time of administration of the medication pre-printed on the form. When the medication is actually administered to the patient, the health professional or aid initials the recommended time and records the actual time of administration. The medications are listed in groups (i.e., scheduled medications, including "one-time" orders and p.r.n. medications). The MAR is produced usually every 24 hours by the pharmacy department, disseminated to the patient care areas, and placed in the chart for daily use. A similar listing of prescribed medications is usually maintained in a patient's outpatient chart.

Referrals

Whenever a formal referral takes place, an order (often on a separate, pre-printed form) is generated and placed in the chart. It is often kept in a separate section of the chart, readily identifiable.

Self-Monitoring Forms

Many facilities have a self-care program for medications, particularly with patients who are going out of the facility "on pass," intending to return in a day or so, or learning to self-administer their medication regimen upon discharge. Patients will document their medication use in a manner similar to the MAR procedures used by health professionals.

Temporary Information

Different types of temporary information are placed in charts to assist clinicians with care. Preliminary laboratory results, initial diagnoses from informal consults, and recommendations made by pharmacists to change therapy or follow a policy are all examples of temporary information that does not necessarily become a part of the permanent record. Once the permanent report or progress note is placed in the chart, the temporary documents are discarded.

NAME OF HOSPITAL
MEDICATION ADMINISTRATION RECORD: SCHEDULED AND PRN MEDICATIONS

INJECTION SITE CODE

A (R)Deltoid	H (L) Upper Quad
B (L)Deltoid	I (R) Lower Quad
C (L)Lat. Thigh	J (L) Lower Quad
D (R)Lat. Thigh	K (L) Glutial
E (R)Ant. Thigh	L (R) Glutial
F (L)Ant. Thigh	M(L) Ventro-Glutial
G (R)Upper Quad	O (R) Ventro-Glutial

DIAGNOSIS:

ALLERGIES:

GENERATED:
FOR PERIOD:
THROUGH:

START	STOP	MEDICATION	ORDER#	07:01-15:00	15:01-23:00	23:01-07:00
1-5	1-12	AMPICILLIN 250 MG CAPSULES 250 MGS EVERY SIX HOURS	1267904	1200	1800	2400 0600
1-5	1-12	DYAZIDE CAPSULES 1 CAPSULE AT 9AM	1267907	0900		
1-5	1-12	GLUCOTROL 2.5 MG TABLETS ONE TABLET EVERY 12 HOURS	1267908	0900	2000	

INITIALS	NAME & PROFESSIONAL DESIGNATION	INITIALS	NAME & PROFESSIONAL DESIGNATION	INITIALS	NAME & PROFESSIONAL DESIGNATION	INITIALS	NAME & PROFESSIONAL DESIGNATION

Figure 6-2A. Example of a medication administration record for scheduled and p.r.n. medications.

NAME OF HOSPITAL
INTRAVENOUS, STAT, AND ONE-TIME MEDICATION ADMINISTRATION RECORD

INJECTION SITE CODE

A (R)Deltoid	H (L) Upper Quad
B (L)Deltoid	I (R) Lower Quad
C (L)Lat. Thigh	J (L) Lower Quad
D (R)Lat. Thigh	K (L) Glutial
E (R)Ant. Thigh	L (R) Glutial
F (L)Ant. Thigh	M(L) Ventro-Glutial
G (R)Upper Quad	O (R) Ventro-Glutial

DIAGNOSIS:

ALLERGIES:

GENERATED:
FOR PERIOD:
THROUGH:

START	STOP	MEDICATION	ORDER#	07:01-15:00	15:01-23:00	23:01-07:00
1-5	1-12	DEXTROSE 5%/0.45 NORMAL SALINE 1267909 I.V. INFUSE AT 125 MLS/HR (1000 MLS)		0800	1600	2400
1-5	1-6	WARFARIN 2.5 MG TABLETS ONE TABLET AT 5 P.M.	1267905		1700	
1-5 STAT		MORPHINE SULFATE INJECTION 10 MGS I.V. NOW FOR PAIN	1267915			

MEDICATION * DOSAGE * RT OF ADMIN.	GIVEN		NURSE INITIAL	MEDICATION * DOSAGE * RT OF ADMIN.	GIVEN		NURSE INITIAL
	DATE	TIME/SITE			DATE	TIME/SITE	

INITIALS	NAME & PROFESSIONAL DESIGNATION	INITIALS	NAME & PROFESSIONAL DESIGNATION	INITIALS	NAME & PROFESSIONAL DESIGNATION	INITIALS	NAME & PROFESSIONAL DESIGNATION

Figure 6-2B. Example of medication administration record for intravenous, STAT, and one-time medication orders.

THE PHARMACY RECORDS

Prescription Records—Outpatient Practice

The prescription is the primary form of communication between the pharmacist and the practitioner who is initiating treatment on the patient with prescription drugs or the use of prescription devices. The prescription is the vehicle by which a patient chooses care when in need of prescription drug management. The prescription is provided to the pharmacist in written form; handwritten, generated from a printer or fax machine, or electronically transmitted to the pharmacy. The prescription is the legal order for prescription medication or other items in the outpatient setting, including skilled nursing facilities (**Figure 6-3**).

Medication Orders—Inpatient Practice

When a physician or other authorizing prescriber prescribes the patient's medications while in the hospital setting, they do so on order forms usually entitled "Physicians Orders." The medication order is the legal order for prescription and over-the-counter medications prescribed in the inpatient setting.

The Patient's Profile—All Settings

The Patient's Profile is the medical chart equivalent document for the pharmacist. It is maintained in all practice settings. Its purposes and uses are the medical chart equivalent for the pharmacist and the pharmacy staff serving the patient. Therefore, you will see much more information than that provided by a prescription or medication order alone, depending upon the quality and breadth of pharmacy services offered. The profile may serve as the record of care provided to the patient when served by the pharmacists and technicians.

Almost all pharmacy settings are computerized today. As a result, the pharmacist (or pharmacy clerk or technician depending upon both the practice model and state rules and regulations) will enter prescription or medication orders into the pharmacy computer system. A computer-based medication profile is created from the order entry process. Numerous settings have expanded to have both physicians and prescribers enter the prescription or medication order; however, this is not yet a standard of practice.

Most prescription records are on paper, as originally written by the prescriber. The profile is commonly observed as several computer screens reflect the range of patient data within the pharmacy computer system, the Medication Administration Record (MAR) summarizing the medication orders in the inpatient setting, or the Medication Record summarizing the prescriptions in the outpatient setting. The profile is stored in the pharmacy computer system, with supplementary medication orders or prescription records in paper files. When the profile is viewed on the computer screen, it is common for several computer windows to reflect detailed information such as medication name, strength, dose and form, route of administration, frequency of administration, and start and end dates. Additional information is displayed to assist the pharmacist with drug regimen review at the time of order entry. Two examples of this regimen review, which commonly result in followup, may include assessment of the patient's medication order against the acceptable dosing range (minimum–maximum dose) or determining the presence of a clinically significant drug interaction. Biographical, financial/insurance data, and consent forms are also part of the profile. Throughout the cases examples of how the profile varies in content illustrate these differences.

Pharmacists' Notes

Pharmacists' Notes are similar to the section entitled Progress Notes or Nursing Notes in the medical chart. This section is where problem identification, care plan development, and documentation of care provision occur. The Progress Note is typically organized as such.

Problems or Complaints

Depending upon the clinical setting, patients may present at a scheduled or drop-in appointment with a pharmacist, or they may initiate a conversation with the pharmacist. Often patients in a retail setting initially present with clinical signs or symptoms resulting in a complaint.

Physical Functioning and Behavioral/Mental Status

The patient's ability to function independently is an important assessment of the pharmacist. Pharmacists use specific tools, such as activities of daily living (ADLs), or the mini-mental status examination (MMSE), to assist in this assessment.

```
Joyce Miller MD                          DEA No. AC 1269478
Don Hancock, M.D.                        DEA No. AD 3497682

              Metropolitan General Family Medicine Clinic
                         1234 Detroit Avenue
                        Detroit, Michigan 48169
Rx



Refills: ____
_____        _____
Dispense as Written             May Substitute Generic/Therapeutic
                                Equiv.
```

Figure 6-3. Example of a traditional, handwritten prescription blank commonly used in outpatient settings.

Physician Examination and Assessment

A review of systems approach may be employed by the pharmacist to gather greater clinical insight. Pharmacists also employ limited, focused physical assessment skills to determine clinical problems and assess response to drug therapies. Pharmacists in community settings also provide blood pressure cuff devices and body temperature measurement devices to assist patients with home monitoring activities.

Laboratory Data and Assessment

Clinical laboratory test results are sometimes ordered or requested by pharmacists who perform drug therapy monitoring and dosing adjustments. However, the consumer home testing market has made the pharmacy a central place for purchase. Individuals are now self-monitoring their diabetes through blood sugar testing strips and monitors, lipid management through cholesterol measurement, and diagnostic pregnancy testing and ovulation prediction kits. Many pharmacists have established practices to help patients select and properly use and interpret the diagnostic and monitoring tests.

Medication-Use Evaluation

This evaluation is conducted on patients whenever they approach a pharmacist for drug therapy-related care. Chapter 8 will take us through the clinical reasoning process that both identifies drug-related problems and conducts the medication-use evaluation. These results are documented in the profile. Patients may receive brief, meaningful evaluations and feedback from the pharmacist, with a care plan successfully designed and implemented in episode of care. On the other hand, pharmacists may have multiple, scheduled visits with patients to optimize drug therapy and patient care.

Medication Adherence/Compliance History

The prescription records provide a unique history of medication use. The pharmacist has a unique dataset—knowing what prescription medications have been filed, when they were filled, and whether the patient has maintained a continuous refill history. Evaluation of these records provides the pharmacist with insight about the medication-use pattern of the patient.

Care Plans

The pharmacist evaluates these problems and develops an overall care plan. The plan may be limited in focus on one problem or activity or comprehensive to include multiple goals, alternative treatments with proxy outcome measures to monitor, and patient education plans to achieve goals.

- *Drug therapy problems*. Evaluation of the previous information and consultation with the patient leads the pharmacist to identify the patient's drug therapy problems. They are recorded in the patient's profile.
- *Interventions*. Some drug-related problems require recommendations to other care providers for an alteration or change in the drug therapy approach. Recommendations might include changing the drug entirely or modifying the regimen to optimize the patient's outcome individualized to the lifestyle and personal considerations of the patient.
- *Patient education*. Pharmacists care plans usually involve a structured form of patient education. Common plans include proper drug use, monitoring devises and testing kits, and therapeutic intervention with patient re-education.

Documentation of Care

The patient profile should document all aspects of a pharmacist's care plan and provision. This documentation of care is necessary for ongoing continuity of care, determination of a patient's progress, and for reimbursement of patient care services.

Consults

If a patient is referred by another practitioner for a pharmacist consultation, you may record the assessment and findings in consultation notes in the profile.

PROFESSIONAL CONDUCT ISSUES RELATED TO PATIENT CONFIDENTIALITY

The patient medical chart is a legal document of the health services provided to the patient during hospitalization; it belongs to the hospital. However, the information contained in the chart belongs to the patient and, therefore, is private. This same arrangement is true for the patient profile and prescription records of the pharmacy. As health care providers, pharmacists have access to this information and must ensure that the patient's right to privacy is not violated. In 1974, Congress passed Public Law 93-579, or the Privacy Act of 1974, to preserve this individual right to privacy. In many hospitals, this law is used as a framework for policies on patient confidentiality. In short, the law states that any federal agency maintaining records on individuals must permit them to know what records are being kept and how the information is being used. The law gives individuals access to their records and permission to have a copy. Individuals also have the right to correct or amend the records.

The Privacy Act requires that the data be collected for a specific purpose. If the information is to be used for other purposes, the law requires written consent by the individual.

State laws and professional codes of ethics also protect patient privacy. You should be familiar with your own state's privacy legislation and the codes of pharmacy practice.

Patient confidentiality is part of the right to privacy. By designating information as confidential, the right to privacy is recognized. Patients trust that information about them will be kept private and confidential. Confidentiality gives patients the right to indicate what information will be available and to whom. In fact, patient consent must be obtained before patient information can be released to outside parties. At admission, patients are asked to sign an "Authorization to Release Medical Information." This statement authorizes the hospital to release information to named parties. The patient must specifically authorize release to anyone else. These same authorizations are now being used in community pharmacy practice since the enactment of HIPAA.

The ASHP policy on nondiscriminatory pharmaceutical care states, in part, that "all patients have the right to privacy, respect, confidentiality, and high-quality pharmaceutical care" and that "pharmacists must always act in the best interest of individual patients while not placing society as a whole at risk." The American Pharmacists Association (APhA) Code of Ethics makes a similar statement: "A pharmacist should respect the confidential and personal nature of professional records; except where the best interest of the patient requires or the law demands, a pharmacist should not disclose such information to anyone without proper patient authorization."

Corporate Policies

Now that you have a general understanding of the legality and professional ethics of privacy and confidentiality, let us address the specific directives of your organized health care setting or community pharmacy. Each organization has a policy on patient confidentiality and release of information that is specific to that organization, but all policies serve the same purpose: to guarantee patients access to their own medical information while maintaining their privacy and monitoring the release of that information to other individuals.

How do you orient your practice so that you use the information available with discretion and respect for a patient's rights? The basic rule is to be constantly vigilant. Suppose that you are reviewing the patient chart of Mrs. Jan Smith at the desk in the hallway outside of her room. You are reading the History and Physical section of her chart, which mentions that she had an abortion 3 years ago. Because her height is not noted anywhere in the chart, you go to Mrs. Smith's room to ask her. However, you leave the chart open to the History and Physical section instead of closing it and returning it.

While you are talking with Mrs. Smith, her mother, who is unaware of her daughter's abortion, comes to visit. When she notices that you are in her daughter's room, she sits down at the desk to wait for your departure. She sees the open chart and discovers that her daughter had an abortion. You have, however inadvertently, disclosed information that the patient did not want known.

A similar situation could occur with computerized information. A health care professional may access patient information from a computer on the nursing station and leave the unit without signing off from the data screen. Patients, visitors, and other people may walk by the computer and read the screen. Again, patient confidentiality is compromised.

Occasionally, a patient's family members or visitors may ask to read the chart or may pull it from its storage shelf and begin skimming. Allowing these people access to the medical chart also breaches patient confidentiality, unless authorized by the patient, hospital, and physician.

The above examples illustrate negligent uses of a patient's medical chart. It is also possible to use the information in a fashion not considered negligent but which is still improper. This problem often occurs during verbal discussions in public places. You now know that Mrs. Smith had an abortion 3 years ago. While working in the satellite pharmacy, you casually mention this fact to a fellow pharmacist during a discussion of the abortion rights movement. Although the other pharmacist has access to patient medical charts, he has no professional reason to know about Mrs. Smith's abortion. Therefore, you have breached her right to confidentiality. The same principle is involved if you discuss Mrs. Smith's medical history with her family or visitors. She has the right to limit the information that they may know, and you must respect that right.

Discussion of patient information in public places, even when among appropriate health professionals, also violates patient confidentiality. Such discussions should never occur in hospital elevators, in the cafeteria, or at social gatherings.

In all of these examples, failure to observe patient confidentiality occurred because personal information was released without the patient's consent. Health care professionals can never be too careful when protecting a patient's privacy and preserving confidentiality.

SUMMARY

The patient's medical chart or patient profile provides a key source of information in the provision of care. The chart or profile represent common vehicles to document care and track the monitoring of the patient's progress. Other uses for the patient's record aid research initiatives or public health statistics. However, any use of the patient's record must be consistent with the Privacy Act of 1974 and the Health Insurance Portability and Accountability Act of 1996 (HIPAA).

CASES

See pages 103–111 for cases.

Case 1: *Lauren Smith brings a prescription to Nasir Jabr, PharmD, after seeing Dr. Miller.*

(Nasir Jabr sees Lauren approaching.)

Nasir Jabr: "Hello Lauren. What may I do for you?"

Lauren: "Well, I wanted to thank you Nasir. Dr. Miller was very good. But I have a few problems that I was unaware of. You were right; I have a urinary tract infection. So I brought my prescription for you to fill."

(Nasir takes the prescription and hands it to Joe, the Pharmacy Technician.)

Nasir Jabr: "Joe, would you please set this up for me while I speak briefly with Ms. Smith? Thank you. Lauren, come around to this counseling area over here so that we can speak with some privacy." (She looks slightly relieved.)

(Nasir shakes her hand. He notices that it is cold to the touch and a little "clammy"—perspiring.)

Nasir Jabr: "Lauren, I have started a patient profile for you here at the pharmacy (**Figure 6-4**). When patients come in for care and advice, we establish a record, just like in the physician's office or in the hospital. May I ask you a few more questions so that I can have a complete record? It should help both of us in the future."

Lauren: "Sure."

(While Nasir and Lauren are speaking, Nasir notices that she appears a little tired and slightly pale.)

Nasir Jabr: "What did Dr. Miller tell you your medical problems were in addition to the urinary tract infection?"

Lauren: "Well, she really surprised me because she suspected that I have hypertension! The nurse had taken my blood pressure and it was 148/100. I was so shocked, I didn't really say anything! Then she said something about my birth control pills and the smoking, too. I am not exactly sure. Oh, and I forgot to tell her about the Advil."

Nasir Jabr: "I would like to ask you a few more questions, then I would like to explain what I believe Dr. Miller was trying to let you know. Is that okay?"

Lauren: "Yes."

Nasir Jabr: "What birth control pills are you taking?"

Lauren: "Well…I am not. I am using the patch."

Nasir Jabr: "How long have you been on this?"

Lauren: "Just a year. Before that I took Lo-Ovral for 2 years."

Nasir Jabr: "Describe how you take your Advil."

Lauren: "I usually take three or four tablets whenever I have pain or discomfort."

Nasir Jabr: "How often do you have pain or discomfort?"

Lauren: "Well… I have three to four headaches a week…some of them are pretty bad."

Nasir Jabr: "Tell me more details about how you use the Advil."

Lauren: "Well, I usually wait until my headaches are pretty bad before I take any of it. But it seems like I always need to take it."

Nasir Jabr: "Can you describe the headaches for me?"

Lauren: "I usually get pain in my forehead area, but sometimes it seems like it's also in my eyes."

Nasir Jabr: "Does it get worse when you lean forward?"

Lauren: "No, not really."

Nasir Jabr: "Does anything in particular seem to cause the headaches?"

Lauren: "I can't really identify anything. They do seem to get worse around my period though."

Nasir Jabr: "How many packs of cigarettes do you smoke a day?"

Lauren: "Probably one or two. It just depends on how busy I am that day. I wish I never started."

Nasir Jabr: "Have you ever been told that you have any allergies?"

Lauren: "No."

Nasir Jabr: "Allergies to medications?"

Lauren: "No."

Nasir Jabr: "Is there anything else that you might want to tell me about?"

Lauren: "I can't think of anything. How do I use the medication Dr. Miller prescribed?"

Nasir Jabr: "Let me go check the prescription so that I can show it to you while I am explaining what you need to do. Could I have Joe take your blood pressure while you are waiting?"

continued

Case 1: *Lauren Smith brings a prescription to Nasir Jabr, PharmD, after seeing Dr. Miller. (cont'd)*

Lauren: "Sure. I didn't know pharmacists did this sort of thing!"

Nasir Jabr: "Yes. We are developing programs in community practice to help our patients with medication management. I am very glad you wandered in to see us. It will just be a moment."

(Joe, Pharmacy Technician, takes Lauren's blood pressure. It reads 150/102. Joe tells Nasir. Nasir returns to Lauren with the prescription.)

Nasir Jabr: "Lauren, this is an antibiotic; the name is 'trimethoprim–sulfamethoxazole.'"

(Nasir opens the container and shows her the oblong white tablets. He recaps the bottle and hands it to her so that she can read the instructions while he is explaining them.)

Nasir Jabr: "Lauren, you need to take two tablets right away, then take one tablet two times a day until they are all gone. This should take 7 days. Do you have any questions so far?"

Lauren: "No. I understand."

Nasir Jabr: "It is very important for you to finish all of the tablets, even after you are feeling better. You will start experiencing less pain, and will likely be pain free within 2 days of starting the antibiotic. It is also important that you drink plenty of liquids; water is best. This will help clear the bladder of infection."

Lauren: "Okay."

Nasir Jabr: "Let's move on to the other concerns. Your blood pressure reading here is 150/102, which is high. You have multiple reasons for a high blood pressure. Birth control pills have been shown to increase blood pressure. Smoking contributes to increased blood pressure. And frequent use of medications, known as nonsteroidal anti-inflammatory drugs, also increases blood pressure. That is your Advil. I offer a smoking cessation program and a hypertension management service in cooperation with a few of the physicians in the area. Dr. Miller is one of them. I wanted you to be informed of this option. In the meantime, I would like you to stop back in a week. We would be happy to check your blood pressure again, and you can tell me how everything is going. How does that sound?"

Lauren: "Sounds okay…I do have a question though. Does the birth control patch cause high blood pressure also? Or is it just the birth control pills?"

Nasir Jabr: "Well, that is an excellent question. Why don't I investigate the correct answer to that question and have an answer for you when you stop by next week?"

Lauren: "That would be great. Thanks for everything Nasir."

Nasir Jabr: "My pleasure. If you would check out with Joe, you will be all set. Please call or stop by if you have any other questions."

(Nasir writes a pharmacy progress note in Lauren's Pharmacy Profile.)

CASE 1: SPECIFIC QUESTIONS

1. Review the case details provided to you about Lauren Smith in Chapters 1–6. Establish the data needed for her patient profile by completing the details that you can to make one comprehensive pharmacist's database using the Patient's History Form–Pharmacist's Recommendations/Plan (Figure 5-1).

Pharmacy Profile for:

Patient:	Smith, Lauren		New Patient	Print	Close Record

Demographic	OTC / Allergy		Insurance	Diagnosis	Contacts
General Health	Care Plans	Surveys	Account Status		Current Therapy
General Information	Illnesses	Systems Review	Vital Signs		Lab Values

Pharmacist's Progress Note: Date: 02-02

LS referred to Dr. Miller by NJ on 02-01 for evaluation of probable UTI. LS presented today with co-trimoxazole prescription. Upon brief history and examination the following was noted:

S: LS reports BP at physician's 148/100; using birth control patch after 2 year history of Lo-Ovral; 3-4 Advil 200 mg tablets 3-4 x per week for headaches – characterized by frontal discomfort and occasional periorbital pain; 1-2 ppd cigarettes. Denies allergy to medications.

O: BP 150/102 seated (repeated here)

A: UTI, probable essential HTN worsened by NSAID use and nicotine addiction - increased risk of thromboembolic events and elevated BP and headaches – symptoms consistent with sinus headache – likely in need of a decongestant rather than Advil.

P: Dispensed co-trimoxazole and counseled to consume water, take to completion. Offered smoking cessation and hypertension management service. Research her question, "Does birth control patch affect BP also?" Asked her to visit in one week for follow-up.

Nasir Jabr, Pharm.D.

Figure 6-4. Computerized pharmacy profile for patient Lauren Smith.

Case 2: *Christine Johnston reviews Eduardo Montanez's clinic record and laboratory findings.*

Christine Johnston reviews the clinic records of Eduardo Montanez. She focuses on a summary note about Mr. Montanez prepared by Dr. Mattis, his primary physician (**Figure 6-5**). She also reviews the laboratory data obtained when he visited with her at the clinic (**Figures 6-6** and **6-7**).

CASE 2: SPECIFIC QUESTIONS

1. Review the case details provided to you about Eduardo Montanez in Chapters 1–5, and the clinic summary note and laboratory reports that follow. Establish the data needed for her complete patient profile by completing the details that you can into one comprehensive pharmacist's database using the Patient's History Form–Pharmacist's Recommendations/Plan (Figure 5-1).

HEART OF TEXAS SYSTEM CLINICS		Patient Identification (Stamp)

HEART OF TEXAS SYSTEM CLINICS

PROGRESS NOTES

Patient Identification (Stamp)
Name: **Eduardo Montanez**

Reg.No. **16254**

Location: **Main Clinic**

Date: **09/15/03**

	Age	Sex
V S	Weight _____	Height _____
I I		
T G	B/P _____	Temp _____
A N		
L S	Pulse _____	Resp. _____

Leukocytes _____

Nitrite _____ ph _____

Protein _____ Glucose _____

Ketones _____ Urobilinogen _____

Bilirubin _____ Blood _____

Hct __12__ Preg. __N/A__ Hemocult _____ Strep _____ Other

UA Micro: WBC _____ RCB _____ WBC _____ Epis _____ Bacteria _____

Appt. ___X___ Call/Walk In _____ Primary Physician ___**Dr. Mattis**___ /Staff _____

Date: 9-15-03

1:30 p.m.   EM is a 68 year old Hispanic male who is here for a routine check up for his diabetes mellitus. He presents with thirst, hunger and increased urination.

PMHx: diabetes mellitus type II x 15 years known
           Dyslipidemia; 10 years

PMI: DM, Dyslipidemia, pain and discomfort in legs – probable neuropathy 2° to long standing Diabetes

SH: Lives with daughter-in-law, Maria and his son. Dependent upon son for medical coverage. EtOH- 5-6 beers a day; denies smoking

PE: V.S. BP – 145/89 HR – 60 Resp 18/min.

ROS: HEENT: Poor vision – no corrective lenses – refuses care.
          NECK: supple, no JVD, carotids 2/2. Trachea is midline
          CARDIAC: regular rate and rhythm, S_1 and S_2, no S_3 no S_4.
          ABDOMEN: no distension or organomegaly
          GI/GU: polydypsia, polyphagia, polyuria
          RECTAL: guaiac negative
          NEURO: alert and oriented x 3. Pedal pulses dull.

LABS: Fasting Blood Sugar = 218; trace protein in urine; $HgbA_1c$ = 12 mg%, total chol = 220.

MEDS: Diabenese 125 mgs po qd; tolazamide 250 mgs po qd; Mevacor 20 mgs at evening meal;
           Tylox for leg pain –take 1 q 4 hrs prn.

IMPRESSION: EM has poorly controlled diabetes. Probable cause for elevated cholesterol. Provided home blood glucose meter and taught daughter to monitor blood sugar every day. Instructed to bring readings in next clinic visit in 3 months. Recommended optometry evaluation to EM and daughter.

Dr. Mattis
_____
Signature

2:30 p.m.   Clinic no show on 12/22/03

Dr. Mattis
_____
Signature

Figure 6-5. Summary note of past medical history for patient Eduardo Montanez.

Laboratory Test - STAT Request			
UA DIP STICK			Date Requested **06/12/04**
cloudy		Color/Appearance	
	Neg.	Glucose	
	Neg.	Bilirubin	
	Neg.	Ketones	
1.020	1.003-1.030	Specific Gravity	
	Neg.	Blood	
	4.5-8.0	pH	
2++	Neg.	Protein	
	Norm.	Urobilinogen	
	Neg.	Nitrite	
	Neg.	Leukocytes	
UA MICROSCOPIC			
N/A		WBC/HPF	
N/A		RBC/HPF	
N/A		Mucus	
N/A		Renal Epith/HPF	
N/A		Squamous Epith/HPF	
N/A		Bacteria	
N/A		Crystals	
N/A		Casts/HPF	
URINE PREGNANCY			
N/A			

Chart No. **16254** Doctor: **Mattis** Patient: **Eduardo Montanez**

Figure 6-6. Urinalysis test results for patient Eduardo Montanez.

MISCELLANEOUS LAB RESULT – STAT REQUEST PROGRESS NOTES			Patient Identification (Stamp)
			Name: **Eduardo Montanez**
			Reg.No.**16254**
Hemoglobin A$_1$c	12.5 mg%	(normal range: 4-6 mg%)	Location: **Main Clinic**
Blood glucose	220 mg/dL	(normal range: 80-120	Date: **06/12/04**

Figure 6-7. STAT laboratory test request for patient Eduardo Montanez.

Case 3: *Luisa Rodriguez reviews Huong Tran's admission note from the physician.*

Luisa Rodriquez goes to the chart to review the details of Huong's admission (**Figure 6-8**). She also looks to see what the admitting orders are from Dr. Mooris (**Figure 6-9**).

CASE 3: SPECIFIC QUESTIONS

1. Review the case details provided to you about Huong Tran in Chapters 1–6. Establish the data needed for her patient profile by completing the details that you can into one comprehensive pharmacist's database using the Patient's History Form–Pharmacist's Recommendations/Plan (Figure 5-1).

Memorial Hospital and Health System		Patient Identification (Stamp)

Memorial Hospital and Health System

PROGRESS NOTES

Patient Identification (Stamp)

Name: **Huong Tran**

Reg.No. **2364590**

Location: **5W Pediatrics**

Date: **04-02-04**

Age: 8 years old	Sex: Male	VITAL SIGNS:	
Weight _40 kg_	Height _5'_	B/P _110/70_	Temp _98.6°_
Pulse _85_	Resp. _18_		

4-2-04 Admit to 5W Pediatrics:

HT is an 8 yom who presented to the ER with moderate to severe asthma exacerbation. 3x in 2 weeks. His FEV was 60% - Was treated with two courses of - albuterol 8 puffs in 10 minutes/ repeat every 20 minutes until breathing normal. Solu-medrol 40 mgs IV. Pharmacist used spacer device and assisted HT with albuterol use.

Mother and father present – non-English speaking Vietnamese descent. Only child can speak and translate English for himself and parents. No additional relatives or immediate care takers.

Will follow-up in afternoon…

Dr. Mooris
Signature

Figure 6-8. _Brief admission note in the progress note section for patient Huong Tran._

START DATE →	DATE 04-02-04	TIME 1500	I CERTIFY THAT THE ADMISSION OF THIS PATIENT IS MEDICALLY NECESSARY

PHYSICIAN'S ORDERS:

Admit to hospital:

Acute exacerbation of asthma

1. V.S. every 4 hours for 24 hours
2. Albuterol metered dose inhaler – 2 puffs every 4 hours while awake.
3. Pharmacist consult – medication history and education on Metered dose inhaler
4. Solu-medrol 40 mgs IV q 6 hours for remaining 24 hours – DC at 1500 on 04-03-04.
5. Start D5/0.25NS at 30 mls/hour starting at 1600.
6. Labs in a.m. – CBC, chem-20, PT, PTT
7. Social work consult – need for assistance with medical coverage And comprehensive discharge plan.
8. Request Vietnamese interpreter for family.

Dr. Mooris
Signature/pager no 0693

Memorial Hospital and Health System

ADDRESSOGRAPH IMPRINT HERE

Name: **Huong Tran**

Reg.No. **2364590**

Location: **5W Pediatrics**

Date: **04-02-04**

ALLERGIES AND SENSITIVITIES:

1. **Penicillin – rash and itching**

2.

*A GENERICALLY OR THERAPEUTICALLY EQUIVALENT DRUG AS APPROVED BY THE PHARMACY COMMITTEE MAY BE DISPENSED UNLESS OTHERWISE SPECIFICALLY STATED.

Figure 6-9. _Hospital admission orders for patient Huong Tran._

Case 4: *Michael Jones, RPh, MS, reviews Samuel Robinson's medical record and other sources of information.*

Michael Jones goes to the nursing station area where the patient's medical record and medications from home are located (Medications brought from home are not allowed to be administered in the hospital per policy and are stored under lock and key and returned to the patient upon discharge). He decides to first review the Nurses Admission Database and the Laboratory Test Order Form (**Figures 6-10 and 6-11**). He knows that this form contains much of the demographic and economic information. He examines the medications in the bag from home and finds the following:

Synthroid 120 mcg every day.
Warfarin 5 mg orally every day Monday through Saturday.
Vitamin E 1,000 I.U. orally every day.

Digoxin 0.25 mg orally every day.
Clonidine 0.05 mg orally every day.
Hydrochlorothiazide 25 mg orally every day.
Dofetilide 250 mcg orally two times a day.
Aspirin 81 mg orally every day.

After looking at all of these sources of information, he determines that there is a discrepancy between the Nurses Admission Database and the medication container for warfarin about the daily dose. He is concerned about the dosing of warfarin that needs to be initiated in the hospital. He also notes that the vitamin E is 1,000 I.U.s —and that this is a pretty large dose. The bottle containing Synthroid is nearly full, even though the date on the medication label of the bottle is from 3 months ago.

CASE 4: SPECIFIC QUESTIONS

1. Identify two other information sources that Michael Jones might use to determine what the correct regimen for warfarin was supposed to be just prior to Mr. Robinson's admission to the hospital.

GENERAL ASSESSMENT QUESTIONS

1. Describe five common uses for the medical chart.
2. Describe the differences between subjective and objective information.
3. How does the Privacy Act protect a patient's confidentiality?
4. What action should you take as a pharmacist when a patient's medication order or prescription is difficult to read or unclear in its intent?
5. If you wanted to audit several medical charts for patients to gather data about a pharmacy program's effectiveness (you do not intend to publish this), would you need to seek each patient's consent before you did it?

ASSIGNMENT

1. Contact the director of pharmacy in your community hospital. Ask the director to describe the characteristics of the medical record at his or her hospital. Is it all paper, all electronic, or a mixture of both? Do they use an electronic medication administration record (MAR)? Do pharmacists document their patient care activities in the medical records? What section?
2. Speak with a hospital pharmacist in your community. Ask about the process to transmit orders from the patient's chart to the pharmacy. Describe this process.
3. Contact a pharmacist in your local community pharmacy. Ask the pharmacist to describe the characteristics of the pharmacy patient profile at his or her pharmacy. Is it all paper, all electronic, or a mixture of both? Do they document patient care activities on the pharmacy profile?
4. Speak with a community pharmacist in your community. How do orders get transmitted from the physician's office to the pharmacy? Describe the various methods.

REFERENCES

1. Rakel E. Essentials of family practice. Philadelphia, Pa: W.B. Saunders; 1993.

2. Shepherd MF. Module 1: Reviewing patient medical charts, in ASHP Clinical Skills Program—Advancing Pharmaceutical Care. Bethesda, MD: American Society of Health- System Pharmacists, Inc.; 1992.

NURSING ADMISSION DATABASE   NOTE: ENTRIES DOCUMENTED IN PENCIL ARE NOT CONSIDERED PART OF THE PERMANENT RECORD.   (TRANSCRIBE IN PEN)

A. ADMISSION INFORMATION

ADMISSION DATE: _____ TIME: _____ ☐ A.M. ☐ P.M.

ADM. FROM: _____ VIA: _____

REASON FOR ADM.: _____

ANTICIPATED DISCHARGE DATE: _____

CONTACT IF NECESSARY:

REL.: _____ PHONE (H) _____ PHONE (W) _____

REL.: _____ PHONE (H) _____ PHONE (W) _____

PERSONAL BELONGINGS/HEALTH AIDES: ☐ DENTURES ☐ GLASSES
☐ PACEMAKER ☐ PROSTHESIS ☐ WALKING AIDS
☐ CONTACT LENSES ☐ HAIRPIECE ☐ HEARING AIDS

PT./FAMILY INSTRUCTED: ☐ INTERCOM ☐ BATHROOM ☐ LIGHTS
☐ MEALTIMES ☐ CHAPLAINCY SVC. ☐ HELPLINE
☐ SMOKING PLICY ☐ BED CONTROLS ☐ VISITNG HOURS
☐ JEWELRY (LIST INDIVIDUAL ITEMS, STATE BRAND NAMES IF APPLICABLE): _____

☐ MONEY (ENCOURAGE NO MORE THAN $20) AT BEDSIDE: $ _____

INFORMATION OBTAINED FROM: _____

ORGAN DONOR: Completed by R.N. Ask only adult patients admitted to adult medical/surgical Units.

ARE YOU AN ORGAN DONOR? ☐ YES ☐ NO

ORGAN(S) DONATED: _____

SMOKE: ☐ YES ☐ NO   HOW MUCH? _____

ALCOHOL: ☐ YES ☐ NO   HOW MUCH? _____

SUBSTANCE ABUSE: ☐ YES ☐ NO   HOW MUCH? _____

ALLERGIES/SENSITIVITIES – TYPE & REACTION: _____

PLACE ALLERGY INFORMATION ON ARMBAND AND M.A.R.

RELIGION: _____

The above information has been explained to me. It is accurate and I understand. I also understand that I have been advised the hospital is not responsible for valuable kept at bedside.

PATIENT/FAMILY SIGNATURE   UNIT PERSONNEL

RISK/FALL ASSESSMENT: ☐ NOT AT RISK ☐ AT RISK
IF AT RISK, COMPLETE RISK/FALL ASSESSMENT SHEET

PRE-ULCER ASSESSMENT: ☐ NOT AT RISK ☐ AT RISK
IF AT RISK, COMPLETE PRE-ULCER RISK ASSESSMENT SHEET

B. PHYSICAL PROFILE

ADMISSION VITAL SIGNS: BP _____ T _____

P _____ R _____ HEIGHT _____ WEIGHT _____

DIET: _____

MEDICATIONS: (DISPOSITION ☐ HOME ☐ PHARMACY ☐ OTHER _____

HISTORY OF PRESENT ILLNESS: _____

PAST MEDICAL HISTORY: (MAJOR ILLNESSES, SURGERIES, OTHER TREATMENTS, FAMILY HISTORY, NEUROLOGICAL, MUSCULOSKELETAL, ARDIOVASCULAR, GI, RENAL, RESPIRATORY, AND ENDOCRINE CONDITIONS. INCLUDE DATES)

C. DISCHARGE PLANNING CRITERIA

The following are High Risk Criteria for discharge planning, check all that apply:

☐ AGE OVER 65
☐ TRANSFERRED FROM A NURSING HOME
☐ FOLLOWED BY COMMUNITY AGENCY PRIOR TO ADMISSION
☐ HISTORY OF REPEATED ADMISSIONS
☐ ELDERLY PATIENT WHO LIVES ALONE
☐ ALTERED MENTAL STATE
☐ HISTORY OF DRUG OR ALCOHOL ABUSE
☐ NO FAMILY MEMBERS AVAILABLE TO PT.
☐ NO METHOD OF PAYMENT
☐ FINANCIAL DIFFICULTIES REQUIRING INTERVENTION
☐ HIGH LEVEL OF ACUITY WITH POOR PROGNOSIS
☐ VICTIM OF ABUSE OR NEGLECT
☐ ADM. DIAGNOSIS OF FAILURE TO THRIVE OR LIFE-THREATENING ILLNESS
☐ NONCOMPLIACNE
☐ HISTORY OF PHYSICAL OR MENTAL ABUSE
☐ DIAGNOSIS REQUIRING FOLLOW-UP TREATMENT, TEACHING OR REFERRAL

ADL'S: ☐ INDEPENDENT ☐ DEPENDENT – SPECIFY: _____

LIVES WITH: _____

SUPPORTIVE FAMILY: ☐ YES ☐ NO

PRIMARY CAREGIVER: _____

	INITIAL SCREENS OBTAINED
☐ NO REFERRALS NEEDED	
PT./FAMILY SVCS.	☐
NURSING CONSULTANTS	☐
PT/OT/ST	☐
DIETARY	☐
FINANCIAL COUNSELOR	☐

ADM. NURSE SIGNATURE: _____

NAME	AGE	SEX	M.D.
DATE ADMITTED	ROOM/BED		

Figure 6-10. Nurses admission database for patient Samuel Robinson.

REQUIRED PATIENT INFORMATION

Last Name   First Name   Middle Initial
| R | O | B | I | N | S | O | N | | | S | A | M | U | E | L | | | | | | | | | | |

Date of Birth
| 1 | 1 | | 2 | 3 | | 1 | 9 | 2 | 8 | Sex X M ☐ F Patient I.D. 02946372_____

SSN
| 6 | 8 | 0 | | 1 | 2 | | 3 | 9 | 2 | 7 | Phone: _(901)_468-4832_____

Bill To: ☐ Our Account (No further information is needed).
        X Patient Insurance (The following must be completed or your account will be billed.)

Patient's Marital Status (Circle One): S M D W ⟲

Responsible Party
    Name | | | | | | | | | | | | | | | | | | | | |
    Address | 1 | 3 | 6 | 2 | M | O | C | K | I | N | G | B | I | R | D | | L | A | N | E | |
    City | B | I | L | O | X | I | | | State | M | S | Zip | 7 | 8 | 0 | 2 | 3 |

    SSN | | | | - | | | - | | | | | Relationship to Patient:____SELF__

Primary Insurance Information
    Insurance Co. Name | | | | | | | | | | | | | | | | | | | | | | |

    Address | | | | | | | | | | | | | | | | | | | | | | | |

    X Medicare ☐ Medicaid ☐ Insurance No. | | | | | | | | | | | | | | | |

    Group No. | | | | | | | | | | | | | | | | | | |

Primary Care Physician (if other than ordering physician)_____
Secondary Insurance Information: Attach separate sheet
Check if this incident involves: ☐ Worker's Comp ☐ Litigation
Are ABN's, Referrals or Waivers needed for this billing? X No ☐ Yes (Attach Copy)

MEMORIAL HOSPITALS AND HEALTH SYSTEMS

Specimen Information
Collection Date:__ _/__ _ /_ _ _ _ Time: ___ ☐ PM☐AM
IF APPLICABLE

☐Fasting X Therapeutic Drugs Phlebotomist's ID_____

Time of last dose:___PTAdmit_____ ☐ AM ☐ PM

Handling:☐ Room Temp ☐ Refrigerated
         ☐ Frozen   ☐ Spun-Down
☐ Perform STAT
   ☐ Phone Results to_____
   ☐ Fax Results to #_____

Diagnosis #1 CHF	Diagnosis #2 DVT prophy	Diagnosis #3	Acct No.	Fin Class	Specimens Rcvd	Bar Code Label

1	2	3			1	2	3			1	2	3			1	2	3				1	2	3				1	2	3	

Panel Tests (Defined on Back)

	Basic Metabolic (S)	x		Lipid (S)		x		Hemoglobin A₁C(L)		x		TSH (S)		Microbiology/Virology*
x	Basic Metabolic (S)	x		Lipid (S)		x		Hemoglobin A1C(L)		x		TSH (S)		Microbiology/Virology* (Use line provided to identify source)
x	Comprehensive (S)			Obstetrics*(R,L,S)				Hemogram (incl. plt/no diff) (L)				Uric Acid		
	Electrolytes (S)	x		Renal Function (S)				Hepatitis A IgM Ab(S)				Urinalysis (w/o		AFB Culture_____
	Hepatic (S)							Hepatitis B Core Ab (HBcAb) (S)				microscopy)* U		Anaerobic Culture_____
Individual Tests								Hepatitis B Survace Ab (HBsAb) (S)		**Additional Tests**				Chlamydia PCR_____
x	Albumin (S)							Hepatitis B Surface Ag (HBsAg)* (S)						Gonorrhea PCR _____
	Alkaline Phosphatase (S)							Hepatitis C AB (HCV Ab) (S)						Chlamydia Culture_____
	ALT (SGPT) (S)							HIV-1/HIV-2 Abs (Consent Form Required)* (S)						Gonorrhea Culture_____
	ANA (Anti-nuclear AB) (S)							Lead ☐ Venous (T)☐ Capillary (LM)						C. Difficile Toxin_____
	AST (SGOT) (S)							Lymph Immune Markers (1L) Room Temp Draw M-Th: call for STAT PICK-UP						Fungus Culture_____ Giardia Antigen_____
	Bilirubin, Direct (S)							Mononucleosis Screen (S)						Herpes Culture _____
	Bilirubin, Total (S)							Occult Blood (Source)_____						Influenza A Antigen_____
	BUN (S)							Phosphorus (S)						Ova & Parasites_____
	Calcium (S)							Potassium (S)						Respiratory Culture _____
	CBC (incl. hemogram/plt/diff)*(L)				x			Prealbumin (S)						RSV Antigen_____
	Cholesterol, HDL (S)							Protein, Total, Serum (S)						Stool Culture _____
	Cholesterol, LDL Direct Measure (S)							Protein, Total, Urine (U or 24U)						Stool Rotavirus Antigen____
	Cholesterol, Total (S)							PSA (Medically Indicated) (S)						Throat, Beta Strep Culture___
	Creatinine (S)							PSA (Screening) (S)						Rapid Strep Screen, Throat____
	Creatinine Clearance (S, 24U)				x			PT (Pt. on Coumadin XYes ☐ No) LB)						Viral Culture_____
	Digoxin (R)							PTT (Pt. on Heparin ☐Yes ☐ No) (LB)						Agent_____
	Electrophoresis (includes interpretation) Hemoglobin L Serum R Urine U or 24 U							Rheumatoid Factor (S)						Wound Culture_____
								Rubella (S)						Urine Culture _____ Method of collection
	GGTP (S)							Sedimentation Rate (ESR) (L)						
x	Glucose (S)							Sodium (S)						Other Culture _____
	Glucose Tolerance (Pregnant? Yes/No) (S)							Syphilis Serology *(S)						Total No. of Tests Checked
	HCG Qualitative (S)							Triglycerides (S)		L=Lavender Top Tube (EDTA) LM=Lavender Top (EDTA)				LB=Light Blue Top Tube (Sodium Citrate)(Tube must be completely full)
	HCG Quantitative (S)							Triple Screen [complete form]		R=Red Top Tub (Plain Clot) S=Spun Unopened Barrier Tube (SST)				T=Tan Top Tube (K2 EDTA 5.4 mg) U = Random Urine 24U =24 HR Urine Collection

Figure 6-11. Laboratory test order form for patient Samuel Robinson.

3. Mason NA, Shimp LA. Module 2: Building a pharmacist's patient database, in ASHP Clinical Skills Program—Advancing Pharmaceutical Care. Bethesda, MD: American Society of Health-System Pharmacists, Inc.; 1993.

4. Shimp LA, Mason NA. Module 3: Constructing a patient's drug therapy problem list, in ASHP Clinical Skills Program—Advancing Pharmaceutical Care. Bethesda, MD: American Society of Health-System Pharmacists, Inc.; 1993.

5. Jones W, Campbell S. Module 4: Designing and recommending a pharmacist's care plan, in ASHP Clinical Skills Program—Advancing Pharmaceutical Care. Bethesda, MD: American Society of Health-System Pharmacists, Inc.; 1993.

6. Frye CB. Module 5: Monitoring the pharmacist's care plan, in ASHP Clinical Skills Program—Advancing Pharmaceutical Care. Bethesda, MD: American Society of Health Systems Pharmacists, Inc.; 1993.

7. Galt KA. Module 1: Drug information: analyzing and recording a drug information request, in ASHP Clinical Skills Program—Advancing Pharmaceutical Care. Bethesda, MD: American Society of Health-System Pharmacists, Inc.; 1994.

8. Smith GH, Norton LL, Ferrill MJ. Module 2: Drug information: evaluating drug literature, in ASHP Clinical Skills Program—Advancing Pharmaceutical Care. Bethesda, MD: American Society of Health-System Pharmacists, Inc.; 1995.

9. Galt KA, Calis KA, Turcasso NM. Module 3: Preparing a drug information response, in ASHP Clinical Skills Program—Advancing Pharmaceutical Care. Bethesda, MD: American Society of Health-System Pharmacists, Inc.; 1995.

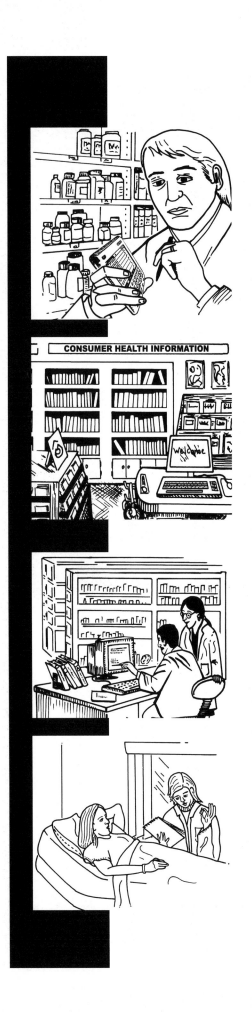

CHAPTER 7

Gathering Drug Information and Evidence

"Science is taught as if its facts were somehow superior to the facts in other scholarly disciplines, even though every field of science is incomplete."

Dr. Lewis Thomas

Chapter Outline:

Objectives / To be able to understand:

1. the drug information needs in the context of the patient care situation;

2. a timeframe for responding to a drug information need;

3. a drug information request to assist you in selecting appropriate information resources;

4. the depth of information for the response required;

5. a strategy for accessing patient-specific information for response to a drug information request;

6. effective listening skills when gathering information;

7. the use of drug information for care provision and administrative uses;

8. the relevant patient-specific data needed to respond to information requests in an appropriate clinical context;

9. reliable information sources to consult for drug information requests;

10. the characteristics of primary, secondary, and tertiary drug information sources; and

11. drug information resources to determine their relevance in meeting your needs.

Purpose: The purpose of this chapter is to assist you in understanding and developing the drug information skills you need to provide patient care.

You will be introduced to the skills needed to respond to information requests from patients and other providers and gain a working knowledge of available resources. Selecting accurate and relevant information for use in a timely manner is the key to this area of practice expertise.

DETERMINING THE PATIENT'S CARE NEEDS

One of the most common professional services you provide as a pharmacist is expert information about drug therapies and treatments. To do it well, you must distinguish between serving as an expert information resource (such as a medical librarian) and providing a clinical recommendation. Discerning between these two services is critical to meeting the needs of the patient, health care professional, or other requester.

To use your expertise correctly, you must first understand the request. You must determine what information is really needed rather than simply what is asked. If you answer a request without knowing how the information will be used, you will waste essential time, provide unnecessary or insufficient material, and possibly cause unintentional harm. By using an organized approach to ask the right questions and also record your data, you will learn how to provide valuable drug information. To accomplish this task, you need expert knowledge about the various types of drug information sources and how to search them productively. These sources are described later in the chapter along with the searching strategies needed to use them effectively. The remainder of this chapter will focus on the approach itself. Our assumption is that the requestor is seeking your expert knowledge and recommendation for a patient who needs care. (Chapters 8–11 will illustrate how to integrate the use of expert information into clinical skills for patient care.)

Origins of Drug Information Requests

Requests for information come from people with a wide range of backgrounds and in a multitude of settings. Such requests commonly originate from physicians, nurses, patients, the public, and other pharmacists. Requests also come from other health professionals such as physical or respiratory therapists, dietitians, psychologists, and social workers. When you receive a request, you should first note the date and time that you received it, who you received it from, and the route of communication by which it was received (telephone, in writing, or in person). Documentation assists you in "keeping track" of the circumstances surrounding a request and in meeting the turnaround time required for a useful response. You should obtain the name and phone or fax

number of the individual requesting information. By also knowing this individual's professional background, you can sometimes determine the complexity of the information required. Be sure to ask the affiliation and title of the individual so you can reply in writing, if required. It takes a few extra minutes to gather this information; however, it may make the difference in accurately and promptly responding. The process becomes efficient once you have established professional relationships with your patient or health care colleagues.

Physicians, Technicians, and Other Professionals

Compared to requests from other professionals or patients, physicians often require more extensive knowledge and literature support to substantiate a response. For example, imagine that you are in the outpatient pharmacy when you receive a telephone call from a psychiatrist. He states, "I'm trying to write a discharge prescription for Mr. Cook on 3B. What is the maximum dose of propranolol I can give him?"

To answer this question correctly, you will have to gather patient-specific information such as indication for use, age, concurrent diseases, and other medications being taken. Your response may include advice not only on dose but also on route, frequency of administration, duration of therapy, and caution for patients with diabetes and/or pulmonary disease. Be prepared to discuss other alternatives if your conversation results in a change in care. If your response requires multiple references, inform the physician about them.

Conversely, answers to some questions may require only your professional knowledge. Suppose that a nurse stops you in the hallway to ask, "Is it possible for patients who are on captopril to get hypotension?" The nurse further explains that an elderly black male patient was started on captopril 25 mg po q 8 hr 5 days ago, and his blood pressure was 90/54 this morning. You probably will not need to substantiate your response to this information request with additional expert resources. Your clinical knowledge and experience should suffice.

Pharmacy technicians often seek information from pharmacists to advance their own knowledge and to confirm the correct way to perform tasks. However, when a technician requests information for someone else, you should provide this information directly to that individual. Technicians may need your assistance to determine when an information request is within their scope of practice. Patients usually ask questions to clerical staff who then come to you for answers. Educate them to direct patient questions to you (or another pharmacist) so that you can determine the true nature of the request and your ability to answer it.

Health care administrators, who may or may not have training as health care providers, frequently ask drug information questions. You need to identify the professional's level of knowledge before formulating your response.

Caution should be used when responding to requests from lawyers, journalists, or health care administrators from other organizations. Although this text is intended to develop your skills in answering patient-specific requests, there are a few valuable points to remember. You are not required to respond. It is important to assess whether you even have the right to respond to these requests with any level of disclosure. They may be seeking information that violates a patient's rights or is proprietary. You should always check with the patient or his or her representative even if you have the right to respond. Similarly, you should check with the appropriate individual in your organization if the request is of a proprietary nature. You should establish the motive for initiation of the request. In general, your primary responsibility is to protect the rights and proprietary information of the patients and/or health care organization you are serving.

The individuals to whom you commonly provide drug information and the frequency of such requests depend on your practice setting and your primary practice responsibilities. If you are a hospital staff pharmacist, you frequently respond to requests from other health professionals, administrators, and technicians. If you participate in medication history taking, discharge counseling, and drug therapy monitoring in a decentralized setting, you often answer questions from patients and caregivers directly. Pharmacists in ambulatory, home care, and extended care settings frequently respond to drug information requests from patients and caregivers as well as professional staff.

Patients

Information requests from patients usually are specific to themselves or to a personal friend or relative. Patients may be asking for information only. However, patients frequently seek advice or affirmation on a directive given by another provider. In all cases, you must understand the nature of the patient's request before responding.

For example, suppose that you are counseling a male patient about discharge medications. He asks, "Is it okay to take my warfarin in the morning when I come home from work instead of at 5 p.m.? I know that the doctor told me to take it at 5 p.m., but that's when I'm asleep. I start my evening shift at 9 p.m. and work until 7:30 a.m. I usually sleep from noon to 8 p.m. The physician was in such a hurry that I didn't want to interrupt her and ask about it."

To respond to this patient's request, you must evaluate his total drug therapy regimen for interactions, determine an appropriate schedule for drug administration, and counsel him on all medications. This seem-

ingly simple question is actually a request for information and advice that may differ from his physician's instructions.

Requests for information may come via telephone, in person, in writing, by facsimile, or through electronic mail. All requests, regardless of source or route, should be treated professionally and followed through to completion.

Gathering the Background Information into a Patient-Specific Database

When researching a patient-specific request, you must obtain precise patient data to respond appropriately to the clinical circumstances. Moreover, the efficiency of your search will be improved. Different kinds of patient-specific data are needed for different classifications of drug information requests. A general or basic set of data about a patient is required for all of these requests. Information that you should always seek includes patient name, age, height and weight, gender, race, diagnoses, allergies/intolerances, any present and past medical history, relevant laboratory data, and the physical location of the patient. These data may be obtained through the patient encounter, use of the medical chart, pharmacy records, pharmacy patient profile, laboratory data, professionals caring for the patient, or family members and caregivers who are not health care professionals (**Figure 7-1**).

The patient database you assimilate to answer this request should provide you with enough information so that you can individualize your response and determine the urgency of care. If not readily available, gather as much information as you can before making a recommendation. If you do have access and sufficient time, retrieve additional data from the available sources. **Appendix 7-1** illustrates patient-specific data to collect, depending on the classification of the request. Although these examples may not be all inclusive, they convey the types of questions you should review.

Formulation of the Actual Question and Timeframe for Response

You should accurately restate the actual drug information need and timeframe required for a response based upon your background information. It will guide the remainder of your information search. When a request is received, you might assume that the information needs are immediate. This assumption can be frustrating if the answer requires great depth. But even in this situation, you should not provide a substandard answer. Instead, you should gather sufficient background information to feel as confident as possible about your response within the amount of time available.

DRUG INFORMATION WORKSHEET

Date/Time Received_____ Person Receiving_____ How Received (phone, visit, etc)_____

Requester or Source Information

Name_____
Affiliation _____
Title_____

How to Reach_____
Phone #_____
Pager# _____
Fax #_____
Address_____

Who Requested (check one)
❑ MD   ❑ MD Student   ❑RN   ❑Patient
❑Physical/Respiratory Therapy   ❑ Nutrition Support   ❑Secretary/Ward Clerk   ❑Other_____

Classification of Request

❑ Adverse Drug Reaction (ADR)
❑ Availability
❑ Compatibility/Stability
   (Chemical, Pharmaceutical, Sorption, Solubility, etc)
❑ Compounding/Formulation
❑ Dosage/Schedule
❑ Drug Interactions
   (Drug-Drug, Drug-Lab, Drug-Disease , Drug-Food)
❑ Drug of Choice/Therapeutics/Pharmacology
❑ Identification
❑ Method of Administration

❑ Pharmacoeconomics
❑ Pharmacokinetics
❑ Pregnancy/Lactation/Teratogenicity
❑ Poisoning/Toxicology
   (Environmental, Exposure, Occupational, Mutagenicity,
    Carcinogenicity)
❑Odd Drug Entities and OTCs
   (Investigational, Orphans, Foreign Drugs, Chemical Substances
    Homeopathic Remedies, Vitamin Substances, Herbs, etc.)
❑ Other _____

Patient Data

Name_____ Patient ID_____
Age_____ years_____ months   Height ____ ft ____in
Gender ❑male   ❑female   Weight____ lb ____ kg
Race_____
Diagnosis _____   Allergies/Intolerances_____
Pertinent Medical History/Problem List_____
_____
Pertinent Medication History_____
_____
Pertinent Laboratory Values_____
_____
Miscellaneous Information_____
_____

Room/Bed Number or Location_____
Setting (e.g., inpatient or outpatient)_____

The Request, Actual Drug Information Need, and Time Frame for Response

Original Questions/Notes_____
_____
_____
_____

Figure 7-1. Sample drug information worksheet to research, respond to, and document the responses to a drug information request. *(cont'd)*

Clear Statement of Actual Drug Information Need _____
_____
_____
_____
_____
Time Frame Required for Response_____

Record of Search/Notes
_____
_____
_____
_____
_____
_____
_____
_____
_____
_____
_____
_____
_____

Clear Statement of Response

Clear Statement of Response_____
_____
_____
_____
_____
_____

Response Written: ____documented in chart ____ memo   Response Oral: ____telephone follow-up ____ face to face

Outcomes

General:	Patient-Specific:
☐ More information requested	☐ More information requested
☐ Recommendation accepted	☐ Recommendation accepted
☐ Recommendation rejected	☐ Recommendation rejected
☐ Requester will call back with results / additional requests	☐ Requester will pass information on to patient
☐ Contributed to policy development	☐ Patient education provided
☐ Standard of practice (upheld or improved)	☐ Clinical Impact (+ / - / neutral)
☐ Improved efficacy	☐ Positive patient relations
☐ Improved compliance	☐ Estimated cost impact
☐ Assured safety	☐ None or
☐ Prevented potential medication error	☐ $_____; Describe:_____
☐ Prevented potential ADR	
☐ Estimated cost impact	☐ Probably life saving
☐ None or	☐ Other_____
☐ $_____; Describe:_____	
☐ Other_____	

Figure 7-1. Sample drug information worksheet to research, respond to, and document the responses to a drug information request.

Classification of Request

Next, you should classify the request using your organizational or personal classification scheme and identify how to access additional information. Classification will help you to determine your information resources for collecting patient-specific background information and literature data. Although organizations may have different classification systems, use of a systematic approach helps you to be thorough and less likely to overlook relevant resources. By classifying the request, you can determine what (1) further background information or patient history to gather, (2) preliminary reference sources to search, and (3) type and complexity of response to provide.

Appendix 7-1 provides a classification scheme that is commonly used in practice. For example, imagine that a nurse asks, "Does captopril cause hypotension?" After clarifying that the question is specific to a particular patient, you could classify this request in two categories: adverse drug reaction (ADR) and drug of choice/therapeutics/pharmacology. But because your response could result in changed drug therapy, you would need to gather more background information. The more complex or general the question, the more likely that multiple categories will apply.

Searching Strategy

Classifying a request directs you to the appropriate references to search. Sources such as the captopril product insert and a tertiary drug information text may answer the nurse's request. Since this request is patient specific, you also will need information about the time order of events, frequency and severity of the patients' presentation, and usual management approaches. Specialized information resources about adverse reactions and general therapeutics texts for management guidelines will be essential. Moreover, you may be required to consult the medical literature and then evaluate the studies or case reports. A description of drug information sources and their characteristics is provided in **Appendix 7-2**, Literature and Web Site Search Matrices. This description provides you with a quick decision tool for selecting the appropriate drug information sources based upon your classification. If you classify a request but information in that category is insufficient or inappropriate, you should reevaluate the classification. Be sure to find the best category(ies) to get the information you need.

The correct order of searching for answers to questions, once classified, is to start with tertiary general references, then tertiary specialty references. If these sources do not provide adequate information, you should search secondary, then primary resources. More details about these reference categories are provided later in this chapter.

Record of Search/Notes

When gathering drug information, you should keep track of your searching strategy and resources. These notes will help you to construct your final response. Furthermore, if a question arises regarding this information, you can efficiently refer to your notes. Be sure to document your personal communications with patients, caregivers, other professionals, and organization representatives (e.g., pharmaceutical company and Food and Drug Administration personnel). Record the names of the individuals you speak to and their phone numbers in case there is need for followup.

Clear Statement of Response

Be sure to record what you tell the requester, including a description of your recommendation. If your recommendations influence the requester to take a particular course of action in patient care, document it on the patient chart and/or the pharmacy profile, whichever is appropriate. If you solicit the feedback and opinion of another colleague or professional, you may also choose to document this source. It is customary to provide the actual recommendation in the patient's chart and to record it in a pharmacy documentation system maintained in many practice settings. If this is the case, you should document the route of communication you used to provide the response (verbally, in writing, or by facsimile). Also indicate if you documented the response in a progress note or patient consultation in the patient's medical chart. If your response is written, attaching a copy may be appropriate.

Figure 7-1 is an example of a documentation form to use for drug information requests. The form may be used for training or documentation purposes. It is organized in a way to help you master the skills of providing a drug information response, based upon a search of the evidence and available resources.

Outcomes

During the provision of care, you should reassess how a patient is responding as a result of your recommendations. If you are unable to observe the outcome directly, contact the original requester for followup.

Access to Additional Information

Patient information may be difficult to obtain if you cannot examine the patient's chart or consult the caregivers or patient. For this reason, you should try to obtain as much patient information as possible from the requester. If the patient is in your same inpatient, clinic, or home care setting, this information may be readily retrievable from current records.

In some situations, however, the patient information you may need is not known or documented. You may be asked, for example, to evaluate whether a patient has developed amitriptyline-induced hepatotoxicity. If baseline liver function tests were never performed, you may be unable to determine the time order of events. If history of use of both alcohol and over-the-counter medication is unknown, you cannot rule out these factors. Furthermore, if the requester is unable to supply you with this information or it is inaccessible, this question cannot be answered satisfactorily.

In your response, therefore, you should explain that you are unable to answer this request but will provide as much information as possible. You also may need to classify this request as nonpatient specific. After the reclassification, you can provide information from the literature about the usual presentation of amitriptyline-induced hepatotoxicity without concluding that this patient experienced it. Furthermore, you may offer information about its management. A determination would be made after discussion with the requester about your limited information. If you decide that the patient should be treated as a "probably" case (patient probably has hepatotoxicity), you should restate the information request and reclassify it. This reclassification will enable you to design a new searching strategy.

Communication Skills for Identifying the Actual Question

Requesters often do not ask for the information they really want or need. Your task then—to search and identify the actual request—is not always straightforward. You must ask questions and listen carefully to learn what you need to know.

Questioning Strategies

Keep in mind that your goal is to clarify the actual question being asked. To assess its context, you must gather sufficient information. You can accomplish this task by using the different questioning techniques interchangeably discussed in Chapter 5: open-ended versus closed-ended questioning, direct versus indirect questioning, and probing.

The amount of trust a person places in you will be established not only by the quality of your information but also by your professionalism, interest, and approach when responding to a request. If you solicit the necessary background information but then provide an answer "whenever you get around to it," your attitude will leave a bad impression and overshadow your hard work.

All of these questioning techniques may be used whether you are communicating with someone in person or over the telephone. However, with phone exchange, you lose most components of nonverbal communication except voice quality. Detailed conversations illustrating these techniques are in the cases at the end of this chapter. Let's examine some representative example questions and the interchange between the pharmacist and the requestor.

"What is the dose of gentamicin?" A pharmacist who works in inpatient care area 5D receives a telephone call from a physician. As illustrated in the following example, questions are asked in an illogical order (i.e., details about the patient's characteristics are obtained before demographic information).

> Physician: "What is the dose of gentamicin?"
> Pharmacist: "Is this question about a patient?"
> Physician: "Yes."
> Pharmacist: "How old is the patient?"
> Physician: "He's a 59-year-old male."
> Pharmacist: "How is his renal function?"
> Physician: "His renal function is fine; no problems."
> Pharmacist: "To determine a dose, I need to know renal function stability and his most recent serum creatinine and BUN."
> Physician: "His renal function has been stable since he was hospitalized 5 days ago. I believe his serum creatinine was 1.2 yesterday, and his BUN was 15.
> Pharmacist: "Well, if his renal function is stable, I estimate his creatinine clearance to be around 68 ml/min. Is he obese or underweight?"
> Physician: "No."
> Pharmacist: "I believe I can make a recommendation. Has he been started on gentamicin yet or will this dose be his first?"
> Physician: "He hasn't started yet. I'd like to start him as soon as possible."
> Pharmacist: "What is this patient's name and room number? I'll review his record and recommend a dose in his chart, if you like."
> Physician: "Would you? Great. The patient's name is Mr. Martin, and he's in room 252 on unit 2D."
> Pharmacist: "Oh, I didn't realize that the patient was on the second floor. Another pharmacist handles those patients; let me give you his name and pager number. In the meantime, I will contact him and review what we just discussed. He'll handle it from there. If you have any questions, you can page him."

In this case, the pharmacist gathered useful information by asking specific questions and probing for the facts to calculate a gentamicin dose. However, the questions were asked in an illogical order. This patient's location, for example, should have been determined at the beginning. Only after the pharmacist spent considerable time collecting information did he learn that the patient was not in his area of responsibility.

Now let us see what happens when a pharmacist does not adequately probe for information.

> Physician: "What is the dose of gentamicin?"
> Pharmacist: "Is this question about a specific patient?"

Physician: "Yes. I want to start him on gentamicin as soon as possible."

Pharmacist: "How much does he weigh?"

Physician: "About 75 kilos."

Pharmacist: "The usual loading dose for a man this size is 1.5–2 mg/kg, if you think he is close to his ideal body weight. His loading dose would be 110–150 mg. You would see a peak serum concentration of 4–10 mcg/ml. Have you calculated his creatinine clearance?"

Physician: "No. I haven't done that yet. But his renal function is stable."

Pharmacist: "His maintenance dose and schedule should be adjusted based on his creatinine clearance. I'll calculate them if you know his serum creatinine. How old is he?"

In this example, the pharmacist again did not establish the actual question. He assumed that the physician wanted him to recommend a dose of gentamicin for this patient. Instead, the pharmacist should have asked probing questions to decide if this patient should actually receive gentamicin. As a result, a dose of gentamicin was recommended. The dose also was not specific to achieve a particular peak/trough concentration based on an infectious disease indication.

Now, look at this same gentamicin dosing question from the perspective of a pharmacist who is inquisitive about its true purpose. The pharmacist demonstrates how to identify the actual question.

Physician: "What is the dose of gentamicin?"

Pharmacist: "Is this question for a specific patient?"

Physician: "Yes. The patient is Mr. Martin in room 252, up here on unit 2D."

Pharmacist: "What type of infection are you treating?"

Physician: "Well, the patient has most likely developed pneumonia. He came in with a pretty rapid onset of symptoms."

Pharmacist: "From what type of setting was the patient admitted? Do you think that he has a community-acquired infection or was he in a nursing home?"

Physician: "Right. He was at his own home. We think the most likely causative organism is strep. His sputum showed many gram-positive cocci in pairs and chains. The culture and sensitivity results are pending for blood culture; however, we want to start treatment empirically."

Pharmacist: "Well, if you truly suspect a community-acquired strep pneumonia, you should start with penicillin. How severe is the infection?"

Physician: "Oh, I'd describe it as moderately severe but progressing. We need to start treatment."

Pharmacist: "Under these circumstances, it is probably best to start with parenteral penicillin therapy. Is the patient allergic to penicillin?"

Physician: "No, there's no documented allergy, and he denies it on history."

In this example, the pharmacist asked pertinent questions to determine why the original request was being made. Moreover, key inquiries about the infection and its origins helped to determine that the original question was not needed. Gentamicin was not the drug of choice in these circumstances, so the pharmacist could recommend more appropriate empiric therapy (i.e., penicillin).

Now, let us evaluate an example of a common occurrence in drug therapy communication. In this example, pharmacokinetic information is needed but not just drug dosing.

Physician: "What is the dose of gentamicin?"

Pharmacist: "Is this question about a specific patient?"

Physician: "Yes. The patient is Mr. Martin in room 252, up here on unit 2D."

Pharmacist: "What kind of infection are you treating?"

Physician: "We've isolated *Pseudomonas aeruginosa* in Mr. Martin's CSF."

Pharmacist: "Is the patient already receiving gentamicin?"

Physician: "Yes, we've had him on high doses of gentamicin and ceftazidime parenterally for 48 hr with minimal response. We're confused because the culture and sensitivity results show that *Pseudomonas* is highly sensitive to gentamicin and ceftazidime. Does gentamicin get into the CSF very well?"

Pharmacist: "No. The problem is that the concentration of aminoglycosides in CSF, whether the meninges are inflamed or not, is low and unpredictable. If the patient needs to achieve therapeutic levels of gentamicin in the CSF, the drug should be administered intraventricularly."

Physician: "I've never been involved in a case where we've had to give a drug intraventricularly. How much does its administration change the dose of gentamicin?"

Pharmacist: "To be honest, it has been a while since I've dosed gentamicin intraventricularly. I know intraventricular administration changes the gentamicin dose, but I don't remember by how much. I'll do some checking, review the patient's records, and then make a recommendation in Mr. Martin's chart, if you'd like."

Physician: "Great. In fact, why don't you page me when you get everything? Since I'm not familiar with this area, I'd like you to go over it with me."

Pharmacist: "Sure, doctor. I'll do it right away and

page you when I'm done. Could you please give me the patient's name and ID number? I'll make sure that the chart and additional patient data are available."

The pharmacist listened to the needs of the requester in this brief but effective discussion. With the first three questions, the pharmacist concluded that the request was patient specific, that the indication for the drug was appropriate, and that the patient had already started gentamicin therapy. By asking the third question, the pharmacist implied, "Why are you calling about dosing information for a patient already receiving the drug?" As a result, the requester offered detailed background information.

The next example again illustrates that the actual question is not expressed in the original request.

> Physician: "What is the dose of gentamicin?"
> Pharmacist: "Is this question about a specific patient?"
> Physician: "Yes. Mr. Martin in room 252 on unit 2D."
> Pharmacist: "Why do you need to know the dose of gentamicin?"
> Physician: "I may have Mr. Martin on too high a dose. Yesterday's urinalysis had casts, and he's starting to dump protein. His urinary output has really dropped off over the last 2 days. Do you think this decrease is related to his gentamicin?"
> Pharmacist: "It's likely. Patients on gentamicin, especially if they are dehydrated, are more susceptible to nephrotoxicity. Nephrotoxicity associated with gentamicin, actually all aminoglycosides, may present as tubular necrosis or increases in serum creatinine and blood urea nitrogen with a drop in the creatinine clearance. The urinary output can drop and protein, cells, and casts may be found in the urine. However, a drop in the urinary output is rarer than nonoliguric elevations in blood urea nitrogen."
> Physician: "I guess I should discontinue the gentamicin. I have alternatives."
> Pharmacist: "A reduction in dosage or discontinuation of therapy usually is recommended. It seems wise to discontinue therapy with reduction in urinary output. If you tell me what alternatives you're considering, I'll recommend one for you."

By asking an open-ended versus a direct question ("Why do you need to know the dose of gentamicin?"), the pharmacist encouraged the physician to offer more background information. The pharmacist then determined that an adverse drug reaction required a change in the management of this patient. Both the patient and physician were better served through this indepth approach to identify the actual information need.

EVIDENCE FROM DRUG INFORMATION SOURCES AND CLINICAL LITERATURE

Drug information sources are the cornerstone to your practice of pharmacy. You are known for your expertise in information provision and its application to patient care as much as for your oversight of the medication-use process. Information sources warranting lifelong familiarity include those used by health care providers as well as those accessed by your patients—commonly referred to as consumer drug information sources.

Characteristics of Drug Information Sources for Health Care Providers

Traditionally, information sources used by health professionals have been classified as primary, secondary, or tertiary, based upon function and format. Having this knowledge of a source governs our searching strategies. With the information technology explosion, other sources have emerged for daily use (e.g., online and handheld computer sources). These forms of information should not result in altering your searching approach, as we will describe in greater detail below. However, they should broaden your scope of inclusion in obtaining up-to-date information.

Types of Health Care Provider Drug Information Sources

Tertiary Sources

Frequently labeled general references, tertiary information sources highlight the widely accepted data from primary literature, evaluate this information, and publish the results. Tertiary sources include textbooks, reference books, handbooks and manuals, compendia, pharmacopoeias, and review articles. Commonly used general references are found in pharmacies, while a broad range of general references have traditionally been available only in drug information centers or health sciences libraries. Tertiary information sources are more limited yet practical for most information needs. One of the growing tertiary resource types is known as systematic reviews. The best known in that category is the Cochrane Collaboration (www.cochrane.org). This international collaboration conducts systematic reviews of health care interventions and publishes them electronically. It is an example of a resource that is not likely to be detected through traditional searching strategies but may provide great utility depending upon your needs.

Another tertiary resource that has emerged as a result of the evidence-based movement in care is the clinical practice guideline. These guidelines provide steps to diagnosing or managing medical problems by integrating evidence with clinical experience. They are typically produced through consensus and published for wider use. Guidelines are usually produced under the direction of professional associations or organizations that come together to provide guidance on approaches to care that have the potential to be relatively standard.

Secondary Sources

Secondary information sources are frequently used to access the primary literature and usually consist of bibliographic citations. Most sources identify citations through a computer or "online" searching process. However, some do exist in print form. They are available as abstracting services, citations, indexes with and without full text, and directories. Secondary sources expedite the retrieval of information in the primary literature but are less current than primary literature. One of the biggest problems in drug information searching is the concept of "time lag." In recent years, the publication rate of primary literature has shortened, and the abstracting and cataloging of the literature into secondary searching sources has shortened considerably. The time lag for most secondary sources is now 4–8 weeks after primary resource publication. This shortened timeline substantially reduces the need to search primary information sources that are indexed in these secondary sources.

Primary Sources

Primary information sources are original published or unpublished works that introduce new knowledge or enhance existing knowledge on a subject. They include research results and case reports as well as evaluative and descriptive studies. Moreover, these sources are the foundation for secondary and tertiary literature. Primary sources provide the most accurate information because they contain the original communication of ideas. However, you cannot efficiently search for specific data, as you must go to each primary source for the needed information. It is important to note that not all primary sources are catalogued into secondary sources. Searching primary literature directly requires high-level skill when the secondary source does not provide sufficient, reliable information.

Online Sources

Online information sources are increasing in quantity and accessible via the Internet. The Internet greatly increases the accessibility of online information sources and the rapidity of retrieval. However, searching online introduces less reliability of the information sources, depending upon the point of access. Using general Internet searching engines (e.g., Yahoo!, Alta Vista, Google, others) usually results in many sources that are not reviewed using traditional peer or editorial review

processes associated with reputable information sources. Therefore, online searching may produce far more *unreliable* sources of information, requiring you to spend substantially more time distinguishing between what is useful and what is not. If the point of access is through a professional secondary online source (e.g., PubMed, Science Citation Index, Toxline, others), you will have only traditional health care resources identified.

Web Sites

What are these nonreviewed information sources? The emergence of web sites is one of the largest growing forms of information. Web sites commonly used by health professionals include those maintained by professional associations, pharmaceutical companies, and special interest groups (see Appendix 7-2).

Availability of Journals Online

Publishing of traditional biomedical journals electronically in a paperless format is emerging as a common format. Costs associated with publishing and housing printed articles are becoming prohibitive for libraries and individuals. As a result, many major medical publishers are providing biomedical journal literature electronically. The format, appearance, and accessibility methods are affected by this medium. Potentially, increased access by individual users is tremendous. But there are no agreed-upon standards or methods to providing these publications electronically, thus most publishers are producing both electronic and print versions. Paperless publishing will become the primary, if not sole, method for publishing.

Another emerging source that has rapidly diffused into practice is the availability of information resources via handheld computers or PDAs. Appendix 7-2 also provides a listing of currently available products. Access to these information sources requires that a handheld device have connectivity to a host computer (connectivity can be accomplished through hot syncing or wireless transmission). Almost all sources are provided on a subscription basis to individuals. However, medical libraries are also sources if you have them in your community and have privileges to use the facilities. The most common form of these products are tertiary references that provide most of the core, basic practice information needed, replacing pocket books and what some call "peripheral brains." They will continue to be popular and diffuse as a standard method for accessing needed core information. The handheld device, when loaded with the appropriate software applications, can also serve as a point-of-care computer to receive primary literature sources and graphical information from secondary sources such as the National Library of Medicine PubMed product and others. Becoming comfortable with the handheld device is a good choice to continue advancing your skills in accessing needed information for routine practice. Increasingly, handheld devices are also being used to access patient information in some settings.

Consumer Drug Information Sources— Your Need to Know

Similar to health professionals, consumers are being bombarded with information via such resources as web sites, computer-based commercials, and direct-to-consumer advertising through all media. But the online global movement has made rapid access to all forms of information possible for consumers just as it has been for health professionals. The ability of consumers to rapidly access information is changing the dynamics of the relationship between health professionals and patients.[22] Consumers access both the publicly available worldwide web as well as proprietary networks such as AOL (America Online). AOL's Health Channel is the most visited proprietary site by consumers. In sum, you must be prepared to deal with the "informed" consumer through these new sources of information.

Selection of Appropriate Drug Information Resources

Selecting Useful Drug Information—Determination of Clinical Relevance

Your primary objective is to find information that is clinically relevant to your patient. Determination of the actual drug information question, patient, and pertinent background data guide you to search selected resources. Factors that alter your searching approach include classification of the request, type of requester, and timeframe and depth of response required. Because of the numerous drug information resources, a skill you should maintain is continuously learning about new sources and updates to the existing sources, and the data that each resource provides.

The Searching Strategy

To find information, you generally should begin with tertiary references, then secondary, and finally primary literature for indepth or extensive answers. To identify potentially relevant information sources, you usually begin a broad search of resources at the tertiary level. You evaluate the information to determine relevance to your specific information need, and focus your efforts within the tertiary sources until you are satisfied. If you determine that the information is not sufficient for your needs, you progress to secondary information sources. Once again, you start with a broad search and narrow it down to potentially relevant resources. You evaluate the content again; if it is not sufficient, move to primary sources.

This systematic approach allows you to learn about the generally accepted information on a particular subject and the key vocabulary terms. By using these terms, you can search secondary sources. If abstracted information is inadequate, the primary literature can be obtained and evaluated.

Online Searching Skills

Because databases have different characteristics, you must attain competency using each database individually to conduct your searches. Common to all databases is 1) the use of the Boolean operator terms "and, or and not"; 2) the use of filters that limit the identification of resources based upon the criteria you select; and 3) a controlled vocabulary. All databases have a hierarchy of terms indexed; some provide a thesaurus for these terms and others do not. It is important that you become skilled at using these features for each database.

Evaluating the Literature for Quality

The skills associated with both determining the quality and reliability of published information is commonly known as critical literature evaluation. A large body of literature exists that describes the skills necessary to evaluate and use published literature.[1–21] Several textbooks are published on this specific subject.[22–26] This chapter will focus on how to identify and retrieve the relevant information needed based upon the patient's needs and the information resource characteristics. However, representative tools to assist you with the skills of critical literature appraisal are presented in **Appendix 7-3**, Drug Information Tools and Checklists.

Reliability of Information—Relationship to Source

A reliable source provides valid, truthful information. Reliability is a concern in both people and in published resources. In the case of persons, reliability varies with the expertise, knowledge, memory, trustworthiness, and motivation of a source. Reliability in published literature is dependent upon these same characteristics. However, an additional quality standard known as peer review is intended to capture questionable reliability. Peer review is a process that depends upon colleagues who have knowledge, training, and experience to critique and recommend inclusion and exclusion of materials and information to ensure accuracy, reliability, and quality. By considering both the source of your data and the circumstance of the relationship, you may assess the value and biases of your information.

Online information sources are of great concern when evaluated for reliability. You must use the same degree of care and concern when evaluating the quality of an

Internet-based information source as you would if it were published in a reliable print source. However, this can be difficult, particularly when you must sort through the large number of resources usually identified. An organization known as Health on the Net Foundation was formed as an approval body to determine the reliability and credibility of information accessed on the Internet that is located through web sites. The organization publishing the web site applies for this approval and is able to post a symbol indicating they have received it. However, this is not a requirement of a web site, and few individuals are probably aware of its existence at this time.

Navigating Unreliable Information from Consumer/Patient Information Sources

Some information obtained by consumers or patients is inaccurate. Increasingly, individuals are accessing a wide range of resources directly that do not have the quality assurances built in like professional resources. Nonetheless, consumers and patients bring this information to you to ask for your advice. You're in a good position to assess the information and make your expert recommendation. Patients are likely very receptive since they were seeking your assistance in the first place. However, if you are approached by a patient who clearly has decided that the information is going to guide his or her behaviors, then you can only advise the patient optimally with your current knowledge and expertise. Other things may be important and helpful to the patient, in addition to the course of action chosen. If you believe harm may come to the individual, you have an ethical obligation to educate the patient with your knowledge and inform him or her of the possible outcomes. The patient will ultimately decide. However, you will have provided essential information to prevent harm from occurring.

Alternative Sources of Information

When you have exhausted your resources and still need additional information or expertise, you should consult your network of alternative resources. This network may consist of experienced colleagues, local experts, or a specialized practitioner. Additional sources may also include

- Poison control centers
- Drug information centers
- Medical librarians and searching services
- Other health care professionals
- Pharmaceutical manufacturers
- Professional associations
- Government agencies

You are always responsible for information that you provide, regardless of the source. Therefore, you must ensure the accuracy of your information. If circumstances allow, you should always request written documentation of any information received orally.

Expert Opinions

At times, there is no published information available to help you answer the questions you have. Experts become a valuable resource to you in these situations. Expert resources are used frequently in the provision of patient care. There is tacit knowledge that we gain through the development of practice expertise. This knowledge is often not transcribed to paper and provided for general use. Experts provide an opinion about the likelihood of an event, or a likely best course of action based upon context and circumstances. When you contact an expert for advice, be prepared to provide as much detail as you possibly can, and inform the expert of the attempts you have already made in your systematic search process for information. These individuals are usually well versed in the published literature, and may be able to point you toward a published source that is valuable, in addition to offering expertise.

SUMMARY

Your skills as a drug information provider directly relate to the development of your practice expertise. Mastering these skills and continuing your competency development with the changing landscape of drug information products and services is an essential lifelong commitment you *must* make to be an outstanding care provider.

CASES

See pages 127–135 for cases.

Case 1: *Nasir Jabr seeks evidence in response to Lauren Smith's question.*

Lauren returns to the pharmacy 1 week later for a followup blood pressure check and a response to her question.

Nasir Jabr: "Hello Lauren; how are you today?"

Lauren: "Well, I'm feeling quite a bit better. That prescription really worked. Thanks for all of your help. Did you find anything out about the smoking and birth control patch?"

Nasir Jabr: "Yes…I was able to evaluate the literature about this medication. As it turns out, the cardiovascular risks are considered the same whether you take birth control pills or use this patch."

Lauren: "What do you mean risk?"

Nasir Jabr: "If you smoke while using either of these forms of birth control, your chances of having a clot form in your bloodstream causing a stroke, heart attack, or problems with your circulation are higher than when you do not smoke."

Lauren: "Well…what is the best thing for me to do?"

CASE 1: SPECIFIC QUESTIONS

Use the Drug Information Worksheet completed by Nasir Jabr and the Pharmacy Profile for Lauren Smith (**Figures 7-2** and **7-3**) to answer the case-specific questions.

1. Did Nasir restate Lauren's question accurately?
2. Were the resources he used appropriate choices in which to find information?

Case 2: *Christine Johnston investigates the evidence about the use of herbal remedies for diabetes based upon her interview with Mr. Montanez and Maria.*

Christine Johnston now has a better understanding of Mr. Montanez. She decides to investigate whether Cactus Flowers (prickly pear cactus) and Yucca root have any effect in diabetic patients. She researches the subject and documents her work on the Drug Information Sheet (**Figure 7-4**).

CASE 2: SPECIFIC QUESTIONS

Use the Drug Information Worksheet completed by Christine Johnston on pages 130 and 131 to answer the case-specific questions.

1. Did Christine Johnston restate the correct questions? Would you have stated them differently?
2. Do you agree with how she categorized this request? How might you have done it differently?
3. Do you agree with the choice of references she selected in her search strategy? What are some of the other choices that might also have worked?

Case 3: *Luisa Rodriguez investigates the ingredients and use of Bai Guo Ye.*

Luisa feels uncomfortable with the remedy that Huong has told her about and does not have many references available about foreign drugs, natural products, or herbs and remedies. She starts her search as shown on the Drug Information Sheet in Figure 7-5.

CASE 3: SPECIFIC QUESTIONS

Use the Drug Information Worksheet completed by Luisa Rodriguez on pages 132 and 133 to answer the case-specific questions.

1. Do you agree with the choice of references she selected in her search strategy?
2. How might experts play a role in helping her find this information?

DRUG INFORMATION WORKSHEET

Date/Time Received 02/02 3 p.m. Person Receiving: <u>N. Jabr</u>   How Received (phone, visit, etc) <u>Visit</u>

Requester or Source Information

Name   <u>Lauren Smith</u>   How to Reach _____ <u>will return in one week</u> _____
Affiliation   <u>patient</u>   Phone #_____
Title_____   Pager# _____
                                                 Fax #_____
                                                 Address_____

Who Requested (check one)
❑ MD   ❑ MD Student   ❑ RN   X Patient
❑ Physical/Respiratory Therapy   ❑ Nutrition Support   ❑ Secretary/Ward Clerk   ❑ Other_____

Classification of Request

X Adverse Drug Reaction (ADR)   ❑ Pharmacoeconomics
❑ Availability   ❑ Pharmacokinetics
❑ Compatibility/Stability   ❑ Pregnancy/Lactation/Teratogenicity
  (Chemical, Pharmaceutical, Sorption, Solubility, etc)   ❑ Poisoning/Toxicology
❑ Compounding/Formulation   (Environmental, Exposure, Occupational, Mutagenicity,
❑ Dosage/Schedule   Carcinogenicity)
    ❑ Drug Interactions   ❑Odd Drug Entities and OTCs
                                            (Investigational, Orphans, Foreign Drugs, Chemical
  (Drug-Drug, Drug-Lab, Drug-Disease , Drug-Food)   Substances
                                            Homeopathic Remedies, Vitamin Substances, Herbs, etc.)
❑ Drug of Choice/Therapeutics/Pharmacology   ❑ Other _____
❑ Identification
❑ Method of Administration

Patient Data

Name <u>Lauren Smith</u>_____   Patient ID_____   Room/Bed Number or Location_____
Age <u>23 years</u>_____ months   Height ____ ft ____in   Setting (e.g., inpatient or outpatient)_____
Gender ❑male   X female   Weight____ lb ____ kg
Race__<u>Caucasian</u>
Diagnosis __<u>UTI, probable HTN, Headaches</u>_____   Allergies/Intolerances_____
Pertinent Medical History/Problem List <u>smokes, elevated BP – underevaluation for essential HTN</u>

Pertinent Medication History___ <u>Uses Ortho-Evra; past use of oral BCP x 2 years; Advil use 3-4x/week; actively using co-trimoxazole starts today for 10 days.</u>_____
Pertinent Laboratory Values_____

Miscellaneous Information_____

The Request, Actual Drug Information Need, and Time Frame for Response

Original Questions/Notes_____   <u>Does birth control patch cause high BP also—or is it just the birth control pills?</u>

Figure 7-2. Drug information worksheet prepared by pharmacist Nasir Jabr to research and respond to Lauren Smith's request. (cont'd)

Clear Statement of Actual Drug Information Need <u>What are the cardiovascular risks associated with the use of Ortho</u> <u>Evra? Does Lauren have other risk factors for negative cardiovascular events as well?</u>

Time Frame Required for Response<u> patient will return in one week</u>

Record of Search/Notes

  Package insert: Ortho Evra contains norelgestromin and ethinyl estradiol – delivered topically and administered once a week. The use of combination hormonal contraceptives is associated with increased risks of s everalserious conditions including myocardial infarction, thromboembolism, stroke, hepatic neoplasia, and gallbladder disease, although the risk of serious morbidity and mortality is very small in health women without underlying risk factors. The risk of morbidity and mortality increases significantly in the presence of other underlying risk factors such as hypertension, hyperlipidemias, obesity and diabetes.   AS A BLACK BOX WARNING: Cigarette smoking increases the risk of serious cardiovascular side effects from hormonal contraceptive use. This risk increases with age and with heavy smoking (15 or more cigarettes per day) and is quite marked in women over 35 years of age. Women who use hormonal contraceptives including Ortho Evra – should be strongly advised not to smoke.

  Micromedex: Women on combination oral contraceptives may experience a modest yet statistically significant increase in blood pressure which returns to normal in 1 to 6 months after cessation (AMA 1991;Woods,1988). The risk of developing hypertension is also r eported to bed 3 to 6 times greater in oral contraceptive users than non users (AMA,1991).

Clear Statement of Response

Clear Statement of Response; Clear that she is at risk because of smoking using the patch. Needs to discontinue smoking.

Response Written: ____documented in chart ____ memo   Response Oral: ____telephone follow-up ____ face to face

Outcomes

General:	Patient-Specific:
☐ More information requested	☐ More information requested
☐ Recommendation accepted	☐ Recommendation accepted
☐ Recommendation rejected	☐ Recommendation rejected
☐ Requester will call back with results / additional requests	☐ Requester will pass information on to patient
☐ Contributed to policy development	☐ Patient education provided
☐ Standard of practice (upheld or improved)	☐ Clinical Impact (+ / - / neutral)
☐ Improved efficacy	☐ Positive patient relations
☐ Improved compliance	☐ Estimated cost impact
☐ Assured safety	☐ None or
☐ Prevented potential medication error	☐ $_____; Describe:_____
☐ Prevented potential ADR	
☐ Estimated cost impact	☐ Probably life saving
☐ None or	☐ Other_____
☐ $_____; Describe:_____	
☐ Other_____	

Figure 7-2. Drug information worksheet prepared by pharmacist Nasir Jabr to research and respond to Lauren Smith's request.

Pharmacy Profile for:

Patient:	Smith, Lauren		New Patient	Print	Close Record

Demographic	OTC / Allergy		Insurance	Diagnosis	Contacts
General Health	Care Plans	Surveys	Account Status		Current Therapy
General Information	Illnesses	Systems Review	Vital Signs		Lab Values

---

Pharmacist's Progress Note: Date: 02-02

LS referred to Dr. Miller by NJ on 02-01 for evaluation of probable UTI. LS presented today with co-trimoxazole prescription. Upon brief history and examination the following was noted:
S: LS reports BP at physician's 148/100; using birth control patch after 2 year history of Lo-Ovral; 3-4 Advil 200 mg tablets 3-4 x per week for headaches – characterized by frontal discomfort and occasional periorbital pain; 1-2 ppd cigarettes. Denies allergy to medications.
O: BP 150/102 seated (repeated here)
A: UTI, probable essential HTN worsened by NSAID use and nicotine addiction - increased risk of thromboembolic events and elevated BP and , headaches – symptoms consistent with sinus headache – likely in need of a decongestant rather than Advil.
P: Dispensed co-trimoxazole and counseled to consume water, take to completion. Offered smoking cessation and hypertension management service. Research her question, "Does birth control patch affect BP also?" Asked her to visit in one week for follow-up.
                                        Nasir Jabr, Pharm.D.

Drug Information Search   Date: 02-03

LS inquiry: Does use of birth control patch carry similar cardiovascular risks when a patient smokes as the oral contraceptives do?
Risk is same with oral contraceptives or patch for those who smoke. (see Drug Information Worksheet)

Figure 7-3. Pharmacy profile for Lauren Smith.

DRUG INFORMATION WORKSHEET

Date/Time Received_____ Person Receiving_____ How Received (phone, visit, etc)_____

Requester or Source Information

Name _My own background question_____ How to Reach_____
Affiliation _____   Phone #_____
Title_____   Pager# _____
    Fax #_____
    Address_____

Who Requested (check one)
❑ MD   ❑ MD Student   ❑ RN   ❑Patient
❑Physical/Respiratory Therapy   ❑ Nutrition Support   ❑ Secretary/Ward Clerk   ❑Other_____

Classification of Request

X Adverse Drug Reaction (ADR)
❑ Availability
❑ Compatibility/Stability
  (Chemical, Pharmaceutical, Sorption, Solubility, etc)
❑ Compounding/Formulation
X Dosage/Schedule
X Drug Interactions
  (Drug-Drug, Drug-Lab, Drug-Disease , Drug-Food)
X Drug of Choice/Therapeutics/Pharmacology
❑ Identification
X Method of Administration

❑ Pharmacoeconomics
❑ Pharmacokinetics
❑ Pregnancy/Lactation/Teratogenicity
❑ Poisoning/Toxicology
  (Environmental, Exposure, Occupational, Mutagenicity, Carcinogenicity)
❑Odd Drug Entities and OTCs
  (Investigational, Orphans, Foreign Drugs, Chemical Substances, Homeopathic Remedies, Vitamin Substances, Herbs, etc.)
❑ Other _____

Patient Data

Name _Eduardo Montanez_____ Patient ID_____   Room/Bed Number or Location_____
Age _68___ years_____ months   Height ____ ft ____in   Setting (e.g., inpatient or outpatient)_____
Gender X male   ❑female   Weight____ lb ____ kg   Race_____Hispanic_____
Diagnosis _Diabetes, dyslipidemia_____   Allergies/Intolerances_____codeine_____
Pertinent Medical History/Problem List_____

Pertinent Medication History_____

Pertinent Laboratory Values_____

Miscellaneous Information_____

Figure 7-4. Drug information worksheet prepared by pharmacist Christine Johnston to research and respond to Mr. Montanez's request. (cont'd)

The Request, Actual Drug Information Need, and Time Frame for Response

Original Questions/Notes_____ See actual below_____

Clear Statement of Actual Drug Information Need: Do Cactus Flowers (prickly pear cactus) and Yucca root____
have any effect in patients with diabetes?_____
Time Frame Required for Response_____

Record of Search/Notes

1. Micromedex – negative, no information available
2. www.naturaldatabase.com   - paydirt! Pricky pear cactus used orally for diabetes. May be possibly effective in the
short-term to reduce blood glucose levels in patients with type 2 diabetes. Single doses can decrease blood glucose levels
by 17-46% in some patgients. Not known if daily use will consistently lower blood glucose levels and decrease HbA1c
levels. Only the broiled stems of the species Opuntia streptacantha seem to be beneficial. Raw or crude stems don't seem
to decrease glucose levels. Some species decrease lipid levels too (I need to investgate this further). Drug interaction
cited with chlorpropamide! Ref cited is: Meckes-Lozyoa M, Roman-Ramos R. Opuntia streptacantha; a coadjutor in the
treatment of diabetes mellitus. Am J Chin Med 1986;14(3-4):116-18. They warn of hypoglycemia being enhanced –
caution probably an oral antidiabetic agent problem in general. Dosing discussed is broiling stems of 100-500 grams daily
is typically used. Wonder how person knows what is 100-500 gms? Will check further. Comment is made that prickly
pear cactus is primary used in Mexican and Mexican-American cultures as part of diet and as a treatment for type 2
diabetes. It is the immature form of the cactus that is used.

Clear Statement of Response

Clear Statement of Response_____ Will discuss this with Maria and Mr Montanez…need to evaluate frequency and
quantity of consumption at next clinic visit._____

Response Written: ____documented in chart ____ memo   Response Oral: ____telephone follow-up ____ face to face

Outcomes

General:	Patient-Specific:
☐ More information requested	☐ More information requested
☐ Recommendation accepted	☐ Recommendation accepted
☐ Recommendation rejected	☐ Recommendation rejected
--	--
☐ Requester will call back with results / additional requests	☐ Requester will pass information on to patient
☐ Contributed to policy development	☐ Patient education provided
☐ Standard of practice (upheld or improved)	☐ Clinical Impact (+ / - / neutral)
☐ Improved efficacy	☐ Positive patient relations
☐ Improved compliance	☐ Estimated cost impact
☐ Assured safety	☐ None or
☐ Prevented potential medication error	☐ $_____; Describe:_____
☐ Prevented potential ADR	
☐ Estimated cost impact	☐ Probably life saving
☐ None or	☐ Other_____
☐ $_____; Describe:_____	
☐ Other_____	

Figure 7-4. Drug information worksheet prepared by pharmacist Christine Johnston to research and respond to Mr. Montanez's request.

DRUG INFORMATION WORKSHEET

Date/Time Received_____ Person Receiving_____ How Received (phone, visit, etc)_____

Requester or Source Information

Name <u>My own background question</u>_____   How to Reach_____
Affiliation _____   Phone #_____
Title_____   Pager#_____
                                                     Fax #_____
                                                     Address_____

Who Requested (check one)
❑ MD   ❑ MD Student   ❑ RN   ❑ Patient
❑ Physical/Respiratory Therapy   ❑ Nutrition Support   ❑ Secretary/Ward Clerk   ❑ Other_____

Classification of Request

❑ Adverse Drug Reaction (ADR)   ❑ Pharmacoeconomics
❑ Availability   ❑ Pharmacokinetics
❑ Compatibility/Stability   ❑ Pregnancy/Lactation/Teratogenicity
   (Chemical, Pharmaceutical, Sorption, Solubility, etc)   ❑ Poisoning/Toxicology
❑ Compounding/Formulation   (Environmental, Exposure, Occupational, Mutagenicity,
❑ Dosage/Schedule   Carcinogenicity)
❑ Drug Interactions   X Odd Drug Entities and OTCs
   (Drug-Drug, Drug-Lab, Drug-Disease , Drug-Food)   (Investigational, Orphans, Foreign Drugs, Chemical Substances
❑ Drug of Choice/Therapeutics/Pharmacology   Homeopathic Remedies, Vitamin Substances, Herbs, etc.)
❑ Identification   ❑ Other _____
❑ Method of Administration

Patient Data

Name <u>Huong Tran</u>_____ Patient ID_____   Room/Bed Number or Location <u>Peds Med</u>
Age <u>8</u> years_____ months   Height _____ ft _____in   Setting (e.g., inpatient or outpatient)_____
Gender X male   ❑ female   Weight_____ lb _____ kg
Race <u>Vietnamese</u>_____
Diagnosis <u>uncontrolled asthma</u>_____   Allergies/Intolerances_____ <u>penicillin</u>_____
Pertinent Medical History/Problem List_____
_____
Pertinent Medication History_____
_____
Pertinent Laboratory Values_____
_____
Miscellaneous Information_____
_____

The Request, Actual Drug Information Need, and Time Frame for Response

Original Questions/Notes_____

Figure 7-5. *Drug information worksheet prepared by pharmacist Luisa Rodriquez to research her need in managing Huong Tran's case.*
(cont'd)

Clear Statement of Actual Drug Information Need _____ What is Bai Guo Ye? Has it been used in the treatment of asthma? What are the effects of this substance on an 8 year old boy? _____

Time Frame Required for Response_____ need information today _____

Record of Search/Notes

_____ 1. Lexi-Drugs on PDA – negative info 2. Pub med – negative info 3. IPA – negative info
_____ 4. Micromedex – negative info 5. www.naturaldatabase.com – bai guo ye is ginkgo extract. "Using ginkgo for asthma and bronchitis was described in the first pharmacopoeia, Chen Noung Pen T'sao, dating to 2600 BC. Reference cited is: Diamond BJ, Shiflett SC, Feiwel N, et al. Ginkgo biloba extract: mechanisms and clinical indications. Arch Phys Med Rehabil 2000;81:668-78. Specific dosing not clear to me.

Clear Statement of Response

Clear Statement of Response_____

_____Response Written: _____documented in chart _____ memo   Response Oral: _____telephone follow-up _____ face to face

---

Outcomes

General:	Patient-Specific:
☐ More information requested	☐ More information requested
☐ Recommendation accepted	☐ Recommendation accepted
☐ Recommendation rejected	☐ Recommendation rejected
☐ Requester will call back with results / additional requests	☐ Requester will pass information on to patient
☐ Contributed to policy development	☐ Patient education provided
☐ Standard of practice (upheld or improved)	☐ Clinical Impact (+ / - / neutral)
☐ Improved efficacy	☐ Positive patient relations
☐ Improved compliance	☐ Estimated cost impact
☐ Assured safety	☐ None or
☐ Prevented potential medication error	☐ $_____; Describe:_____
☐ Prevented potential ADR	
☐ Estimated cost impact	☐ Probably life saving
☐ None or	☐ Other_____
☐ $_____; Describe:_____	

☐ Other_____

Figure 7-5. Drug information worksheet prepared by pharmacist Luisa Rodriquez to research her need in managing Huong Tran's case.

Case 4: *Michael Jones evaluates the literature about the significance of Mr. Robinson's vitamin E use and warfarin.*

Michael Jones checks the Anticoagulation Assessment Guidelines for Pharmacists used in his hospital and identifies the possibility of an interaction with warfarin and vitamin E (see guidelines in case presentation in Chapter 5). When he looks at the guidelines, he realizes that there are several other medications of concern, including synthroid and nonsteroidal anti-inflammatory agents such as aspirin and ibuprofen (Advil). He decides to research them to determine what is appropriate to do in the care of Mr. Robinson. He uses the Drug Information Worksheet to guide him through the process of searching for answers to these questions.

CASE 4: SPECIFIC QUESTIONS

Use the Drug Information Worksheet completed by Michael Jones (**Figure 7-6**) to answer the case-specific questions.

1. Evaluate the conclusion that Michael has drawn about the significance of using vitamin E while taking warfarin. Do you agree with his conclusion? Why or why not?

GENERAL ASSESSMENT QUESTIONS

1. Why is it important to "classify" the subject matter of a drug information question?
2. Once you have classified the question, what is the correct searching strategy? Describe the types of references and order of searching that is generally pursued.
3. What is the purpose of a clinical practice guideline? By what process is it usually developed?
4. What advantages do drug information sources offer when made available on handheld devices?
5. What is the nature of reliable drug information?
6. Explain why experts hold a unique body of knowledge.

ASSIGNMENT

1. Visit a local hospital pharmacy department. Work with a pharmacist to show you the drug information references in the pharmacy department. Include computer-based handheld references.

2. Identify five key references warranting immediate access in your daily practice. Describe the rationale for these choices.
3. Go to the National Library of Medicine PubMed search engine (www.nlm.gov). Complete the tutorial on how to conduct an online search. Be sure to become familiar with the following terms:

> MeSH Terms
> Boolean Operators
> Field Descriptions
> Search limit
> Field tags or qualifiers
> Automatic explosion (explode)
> ISSN (International Standard Serial Numbers)

REFERENCES

1. Osman AD, Sackett DL, Guyatt GH, for the Evidence-Based Medicine Working Group. Users' guides to the medical literature—I. How to get started. *JAMA*. 1993; 270(17):2093–5.

2. Guyatt GH, Sackett DL, Cook DJ, for the Evidence-Based Medicine Working Group. Users' guides to the medical literature—II. How to use an article about therapy or prevention A. Are the results of the study valid? *JAMA*. 1993; 270(21):2598–601.

3. Guyatt GH, Sackett DL, Cook DJ, for the Evidence-Based Medicine Working Group. Users' guides to the medical literature—II. How to use an article about therapy or prevention B. What were the results and will they help me in caring for my patients? *JAMA*. 1994; 271(1):59–63.

4. Jaeschke R, Guyatt G, Sackett DL, for the Evidence-Based Medicine Working Group. Users' guides to the medical literature—III. How to use an article about a diagnostic test. A. Are the results of the study valid? *JAMA*. 1994; 271(5):389–91.

5. Jaeschke R, Guyatt G, Sackett DL, for the Evidence-Based Medicine Working Group. Users' guides to the medical literature—III. How to use an article about a diagnostic test. B. What were the results and will they help me in caring for my patients? *JAMA*. 1994; 271(9):703–7.

6. Levine M, Walter S, Lee H et al, for the Evidence-Based Medicine Working Group. Users' guides to the medical literature—IV. How to use an article about harm. *JAMA*. 1994; 271(20):1615–9.

7. Laupacis A, Wells G, Richardson S et al, for the Evidence-Based Medicine Working Group. Users' guides to the medical literature—V. How to use an article about prognosis. *JAMA*. 1994; 272(3):234–7.

8. Oxman AD, Cook DJ, Guyatt GH, for the Evidence-Based Medicine Working Group. Users' guides to the medical literature—VI. How to use an overview. *JAMA*. 1994; 272(17):1367–71.

DRUG INFORMATION WORKSHEET

Date/Time Received_____ Person Receiving_____ How Received (phone, visit, etc)_____

Requester or Source Information

Name <u>background search for myself</u>_____   How to Reach_____

Affiliation _____   Phone #_____

Title_____   Pager#_____

        Fax #_____

        Address_____

Who Requested (check one)

❑ MD   ❑ MD Student   ❑ RN   ❑ Patient

❑ Physical/Respiratory Therapy   ❑ Nutrition Support   ❑ Secretary/Ward Clerk   ❑ Other_____

Classification of Request

❑ Adverse Drug Reaction (ADR)   ❑ Pharmacoeconomics
❑ Availability   ❑ Pharmacokinetics
❑ Compatibility/Stability   ❑ Pregnancy/Lactation/Teratogenicity
   (Chemical, Pharmaceutical, Sorption, Solubility, etc)   ❑ Poisoning/Toxicology
❑ Compounding/Formulation   (Environmental, Exposure, Occupational, Mutagenicity,
❑ Dosage/Schedule   Carcinogenicity)
X Drug Interactions   ❑ Odd Drug Entities and OTCs
(Drug-Drug, Drug-Lab, Drug-Disease, Drug-Food)   (Investigational, Orphans, Foreign Drugs, Chemical
                            Substances, Homeopathic Remedies, Vitamin Substances,
❑ Drug of Choice/Therapeutics/Pharmacology   Herbs, etc.)
❑ Identification   ❑ Other _____
❑ Method of Administration

Patient Data

Name Samuel Robinson_____   Patient ID_____   Room/Bed Number or Location____347 - 1___

Age_76_years _____ months   Height _____ ft _____in   Setting (e.g., inpatient or outpatient) INPT__

Gender   X male   ❑ female   Weight_____ lb _____ kg

Race_____African American_____

Diagnosis <u>CHF, AF, hypothyroid, HTN, dyslipidemia</u>____   Allergies/Intolerances_____

Pertinent Medical History/Problem List_____

_____

Pertinent Medication History_____

_____

Pertinent Laboratory Values_____

_____

Miscellaneous Information_____

_____

The Request, Actual Drug Information Need, and Time Frame for Response

Figure 7-6. *Drug information worksheet prepared by pharmacist Michael Jones to research his need in managing Mr. Robinson's case. (cont'd)*

Original Questions/Notes_____
_____
_____
_____

Clear Statement of Actual Drug Information Need _____ Patient is taking vitamin E while on warfarin, also has thyroid replacement and baby aspirin. What are the interactions between these agents and the use of warfarin in this elderly man?
_____

Time Frame Required for Response_____ need in 1 hour _____

Record of Search/Notes

_____ 1. Micromedex – Warfarin Monograph – large doses of Vitamin E interfere with vitamin K dependent clotting factors and may lead to enhanced risk of bleeding. Monitor INR closely. Large doses of Vitamin E considered greater than 300 IU's per day. Thyroid replacement in a hypothyroid patient may increase metabolism of clotting factors, thus increasing the anticoagulant effects of warfarin itself. Low dose aspirin in patients on warfarin provokes no more bleeding than with warfarin alone --- another study in Micromedex said that there was a 27% increase in major bleeding episodes after an average of 2.5 years when aspirin around 100 mgs per day was used.

Clear Statement of Response

Clear Statement of Response___ Need to get detailed history from Mr. Robinson. IF he is using the vitamin E a few times a week....probably not a problem. But if its every day...is a problem. He may also not be taking his thyroid ...in that case not a problem yet, but will be when he starts back up. Aspiring is okay._____

Response Written: ____documented in chart ____ memo   Response Oral: ____telephone follow-up ____ face to face

Outcomes

General:
☐ More information requested
☐ Recommendation accepted
☐ Recommendation rejected

☐ Requester will call back with results / additional requests
☐ Contributed to policy development
☐ Standard of practice (upheld or improved)
　　☐ Improved efficacy
　　☐ Improved compliance
　　☐ Assured safety
☐ Prevented potential medication error
☐ Prevented potential ADR
☐ Estimated cost impact
　　☐ None or
　　☐ $_____; Describe:_____
☐ Other_____

Patient-Specific:
☐ More information requested
☐ Recommendation accepted
☐ Recommendation rejected

☐ Requester will pass information on to patient
☐ Patient education provided
☐ Clinical Impact (+ / - / neutral)
☐ Positive patient relations
☐ Estimated cost impact
　　☐ None or
☐ $_____; Describe:_____
_____
☐ Probably life saving
☐ Other_____

Figure 7-6. *Drug information worksheet prepared by pharmacist Michael Jones to research his need in managing Mr. Robinson's case.*

9. Richardson WS, Detsky AS, for the Evidence-Based Medicine Working Group. Users' guides to the medical literature—VII. How to use a clinical decision analysis. A. Are the results of the study valid? *JAMA*. 1995; 273(16):1292–5.

10. Richardson WS, Detsky AS, for the Evidence-Based Medicine Working Group. Users' guides to the medical literature—VII. How to use a clinical decision analysis. B. What are the results and will they help me in caring for my patients? *JAMA*. 1995; 273(20):1610–3.

11. Hayward RSA, Wilson MC, Tunis SR et al, for the Evidence-Based Medicine Working Group. Users' guides to the medical literature—VIII. How to use clinical practice guidelines. A. Are the recommendations valid? *JAMA*. 1995; 274(7):570–4.

12. Wilson MC, Hayward RSA, Tunis SR et al, for the Evidence-Based Medicine Working Group. Users' guides to the medical literature—VIII. How to use a clinical decision analysis. B. What are the recommendations and will they help you in caring for your patients? *JAMA*. 1995; 274(20):1630–2.

13. Guyatt GH, Sackett DL, Sinclair JC et al, for the Evidence-Based Medicine Working Group. IX. A method for grading health care recommendations. *JAMA*. 1995; 274(22):1800–4.

14. Naylor CD, Guyatt GH, for the Evidence-Based Medicine Working Group. X. How to use an article reporting variations in the outcomes of health services. *JAMA*. 1996; 275(7):554–8.

15. Naylor CD, Guyatt GH, for the Evidence-Based Medicine Working Group. XI. How to use an article about a clinical utilization review. *JAMA*. 1996; 275(18):1435–9.

16. Guyatt GH, Naylor D, Juniper E et al, for the Evidence-Based Medicine Working Group. XII. How to use articles about health related quality of life. *JAMA*. 1997; 277(15):1232–7.

17. Drummond MF, Richardson WS, O'Brien BJ et al, for the Evidence-Based Medicine Working Group. XIII. How to use an article on economic analysis of clinical practice. *JAMA*. 1997; 277(19):1552–7.

18. Dans AL, Dans LF, Guyatt GH et al, for the Evidence-Based Medicine Working Group. XIV. How to decide on the applicability of clinical trial results to your patient. *JAMA*. 1998; 279(7):545–9.

19. Richardson WS, Wilson MC, Guyatt GH et al, for the Evidence-Based Medicine Working Group. Users' guide to the medical literature. XV. How to use an article about disease probability for differential diagnosis. *JAMA*. 1999; 281(13):1214–9.

20. Guyatt GH, Sinclair J, Cook DJ et al, for the Evidence-Based Medicine Working Group and the Cochrane Applicability Methods Working Group. XVI. How to use a treatment recommendation. *JAMA*. 1999; 281(19):1836–43.

21. Barratt A, Irwig L, Glasziou P et al, for the Evidence-Based Medicine Working Group. Users' guide to the medical literature. XVII. How to use guidelines and recommendations about screening. *JAMA*. 1999; 281(21):2029–34.

22. Nash DB, Manfredi MP, Bozarth B et al. Connecting with the new healthcare consumer—defining your strategy. McGraw-Hill Companies; 2000.

23. Watanabe AS, Connor CS. Principles of drug information services—a syllabus of systematic concepts. Hamilton, IL: Drug Intelligence Publications, Inc.; 1978.

24. Slaughter RL, Edwards DJ. Evaluating drug literature—a statistical approach. McGraw-Hill Medical Publishing Division; 2001.

25. Khan KS, Kunz R, Kleijnen J et al. Systematic reviews to support evidence-based medicine. Lake Forest, IL: The Royal Society of Medicine Press Limited; 2003.

26. Garrard J. Health sciences literature review made easy. Aspen Publishers, Inc.; 1999.

Appendix 7-1. Representative Questions to Ask for Each Request Classification

CLASSIFICATION and ADDITIONAL PATIENT-SPECIFIC DATA

ADVERSE DRUG REACTION (ADR)

To determine the likelihood of an adverse drug reaction, you must reconstruct facts about the events. You must include subjective and objective clinical information along with a specific description of events, including time sequence, to evaluate the onset and severity. You also must review management approaches to provide appropriate advice for the patient's care.

Representative questions:
- What are signs and symptoms of possible reaction?
- What is severity of reaction? (provide specific description)
- What is temporal relationship between drug administration and reaction?
- What is current medical status of patient?
- What is management plan for patient?
- Was patient exposed to similar or identical substance? (document clinical result)

AVAILABILITY

Frequently, medications that prescribers want to use are not readily available in your institution. Reasons for this restriction may include a controlled formulary management system and budgetary constraints. If alternative therapy is needed, the indication for treatment provides you with recommendations. You probably have available agents within the pharmacologic class that are equally efficacious and have an acceptable side effect profile. For example, you may suggest ranitidine (a "representative H_2 blocker") on your formulary to a physician who wants cimetidine.

Representative question:
- What is indication for treatment? (provide alternatives, if more readily available)

COMPATIBILITY/STABILITY

Many patients are both fluid and electrolyte restricted. These patients may be unable to tolerate exposure to amounts of fluid recommended by usual compatibility and stability guidelines. Sometimes, alternative routes of administration are needed. You must know if the patients are limited, particularly those who are managing complex drug therapy at home. Commonly, home chemotherapy patients require evaluation of their parenteral drug therapy and appropriate combinations of medication to allow administration through one access site. This procedure eliminates multiple intravenous punctures.

Representative questions:
- What are fluid volume and electrolyte restrictions?
- What are available routes of administration?
- What is indication for treatment?
- Is drug self-administered in home?

COMPOUNDING/FORMULATION

Prescribers often are unaware that commercial products are available for older, popular formulations. If a patient has tried a commercial formulation and had a bad experience, you should determine if a compounded product has the same offending substance. This practice is common in dermatology preparations. For example, many patients are allergic or sensitive to wool fat-based products (e.g., lanolin).

Representative questions:
- Are agents available in commercial formulation?
- Did patient use agent? What was result?

DOSAGE/SCHEDULE

The dose range of a drug depends on its indication for treatment. However, new indications for medications may require a different dose and schedule than the original indication. For example, amitriptyline as an antidepressant is dosed at 50–300 mg/day. When it is used for intermittent nocturia, amitriptyline usually is dosed at 10 mg/day.

A specific dose within the range often depends on a patient's ideal body weight or actual body weight (if significantly different from ideal). Other factors include whether the drug is plasma protein bound and whether the dose is affected by organ dysfunction. By determining the extent of renal or hepatic impairment, you usually can recommend a dosage adjustment to suit the patient's needs.

A patient's medication compliance with multiple daily doses can be severely hampered by cognitive as well as noncognitive impairments. Therefore, you should determine the extent of a patient's reading, hearing, and vision damage.

Individual lifestyles also influence recommended times for drug therapy administration, so the dosage schedule should be compatible with your patient's needs.

Representative questions:
- What is indication for treatment?
- What is body weight relative to ideal? (provide lean estimate)
- What is protein or albumin status pertinent to plasma protein-bound drugs?
- Are cognitive impairments limiting compliance?
- Is lifestyle affecting ideal dosing schedule?

DRUG INTERACTIONS

Medicine and pharmacy have volumes of literature on drug interactions and interferences. Each patient case requires evaluation of individual circumstances surrounding the suspected interaction. To determine the likelihood of an interaction, you should identify the patient's exposure to all medications or substances. You also must determine if the size of the doses and sequence of events were within a time period likely to support an interaction.

Many variables, such as drug–disease, drug–food, and drug–laboratory interferences, may contribute to a drug–drug interaction and its significance.

Representative questions:
- What is suspected interaction?
- What are respective doses, durations, and time courses of administration of drugs?
- Is drug interference suspected?
- Is lab interference suspected? (identify specific assay method for laboratory procedure)
- Is disease interference suspected? (document temporal relationship)
- Is food interference suspected? (document temporal relationship between food and medication consumption)

DRUG OF CHOICE/THERAPEUTICS/ PHARMACOLOGY

Treatment recommendations must be based on knowledge of the drug's medical indication and determination of the desired therapeutic endpoints. By also knowing concurrent treatments and medical problems, you can refine your recommendations.

Representative questions:
- What is indication for treatment?
- What are current hepatic and renal functions?
- What is current medication regimen?
- What are current medical problems that may be affected by drug in specific class?

IDENTIFICATION

Seemingly simple identification questions usually are intended to determine what medications a patient is taking and then what the patient should be taking. Reasons for these questions include

- A patient mixed up medications in one container, and the physician or nurse is unable to identify them without labels.
- A patient ingested a large quantity of medication, and the physician must identify the substances.
- A patient wants to take a foreign drug product.

You should know the source, size, shape, and any markings of a product without an identifying name. To identify the drug, you can use a specific reference (e.g., Identidex component of Micromedex) or photographs in the Physicians' Desk Reference. If the product is foreign, its name and country of origin allow you to search foreign product compendiums.

Representative questions:
- What is reason for inquiry? Large amount ingested? Foreign product – need equivalent?
- What are dosage form and appearance characteristics (e.g., size, shape, identifying marks, letters, and numbers)?

METHOD OF ADMINISTRATION

By anticipating limitations that patients may have to a route of administration, you can recommend alternatives. Patients in the home setting, for example, may be better at managing their drug therapy preparation and administration by a particular route.

Representative questions:
- Are any routes of administration prohibitive because of patient-specific limitations?
- Is patient receiving product in home?

PHARMACOECONOMICS

Often, prescribers are unaware of alternative agents that are efficacious but more cost effective. A more readily available alternative may be acceptable if the original treatment request is about a nonformulary drug. For antibiotic use in organized health care settings, the least expensive regimen usually is recommended.

Representative question:
- Is cost-effective alternative available based on patient-specific data?

PHARMACOKINETICS

A question initially posed as a pharmacokinetics request frequently leads to a clinical decision about altering drug therapy. Therefore, you must gather pertinent information about how to interpret specific pharmacokinetic data in your patient. To evaluate the data, you should determine the temporal relationship between the dose administered and the drug concentration. Dosage form and frequency of dosing also may affect your interpretation. To assess the peak serum concentration of a drug, you must select the appropriate time interval when the dose is administered. If a drug is administered more frequently, the trough concentration is likely to be higher. A prescriber who asks for the half-life of Dilantin probably wants to alter dosing for uncontrolled seizures.

Representative questions:
- What are possible routes of drug administration for patient?
- What is organ function in patient?
- What are single and multiple doses in patient?
- What are body fluid drug levels in relationship to dosage form administered and time since last dose?

PREGNANCY

To prevent complications to both a mother and fetus, you should try to avoid the administration of drugs during pregnancy. However, many women consume drugs during the initial phases of pregnancy when they may be unaware of their condition. You should determine how many weeks, or in which trimester, the drug was consumed so you can accurately evaluate teratogenicity data. In many clinical circumstances, administration of a drug is desirable or even necessary during pregnancy. If consumption has occurred, you should document the amount of drug and duration of use to determine the significance of exposure to the mother and fetus.

Questions regarding lactation can be asked for the following reasons:

- Because a baby might have been exposed to a substance through breast milk.
- Because a decision to breastfeed is or is not being made.

As a pharmacist, you need to identify the reason. If an exposure has occurred, you should obtain as much information as possible about clinical presentation.

Representative questions:
- Did patient take drug? (describe dose, route, frequency, and duration)
- In what trimester of pregnancy is patient?
- Are nondrug alternatives available? (if patient has not consumed drug)

Lactation
- Is patient breastfeeding?
- Was baby exposed?
- What are clinical manifestations, if any, in breastfed baby?
- What are time course and sequence of events?

Teratogenicity
- Was fetus exposed?
- Did drug probably cause deformity or abnormality in child?
- What are dose, frequency, route, and duration of therapy?
- What are clinical manifestations?
- What are time course and sequence of events?

POISONING/TOXICOLOGY

The appropriate management of a poisoning requires a good history. The ingested substance provides information about the toxicity of the agent, whereas age and weight indicate the potential severity of an exposure. Moreover, the amount ingested and time passed since ingestion provide information about the symptoms to expect and their management. Ingestion of multiple medications is common and can make management more complex. Sometimes, antidotes and remedies that are administered by well-meaning individuals result in further complications. A patient's clinical presentation, explained in an interview, determines your management of the case.

Representative questions:
- What is accurate identification of drug or substance?
- What was amount of substance ingested? What was package size?
- Were other medications ingested?
- When was substance ingested?
- Were other substances ingested, including alcohol or attempted remedies?
- What was route of administration or exposure?
- Does system history indicate if signs or symptoms are developing?
- What was done to treat patient?

ODD DRUG ENTITIES AND OTCS

Uncommon drug products include medications made in foreign countries, investigational medications, and herbal preparations sold at health food stores. To answer questions about either common or uncommon and prescription or nonprescription products, you must gather specific information about the particular medication. Information for such requests may require specialized information resources and drug literature searches.

Representative questions:

- Is substance commercially available in the United States? A foreign country? Which ones?
- Was substance obtained through participation in a research study? Special request from the government?
- Was product obtained in a health food or natural products store? Herbal market? Chinese apothecary? Homeopathic pharmacy or doctor's office?
- Is substance from a plant source?
- What are other names for substance (if any)?
- Is substance a vitamin?
- Was product obtained by prescription?

Appendix 7-2. Literature and Web Site Search Matrices

Tertiary Literature Matrix

Reference Title and Editor	Request Class ◆	Bibliography	Update	Downloadable to PDA	Publisher
Books and Compendia					
AHFS DI Essentials	a,c,e,f,g,h,i,j,l,o,p,q,r,s	No	No		American Society of Health-System Pharmacists
American Drug Index 2004 Billups NF, Billups SM, eds.	b,d,k,r	No	Annually	No	Facts and Comparisons
American Hospital Formulary Service Drug Information	a,c,e,f,g,h,i,j,l,o,p,q,r,s	No	Annually with four supplements	No	American Society of Health-System Pharmacists
Applied Pharmacokinetic: Principles of Therapeutic Drug Monitoring Evans WE, Schentag JJ, Jusko WT, eds				No	Applied Therapeutics, Inc.
Applied Therapeutics: The Clinical Use of Drugs Koda-Kimble MA, Young LL, Kradjan WA, Gugliemo J, eds.	a,e,f,g,h,i,j,l, o,p,r,s	Yes	Ad lib	No	Applied Therapeutics, inc.
Basic Clinical Pharmacokinetics Winter M, ed.				No	Applied Therapeutics, Inc.
Basic Skills in Interpreting Laboratory Data	a,f,g,h,i,o,s	Yes	Ad lib	No	American Society of Health-System Pharmacists
Clinical Guide to Laboratory Tests. Tieta FW ed.				No	Elsevier Science Publishers
Clinical Laboratory Medicine: Clinical Applications of Laboratory Data Ravel R, ed.				No	Mosby
Clinical Pharmacokinetics Pocket Reference	e,l,o	No	Ad lib	No	American Society of Health-System Pharmacists
Clinical Toxicology of Commercial Products: Acute Poisoning Gosselin RE, ed.	a,b,k,q,s	No	Ad lib	No	Lippincott, Williams & Wilkins

Reference Title and Editor	Request Class ◆	Bibliography	Update	Downloadable to PDA	Publisher
Current Pediatric Diagnosis and Treatment Hay WW, Hayworth AR, Levin MR, Sondheimer JM, eds.				No	McGraw – Hill/Appleton Lange
Diccionario de Especialidades Farmaceuticas				No	Medical Economics Company
Drug Facts and Comparisons 2004	a,b,e,f,i,j,k,l,m,o,p,r,s	No	Monthly	Yes eFacts	Facts and Comparisons
Drugs in Pregnancy and Lactation: A Reference Guide to Fetal and Neonatal Risk Briggs GG, Freeman RK, Yaffe SJ, eds.	a,g,q,s	No	Ad lib	No	Lippincott, Williams & Wilkins
Drug Interaction Facts 2004 Tatro DS, ed.	a,e,f,g,h,i,l,o,p,r,s	No	Quarterly	Yes eFacts	Facts and Comparisons
Drug Prescribing in Renal Failure: Dosing Guidelines for Adults Aronoff GR, ed.				No	American College of Physicians
Red Book 2003 Drug Topics Cohen HE, Medical Economics Staff, eds.				No	Medical Economics Co.
European Drug Index Muller NF, Dessing RP, eds.	b,k,n	No	Ad lib	No	American Pharmaceutical Association
Pocket Guide to Evaluation of Drug Interactions Zuchero FJ, Hogan MJ, Sommer CD, Curran P, eds.	f,g,h,i	Yes	Ad lib	No	American Pharmaceutical Association
Goodman and Gilman's Pharmacological Basis of Therapeutics Hardman JG, LimbirdLE, Gilman AG, eds	a,j,n,o,p,q,r,s	Yes	Ad lib	No	McGraw-Hill Professional
The Sanford Guide to Antimicrobial Therapy Gilbert DN, ed.				No	Antimicrobial Therapy, Inc.
Guide to Parental Admixtures King JC, Catania PN, ed.				No	King Guide Publications, Inc.
Handbook of Clinical Drug Data Anderson PO, Troutman WG, Knoben JE, eds.	a,e,f,j,l,o,p,q,r	Yes	Ad lib	No	Drug Intelligence Publications
Handbook of Nonprescription Drugs Berardi R, DeSimone EM, et al eds.	b,e,f,g,h,i,j,l,o,p,q,r,s	Yes	Ad lib		American Pharmaceutical Association
Driesbach's Handbook of Poisoning: Prevention, Diagnosis, and Treatment True BL, Driesbach RH, eds.				No	CRC Press – Parthinon Publishers

Reference Title and Editor	Request Class ◆	Bibliography	Update	Downloadable to PDA	Publisher
DrDrugs – Drug Guide for Physicians				Yes	www.skyscape.com FA Davis Company
ePocrates				Yes	www.epocrates.com ePocrates, Inc.
Handbook on Injectable Drugs Trissel LA, ed.	c,e,f,l,m	Yes	Ad lib	No	American Society of Health-System Pharmacists
Hansten Drug Interactions Hansten PD, ed.	a,f,g,h,i	Yes	Ad lib	No	Facts and Comparisons
Harriet Lane Handbook: A Manual for Pediatric House Officers Gunn VL, ed.	a,e,j,l,p,q,r	No	Ad lib	Yes	W B Saunders and Co.
Harrison's Principles of Internal Medicine Braunwald E, et al, Eds.				Harrison's on-line	McGraw Hill Publisher
iFacts				Yes	www.skyscape.com Facts and Comparisons
Imprex Collier WA, ed.		No		No	American Pharmaceutical Association
Index Nominum By Swiss Pharmaceutical Society		No		No	CRC - Press
Interpretation of Diagnostic Tests Wallach J ed.				No	Lippincott, Williams & Wilkins
Lexi-Drugs Platinum for Palm OS				Yes	www.lexi.com Lexi-comp, Inc.
Lexi-Interact for Palm OS				Yes	www.lexi.com Lexi-comp, Inc.
Manual of Antibiotic and Infectious Diseases: Treatment and Prevention Conte JE, ed.				No	Lippincott, Williams & Wilkins
Martindale: The Complete Drug Reference Sweetman S, ed.	a,b,d,e,f,g,h,i,j, k,m,n,o,p,q,r,s	Yes	Ad lib	No	Pharmaceutical Press
Handbook of Antimicrobial Therapy Abramowicz M, ed				No	The Medical Letter, Inc.
Ellenhorn's Medical Toxicology: Diagnosis and Treatment of Human Poisoning Hathwani B, Ellenhorn MJ, eds.	A,b,f,g,h,o,p, q,r,s	Yes	Ad lib	No	Lippincott, Williams & Wilkins
Merck Index	b,c,d,k,m,n,o,p,s	Yes	Ad lib	No	Publishing Group

Reference Title and Editor	Request Class ◆	Bibliography	Update	Downloadable to PDA	Publisher
O'Neil MJ					
Meyler's Side Effects of Drugs: An Encyclopedia of Adverse Reactions and Interactions. Aronson JK, Dittman S, Dukes MN, eds	a,e,f,g,h,i,l, o,p,r,s	Yes	Annually	No	Elsevier Health Sciences, Inc.
Micromedex				Yes	www.micromedex.com
Altmed Dex ®					
CareNotes ®					
Disease Dex®					
Drugdex ®	a,b,c,d,e,f,g,h,i,j,k, m,n,o,p,q,r,s	Yes	Quarterly		Micromedex, Inc.
Identidex	b,k,m,n	No	Quarterly		Micromedex, Inc.
Poisindex	a,e,k,l,m,n,r,s	Yes	Ad lib		Micromedex, Inc.
Nelson Textbook of Pediatrics. Behrman RE, Kliegman RM, Jenson HB, eds.				No	W. B. Sanders Co.
Patholphysiology and Management of the Newborn. Avery GB, ed.				No	J.B. Lippincott Company
Pediatric Dosage Handbook. Takemato CK, Hodding JH, Kraus DM., eds				No	American Pharmaceutical Association
The Pediatric Drug Handbook. Benitz WE, Tatro DS, eds.				No	Mosby
Pediatric Drug Formulations. Nahata MC, ed.				No	Harvey Whitney Books Company
2003 Pediatric Red Book: Report of the Committee on Infectious Diseases				No	American Academy of Pediatrics
Pharmacotherapy: A Pathophysiologic Approach. DiPiro JT, Talbert RL, Yec GC, Matzke GR, Wells BG, Posey LM, eds	a,e,f,g,h,i,j,l,o,p,r	Yes	Ad lib	No	Appleton & Lange
Pharmacy Law Digest 2004. Fink JL, Keller-Reid K, eds.	NA	NA	Yearly with one update	No	Lippincott, Williams, & Wilkins

Reference Title and Editor	Request Class ◆	Bibliography	Update	Downloadable to PDA	Publisher
Physician's Desk Reference	a,b,c,d,e,f,g,h,i,k, l,o,p,q,r,s	No	Annually	Yes	www.franklin.com Thomson Healthcare
Physicians Drug Handbook				Yes	www.franklin.com Thomson Healthcare, Inc
Pocketbook of Pediatric Antimicrobial Therapy				No	Lippincott, Williams, & Wilkins
Principles and Practice of Infectious Disease Mandel Gl, Bennett JE, Dolin R, eds				No	Churchill Livingstone
Problems in Pediatric Drug Therapy Pagliaro LA, Pagliaro AM, eds.				No	APhA Publications
2003 Red Book: Report of the Committee on Infectious Diseases					American Academy of Pediatrics
Remington: The Science and Practice of Pharmacy Gennaro AR	a,c,d,e,j,k,p,r,s	Yes	Annually	No	Lippincott, William & Wilkins
Stedman's Medical Dictionary	NA	NA	Ad lib	No	Lippincott, William & Wilkins
Tarascon ePharmacopoeia				yes	www.tarascon.com Tarascon Publishing
Textbook of Adverse Drug Reactions Davies A, ed.					Oxford University Press
The Use of Antibiotics: A Clinical Review of Antibacterial, Antifunal, and Antiviral Drugs Kucers A, Hoy JF, Grayson ML, Crowe SM, eds.					Arnold Publications
USP Dictionary of USAN and International Drug Names USP Committee of Revision, eds.					United States Pharmacopeial Convention, Inc.
USP DI, Volume I: Drug Information for the Healthcare Professional	a,b,e,f,g,h,j,l, o,p,r,s	No	Annually	No	Medical Economics
USP DI, Volume II: Advice for the Patient-Drug Information in Lay Language	b,k,n	No	Annually	No	Medical Economics
USP DI, Volume III: Approved Drug Products and Legal Requirements	b,d,k,m	No	Annually	No	Medical Econimics

Reference Title and Editor	Request Class ◆	Bibliography	Update	Downloadable to PDA	Publisher
Clinical Practice Guidelines					
The Agency for Health Care Research and Quality National Guidelines Clearinghouse			http://www.guideline.gov		
Guidelines and Guidelines Practice			http://www.eguidelines.co.uk		
Systematic Review Sources					
The Cochran Library					
The Cochrane Database of Systematic Review					
Database of Abstracts of Reviews of Effects (DARE)					
Health Technology Assessment (HTA) Database					
Collaborative Review Groups (CRGs)					

◆

a. Adverse drug reaction
b. Product availability
c. Compatibility/stability
d. Compounding/formulation
e. Dosage/schedule
f. Drug-drug interactions
g. Drug-lab interactions
h. Drug-disease interactions
i. Drug-food interactions
j. Drug of choice
k. Identification
l. Method of administration
m. Investigational agents
n. Foreign products
o. Pharmacokinetics
p. Pharmacology
q. Pregnancy/lactation
r. Therapeutics
s. Toxicology/poisoning

Secondary Literature Matrix

Data Base	Format▲	CV✹	Unique Features◆	Publisher
AIDSline	a,c	Yes	a,b,c,d,e	National Library of Medicine
BIOSIS (Biosciences Information Service) (Print version – Biological Abstracts)	a,c	Yes	a,b,c,d,e	BIOSIS
Cancerlit	a,c	Yes	a,b,c,d,e	National Library of Medicine
CA Search (Print version – Chemical Abstract)	a,c	Yes	a,b,d	Chemical Abstract Services
Clin-Alert				Science Editors, Inc.
Current Contents: Life Sciences	a,c	No	b,d,e	Institute for Scientific Information
EMBASE (Print version-Excerpta Medica)	a,c,d	Yes	b,d,e	Elsevier Science, Inc.
IDIS (Iowa Drug Information Service)	a,c	Yes	b,d,e	Iowa Drug Information Service
IPA (Print version- International Pharmaceutical Abstracts)	a,b	Yes	a,b,c,d,e	American Society of Health-System Pharmacists
MEDLARS (National Library of Medicine) Medline(Print version- Index Medicus)	a,c	Yes	a,b,c,d,e	National Library of Medicine
Toxline	a,c	Yes	a,b,c,d,e	National Library of Medicine
InPharma	a,b	No	a,b,c,d,e	Adis International Limited
Reactions	a,b	No	a,b,c,d,e	Adis International Limited

▲
a. Bibliography and abstract
b. Staff-generated abstract
c. Published abstract
d. Full text

✹ CV=controlled vocabulary

◆
a. Spotlights abstracts for meetings
b. Covers foreign journals
c. Covers state association journals
d. Emphasizes pharmaceutical literature
e. Emphasizes drug therapy literature

Primary Literature Matrix

Journal Name	Scope▲	Traits/Features✱	PR◆	Publisher
American Journal of Health-System Pharmacy (formerly American Journal of Hospital Pharmacy)	a,b,c,d,e,f,g	1,2,3,4,5,6,7,8,9,10,11,12,13	Yes	American Society of Health-System Pharmacists
American Journal of Medicine	a,b,c,d,e,f,g	2,3,6,10,11,12,13,14	Yes	Excerpta Medica
Journal of the American Pharmacists Association	a,b,c,d,e,f,g	2,3,5,6,8,10	Yes	American Pharmaceutical Association
Annals of Internal Medicine	a,b,c,d,e,f,g	2,3,6,9,11,12,13	Yes	American College of Physicians
Annals of Pharmacotherapy	a,b,c,d,e,f,g	1,2,3,4,5,8,9,10,11	Yes	Harvey Whitney Books Company
Archives of Internal Medicine	b,c,d,e,f,g	3,10,11,13	Yes	American Medical Association
British Medical Journal	a,b,c,d,e,f,g	4,6,7,9,11	Yes	British Medical Association House
Clinical Pharmacokinetics	b,c,g	2,11	Yes	Adis International Limited
Clinical Pharmacology and Biopharmaceutics				
Clinical Pharmacology and Therapeutics	b,c,e,f,g	6,10,11	Yes	Mosby
Drug Information Journal	b,d,e,g	4,6,11,12	Yes	Drug Information Journal
Drugs	b,c,g	2,11,13	Yes	Adis International Limited US: (215) 741-5200
Hospital Formulary	a,b,c,d,e,f	2,3,5	Yes	Advanstar Communications, Inc.
Hospital Pharmacy – Lippincott's	a,b,c,d,e,f	1,2,3,7,8,10, 11,12,13,14	Yes	J.B. Lippincott Company
Journal of Parenteral and Enteral Nutrition	b,c,d,e,f	3,6,9,10,11	Yes	American Society for Parenteral and Enteral Nutrition
Journal of Pediatrics	a,b,c,d,e,f,g	3,4,9,10,11	Yes	Mosby

Journal Name	Scope▲	Traits/Features✳	PR◆	Publisher
Journal of the American Medical Association	a,b,c,d,e,f,g	4,6,7,9,10,11	Yes	American Medical Association
Journal of Pharmacokinetics and Biopharmaceutics				
Lancet	a,b,d,e,f	2,3,4,9,10,11	Yes	Williams & Wilkins
Medical Clinics of North America	c	3,4	No	W. B. Saunders Company
Medical Letter	a,c	2,3	No	The Medical Letter
Morbidity and Mortality Weekly Report	a,b,g	6,11	No	Massachusetts Medical Society
New England Journal of Medicine	b,c,d,e,f,g	2,3,4,6,9,11	Yes	Massachusetts Medical Society
Pharmacist/Prescriber Letter	a,c	2,3	No	The Pharmacists Letter
Pharmacoeconomics	b,c,e,f,g	2,11	Yes	Adis International Limited
Pharmacotherapy	b,c,d,e,g	2,3,6	Yes	Pharmacotherapy Publications, Inc.

▲
a. Medical news
b. Original articles
c. Review articles/grand rounds
d. Case/short reports
e. Editorials/commentaries
f. Letters/correspondence
g. Special Reports

✳
1. Compatability/stability
2. Drug reviews
3. Therapy reviews
4. Primers
5. Drug usage evaluations
6. Official journal of association
7. Question and answer column
8. Continuing education
9. Book reviews
10. Career opportunities/pharmacists
11. Primary studies
12. Administrative topics
13. Agenda/topics-professional meetings
14. Article abstracts from other journals

◆ PR=peer reviewed

Internet-Based Resources Matrix

References	Site Address
National Organizations	
Food and Drug Administration	www.fda.gov
National Library of Medicine	www.nlm.nih.gov
Centers for Disease Control	www.cdc.gov
National Institutes of Health	www.nih.gov
Professional Organizations	
American Society of Health-System Pharmacists	www.ashp.org
American Pharmaceutical Association	www.aphanet.org
American College of Clinical Pharmacy	www.accp.com
American Association of Colleges of Pharmacy	www.aacp.org
American Heart Association	www.amhrt.org
American Diabetes Association	www.diabetes.org
American Cancer Society	www.cancer.org
Representative Pharmaceutical Companies	
Listing of Companies	www.pharminfo.com/phrmlink.html#drugs_RandD
Abbott	www.abbott.com
Bristol Myers Squibb	www.bms.com
Eli Lilly	www.lilly.com
GlaxoSmithKline	www.gsk.com
Merck	www.merck.com
Novartis	www.novartis.com
Pfizer	www.pfizer.com
Professional Practice Resources	
1997 Survey of Internet Clinical Medicine Applications	http://www.medmatrix.org/Info/survey.html
Avicenna	http://www.avicenna.com
BIDS Embase	http://www.bids.ac.uk
Biosis	http://www.biosis.org
Center Watch	http://www.centerwatch.com
Clinical Pharmacology on Line	http://www.cponline.gsm.com
CMA Infobase	http://www.cma.ca/cpgs/
Current Contents	http://www.isinet.com
Docnet Journals	http://www.docnet.org.uk/medisn/journals.html

DoseCalcOnLine	http://www.meds.com/Dchome.html
Drug Interaction Database	http://csmctmto.interpoint.net/davidws/medical.html
Efacts	www.drugfacts.com
Encyclopedia of Human Nutrition	http://apress.gvpi.net
Encyclopedia of Immunology	http://apress.gvpi.net
Frederick L. Ehrman Medical Library	http://library1.med.nyu.edu/Library/ejournal_frames.html
Guidelines and Guidelines Practice	http://www.eguidelines.co.uk
Hardin Meta Directory – Pathology and Laboratory Medicine	http://www.arcade.uiowa.edu/hardin-www/md-path.html
Harrison's Online	http://harrisons.accessmedicine.com
Health Care Information Resources	http://www-hsl.mcmaster.ca/tomflem/top.html
Health services/technology assessment text (HSTAT)	http://hstat.nlm.nih.gov/
HealthAtoZ	http://www.HealthAtoZ.com
Helix	http://www.helix.com
Lexi-Comp On-Line	http://www.crlonline.com
MedHunt Search Engine	http://www.hon.ch/cgi-bin/find?1
Medical Matrix	http://www.medmatrix.org/index.asp
Medical Matrix – Major Journals	http://www.medmatrix.org/Spages/major_journals.htm
Medical Matrix Directory "What's New" Search	http://www.uoeh-u.ac.jp/MML/MMS-e.html
Medical Word Search	http://mwsearch.poly.edu
MedicineNet Medical Dictionary	http://www.medicinenet.com/MAINMENU/GLOSSARY/Gloss_A.htm
Medi-Span Patient Drug Education-PC Healthtough	http://www.healthtouch.com/level1/p_dri.htm
Medscape	http://www.medscape.com
Merck Manual of Diagnosis and Therapy	www.merck.com
Merck Manual of Geriatrics	www.merck.com
Merck Manual of Medical Information – Home Edition	www.merck.com
Multimedia Reference Library – Jonathan Tward's	http://www.docnet.org.uk/medisn/journals.html
National Coordinating Centre for Health Technology Assessment	http://www.hta.nhsweb.nhs.uk/
National Electronic Library for Health	http://www.nelh.nhs.uk/
National Institute for Clinical Excellence (NICE)	http://www.nice.org.uk/
Natural Medicines On-Line	http://www.naturaldatabase.com
OMNI	http://omni.ac.uk
Outlines in Clinical Medicine	http://www.avicenna.com
Patient Handouts	http://www.rxmed.com/handouts.html
PharmWeb	http://pharmweb.net/
Physicians' Online (POL)	http://www.po.com
PubMed	http://www4.ncbi.nlm.nih.gov/PubMed/(Medline)

RXList – The Internet Drug Index	http://www.rxlist.com/
ScHARR-Lock's Guide to the Evidence	http://www.shef.ac.uk/uni/academic/R-Z/scharr/ir/scebm.html
Science Citation Index	http://www.isinet.com
Scientific American Medicine	http://samed.com
SIGN Guidelines	http://www.show.scot.nhs.uk/sign/home.htm
StatRef – Note: a search engine applied to 18 textbooks: Basic and Clinical Pharmacology Color Atlas and Synopsis of Clinical Dermatology Current Diagnosis and Treatment in Orthopedics Current Medical Diagnosis and Treatment Current Pediatric Diagnosis and Treatment Degowin's Diagnostic Examination DSM-IV-TR Griffith's 5-minute Clinical Consult Medical Immunology Mosby's Drug Consult Principles and Practice of Emergency Medicine Review of General Psychiatry Review of Medical Physiology Schwartz's Principles of Surgery Smith's General Urology The ICU Book USPDI Advice for the Patient USPDI Drug Info for the Health Professional	http://online.statref.com
Turning Research Into Practice	http://www.tripdatabase.com
U.S. Pharmacopeia's Education Leaflets Health Answers	http://www.healthanswers.com/health_answers/usp_drug_Search/frames333.htm

Consumer Based Resources

Advice for the Patient: Drug Information in Lay Language - USP DI, Vol. 2: Advice for the Patient – 24th edition.	Published annually, it contains a section on advice to the patient in lay language.	The United States Pharmacopeial Convention, Inc.
Medic Alert Foundation International	Medic Alert bracelets.	Medic Alert Foundation International, P.O. Box 1009, Turlock CA 95381 1-800-344-3226
FDA Consumer	Published monthly, this is an excellent source of health information for the public.	Rockville, MD: HHS Publication No. (FDA) 83-1001. Superintendent of Documents, Government Printing Office, Washington, DC 20402.
The People's Pharmacy - 2. Graedon J. (Ed.).	Written by a pharmacologist, this book for the consumer covers many topics of drug therapy; from drug interactions to selecting a pharmacist	St. Martin's Press, New York, NY 1998.

Appendix 7-3. Drug Information Tools and Checklists

TOOLS FOR CRITICAL LITERATURE APPRAISAL

Several tools are provided here to assist you with learning how to critically evaluate the quality of information sources. Tools provided include:

- Evaluation of tertiary reference sources
- Evaluation of primary reference sources
  - Critical evaluation checklist for general primary literature
  - Checklist of items to include when reporting a randomized trial based upon the Consolidated Standards of Reporting Trials (CONSORT)
  - Checklist of items to evaluate the quality of reports of meta-analysis of randomized controlled trials (QUOROM)
- Evaluation of Internet-searched resources
- Useful web sites and resources for learning more about evidence-based practice

EVALUATION OF TERTIARY OR GENERAL REFERENCES

_____ Author credibility. The authors are reputable, suggesting they are likely to publish more accurate, complete information and contemporary information.

_____ There is a minimal timeframe gap between the coverage of the subject matter and new developments.

_____ Current edition is being used.

_____ There is a bibliography or reference list. The references appear up to date.

_____ The information is easily found and accessible in the general reference.

_____ The indexes and table of contents facilitate rapid discovery of information.

CRITICAL EVALUATION CHECKLIST FOR GENERAL PRIMARY LITERATURE

_____ The journal in which the article appears is considered to be a reputable one.

_____ The title is consistent with the scope of the "summary."

_____ The investigators are considered to be reliable and the study was conducted in a reputable medical center or university teaching hospital.

_____ The location was adequate for the application of good scientific experimental methods.

_____ The objectives and/or hypothesis (i.e., purpose) of the study was well-defined.

_____ Appropriate scientific methods of experimental design were employed for this type of study.

_____ The population sample size was adequate.

_____ The population sample was described adequately.

_____ The subjects were chosen by appropriate means.

_____ Adequate methods and experimental design were used to ensure that the results obtained were valid and free from bias.

_____ The trial was prospective or retrospective.

_____ There were adequate controls established.

_____ Drug and control treatments were allocated to the subjects in a random manner.

_____ Adequate blinding techniques were utilized.

_____ Appropriate considerations for the proper use of the drug were made.

_____ Drug doses and regimens were within the therapeutic range.

_____ The duration of the trial was adequate.

_____ Drugs were used concurrently and were accounted for.

_____ Appropriate considerations were made for the correct measurement of the established parameters of therapeutic efficacy.

_____ Appropriate considerations were made for the correct number and type of observers.

_____ Appropriate considerations were made for the methods of collection.

_____ The measurable parameters were indicative of therapeutic effectiveness.

_____ Factors are known that may influence the parameters measured.

_____ The characteristics of the test methods are used to assess these parameters, and factors may influence the accuracy of the test methods.

_____ Standard measurements are used and are reproducible.

_____ The results are reported accurately.

_____ Side effects were reported, including the nature and incidence of the reactions.

_____ Dropouts were reported, and the precise reasons for their dismissal were given.

_____ There was missing or unreconcilable data.

_____ Appropriate statistical methods were utilized.

_____ Valid conclusions were drawn, i.e., the conclusions of the study were actually supported by the results.

_____ The article does provide a reference list or bibliography to verify footnoted citations.

Adapted from: Watanabe AS, Conner CS. Principles of drug information services: a syllabus and concepts. Drug Intelligence Publications, Inc.; 1978.

Checklist of items to include when reporting a randomized trial based upon the Consolidated Standards of Reporting Trials (CONSORT)[27]

Present	Paper Selection and Topic	Item Number	Descriptor
	Title and abstract	1	How participants were allocated to interventions (e.g., "random allocation", "randomized", or "randomly assigned").
	Introduction and background	2	Scientific background and explanation of rationale.
Methods			
	Participants	3	Eligibility criteria for participants and the settings and locations where the data were collected.
	Interventions	4	Precise details of the interventions intended for each group and how and when they were actually administered.
	Objectives	5	Specific objectives and hypothesis.
	Outcomes	6	Clearly defined primary and secondary outcome measures and, when applicable, any methods used to enhance the quality of measurements (e.g., multiple observations, training of assessors).
	Sample Size	7	How sample size was determined and, when applicable, explanation of any interim analyses and stopping rules.
Randomization			
	Sequence generation	8	Method used to generate the random allocation sequence, including details of any restriction (e.g., blocking, stratification).
	Allocation concealment	9	Method used to implement the random allocation sequence (e.g., numbered containers or central telephone), clarifying whether the sequence was concealed until interventions were assigned.
	Implementation	10	Who generated the allocation sequence, who enrolled participants, and who assigned participants to their groups.
	Blinding (masking)	11	Whether or not participants, those administering the interventions, and those assessing the outcomes were blinded to group assignment. If done, how the success of blinding was evaluated.
	Statistical methods	12	Statistical methods used to compare groups for primary outcome(s); methods for additional analyses, such as subgroup analyses and adjusted analyses.

	Results		
	Participant flow	13	Flow of participants through each stage (a diagram is strongly recommended). Specifically, for each group report the numbers of participants randomly assigned, receiving intended treatment, completing the study protocol, and analyzed for the primary outcome. Describe protocol deviations from study as planned, together with reasons.
	Recruitment	14	Dates defining the periods of recruitment and follow-up.
	Baseline data	15	Baseline demographic and clinical characteristics of each group.
	Numbers analyzed	16	Number of participants (denominator) in each group included in each analysis and whether the analysis was by "intention to treat". State the results in absolute numbers when feasible (e.g., 10 of 20, not 50%).
	Outcomes and estimation	17	For each primary and secondary outcome, a summary of results for each group and the estimated effect size and its precision (e.g., 95% confidence interval).
	Ancillary analyses	18	Address multiplicity by reporting any other analyses performed, including subgroup analyses and adjusted analyses, indicating those prespecified and those exploratory.
	Adverse events	19	All important adverse events or side effects in each intervention group.
	Discussion		
	Interpretation	20	Interpretation of the results, taking into account study hypothesis, sources of potential bias or imprecision, and the dangers associated with multiplicity of analyses and outcomes.
	Generalizability	21	Generalizability (external validity) of the trial findings.
	Overall evidence	22	General interpretation of the results in the context of current evidence.

The CONSORT statement available at: http://www.consort-statement.org.

Checklist of items to evaluate the quality of reports of meta-analysis of randomized controlled trials (QUOROM)

Present	Heading	Subheading	Descriptor	Reported? (Y/N)
	Title		Identify the report as a meta-analysis (or systematic review) of RCTs.	
	Abstract		Use a structured format.	
		Objectives	The clinical question, described explicitly.	
		Data sources	The databases (i.e., list) and other information sources.	
		Review methods	The selection criteria (i.e., population, intervention, outcome, and study design); methods for validity assessment, data abstraction, and study characteristics, and quantitative data synthesis in sufficient detail to permit replication.	
		Results	Characteristics of the RCTs included and excluded; qualitative and quantitative findings (i.e., point estimated and confidence intervals); and subgroup analyses.	
		Conclusion	The main results.	
	Introduction		The explicit clinical problem, biological rationale for the intervention, and rationale review.	
	Methods	Searching	The information sources, in detail (e.g., databases, registers, personal files, expert informants, agencies, hand-searching), and any restrictions (years considered, publication status, language of publication).	
		Selection	The inclusion and exclusion criteria (defining population, intervention, principal outcomes, and study design).	
		Validity assessment	The criteria and process used (e.g., masked condition, quality assessment, and their findings).	
		Data abstraction	The process or processes used (e.g., completed independently, in duplicate).	
		Study characteristics	The type of study design, participants' characteristics, details of intervention, outcome definitions, and how clinical	

			heterogeneity was assessed.	
		Quantitative data synthesis	The principal measures of effect (e.g., relative risk), method of combining results (statistical testing and confidence intervals), handling of missing data; how statistical heterogeneity was assessed; a rationale for any apriori sensitivity and subgroup analyses; and any assessment of publication bias.	
	Results	Trial flow	Provide a meta-analysis profile summarizing trial flow.	
		Study characteristics	Present descriptive data for each trial (e.g., age, sample size, intervention, dose, duration, follow-up period).	
		Quantitative data synthesis	Report agreement on the selection and validity assessment; present simple summary results (for each treatment group in each trial, for each primary outcome); present data needed to calculate effect sizes and confidence intervals in intention-to-treat analyses (e.g., 2x2 tables of accounts, means and standard deviations, proportions).	
	Discussion		Summarize key findings; discuss clinical inferences based on internal and external validity; interpret the results in light of the totality of available evidence; describe potential biases in the review process (e.g., publication bias); and suggest a future research agenda.	

Reprinted with permission from Mohler D, Cook DJ, Eastwood S, et al. Improving the quality of meta-analysis of randomized controlled trials: the QUOROM Statement. The Lancet. Nov. 27, 1999; 354: 1896

The CONSORT statement.available at: http://www.consort-statement.org/evidence/html#quorom

Web Sites and Resources about Applying Evidence-based Practice Skills

ACP Journal Club	http://www.acponline.org/journals/acpjc/jcmenu.htm
Avicenna Home Page (free MEDLINE; registration required)	http://www.avicenna.com
Bandolier	http://www.jr2.ox.ac.uk/Bandolier/band50/b50-8.html
Best Evidence (to order, in the US)	http://www.acponline.org/catalog/cbi/best_evidence.htm?ban
Biomednet (free registration)	http://biomednet.com/
Centre for Evidence Based Medicine, Oxford, England	http://minerva.minervation.com/cebm
Cochrane Library - San Diego	http://www.updateusa.com/clibpw/clibdemo.htm
Cochrane Library – UK	http://www.update-software.com/clibhome/clibdemo.htm
Community of Science: (userid and password required)	http://muscat.gdb.org/repos/medl
Critical Care Critically Appraised Topics:	http://ahsn.lhsc.on.ca
EBM Journal (Evidence-Based Medicine en francais)	http://www.ebm-journal.presse.fr/ebmjournal/
Evidence-Based Medicine	http://www.acponline.org/journals/ebm/ebmmenu.htm
Evidence-Based Mental Health	http://www.psychiatry.ox.ac.uk/cebmh/
Family Practice JC (POEMS):	http://jfp.msu.edu/jclub/jc0496b.htm
Guide to Best Practices	http://www.futurehealthcare.com/pages/guidetobestpractices.htm
Guidelines: National Guideline Clearinghouse	http://www.guideline.gov
Health Information Research Unit, McMaster University, Hamilton, Ontario	http://hiru.mcmaster.ca/
HealthGate Home Page: (registration required)	http://www.healthgate.com

HealthWorld	http://www.healthworld.com/Library/search/medline.htm
Institute for Clinical Evaluative Sciences *Informed*	http://www.ices.on.ca/docs/informed.htm
Knowledge Finder (must be registered user)	http://www.kfinder.com/
Links to journal websites and fulltext journal articles	http://www.pslgroup.com/dg/medjournals. http://www.nthameshealth.tpmde.ac.uk/connect/journals.htm http://www.medmatrix.org/SPages/major_journals.asp http://www.medscape.com/htm
McMaster Health Information Research Unit	http://hiru.mcmaster.ca
Miner Library in Rochester	http://www.urmc.rochester.edu/Miner/Links/ebmlinks.html
Neurosurgery	http://www.brown.edu/Departments/Neurosurgery/EJC/journ.html
NlightN MEDLINE	http://www.nlightn.com
NNT calculators and tools	http://www.shef.ac.uk/~scharr/ir/nnt.html
Oxford Centre for Evidence-Based Medicine	http://cebm.jr2.ox.ac.uk
PalmTop software downloads	http://www.mtco.com/~glwoods/Default.htm
Peds Journal Club	http://pedsccm.wustl.edu/EBJournal_club.html
Preventive Care: Canadian Task Force of Preventive Health Care	http://www.ctfphc.org
SHARR (links to most other EBM sites)	http://www.shef.ac.uk/uni/academic/R/scharr/ir/netting.html
Society for General Internal Medicine Medical SmartSearch (University of Texas Health Sciences Center at San Antonio) website:	http://badgett.uthscsa.edu/cgi-bin/smartsearch.exe?SGIM=YES
University of York/NHS Centre for Reviews and Dissemination (including links to *Effective Health Care* and *Effectiveness Matters*)	http://www.york.ac.uk/inst/crd/dissem.htm
Users guides to evidence based practice	www.cche.net/usersguides/main.asp
Users' Guides to the Medical Literature	http://hiru.mcmaster.ca/ebm/userguid
Web-based Literature Search Hedges	http://www.mssm.edu/library/ebm/ebmhedges.htm

CHAPTER 8

Application of Clinical Reasoning

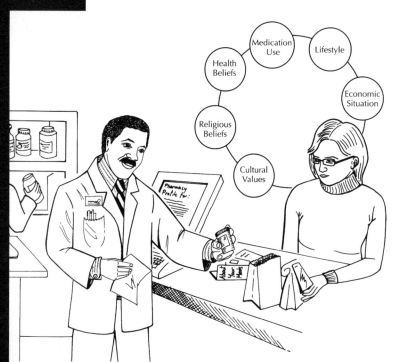

"A medical student asked his attending physician how one acquires clinical judgment. The response was 'from experience.' Then the student asked how to acquire experience. The response was 'from bad clinical judgment.'"

Neal Whitman

Chapter Outline:

Objectives / To be able to understand:

1. how clinical reasoning is used to determine the following:
   a. a patient's health care needs,
   b. a patient's problem list,
   c. the appropriateness of a patient's drug regimen,
   d. an optimal care plan for the patient, and
   e. whether the patient is receiving full benefit of the prescribed drug therapy.
2. how the following factors contribute to clinical reasoning:
   a. empathic reasoning, and
   b. metacognition

3. how the following factors contribute to the quality of clinical reasoning skills:
   a. genuineness as a professional, and
   b. respect towards others
4. evidence-based clinical reasoning.
5. the skills needed for evidence-based clinical reasoning.
6. the skills that you can use to employ empathic, moral, and metacognitive reasoning as well as genuineness and respect for others in the clinical reasoning process.

Purpose: The patient care issues that you need to address should form the basis for your care plan. This chapter will focus on the use of clinical reasoning skills in the pharmaceutical care process.

UNDERSTANDING THE SKILLS OF CLINICAL REASONING

Clinical reasoning is central to delivering professional care to patients. Your ability to use the clinical reasoning process for each patient is what distinguishes you as a professional. Without the use of this reasoning, you become someone who is limited to delivering technically competent service only. Technical competence does not address the moral or empathic needs of the patient in relationship to the pharmaceutical care services that you have a responsibility to provide. If these services are missing, then your purpose as a pharmacist is limited to ensuring technically correct product preparation and dispensing; in other words, only a portion of your professional responsibilities and value to the patient are fulfilled.

Chapter 2 introduced us to the concept of clinical reasoning—the process of expert clinical problem-solving, a dynamic, cyclic, reiterative process in which observation, analysis, synthesis, deduction, induction, hypothesis generation and testing, inquiry-strategy design, and the skills of examination are all interrelated.[1] Figure 2-3 on page 23 shows a representation of the clinical reasoning process. This reasoning, combined with use of evidence, defines your expertise in practice. Chapter 8 will focus on clinical reasoning skills in the pharmaceutical care process.

Important attributes that support your ability to perform clinical reasoning include moral reasoning, metacognition, and empathy as well as display of genuineness in your work and respect for others. The following discussion will address why this is so and what skills you can demonstrate that are consistent with these attributes when delivering care to your patient.

Moral Reasoning

Pharmacists who demonstrate clinical reasoning use moral reasoning skills.[2] What are moral reasoning skills? They are the processes that an individual undergoes to arrive at decisions based upon a concept of right and wrong. The theory that describes moral reasoning in the context of development is Kohlberg's stages of moral development (refer to Box 2-2 on pages 23 and 24). Moral reasoning is a significant determinant of how pharmacists behave; pharmacists with higher moral reasoning skills demonstrate better clinical performance. Research has already demonstrated that when a person in the health professions has more advanced moral

reasoning skills, that individual is most assuredly a high clinical performer.[3,4] These individuals work at being competent and effective as a standard of practice behavior.[5,6] Your moral reasoning skills help you to identify acceptable solutions for a patient.

What moral reasoning skills would you employ? These skills include being aware of your own motivations, abilities, competence, and limitations in order to act on behalf of the patient. Your approach to care requires a commitment to using evidence on behalf of the patient and a commitment to continuing care for that patient. You should get to know as much as you can about the patient in order to understand his or her needs. Maintaining confidentiality about your patient and what you learn in the patient–pharmacist relationship is essential. You have an obligation to inform the patient about what you are going to do or plan to do, while helping him or her reach decisions that are appropriate for the illness and for life. These basic moral skills make you a sound clinical performer.

Metacognition

Metacognition refers to deliberation and reflection during problemsolving. It is the self-monitoring function that tells you how well you are doing in thinking through the patient's problems and possible solutions to consider. It is this ability that is the hallmark of an expert clinician. Metacognition is the main skill in the clinical reasoning process that you must employ to grow and develop professionally. It is the "how" in "how do you clinically problem solve?"

Donald Schon has described the metacognitive reasoning process as reflection-in-action.[7] This descriptive phrase sums up metacognition. Well developed metacognitive skills are observed in expert clinicians. This set of skills is recognized within yourself when you are purposefully positing questions, gathering information iteratively, and testing hypotheses. Metacognition is the constant engagement in this process that makes you aware of the inconsistencies in the patient information or story, the importance of missing data that is not yet understood, or sense of a problem not yet solved, creating in you a feeling of discomfort until resolved. Metacognition is the constant use of reflective skills, which you are aware of, through an iterative experience. You use these skills to develop and consider information, discern its relevance, and then make decisions. It is the cumulative experience of the professional that continually builds and develops with each case, contributing to the ongoing development of these metacognitive skills in each of us. We must purposefully develop our expertise using this approach in order to become better at what we do.

Intuition is not the same as metacognition. Knowing intuitively is to have a direct understanding without reasoning. Intuition can be attributed to the recollection of forgotten facts, to automatic thinking, or to the unconscious processing of a difficult problem. These experiences are not reflective or systematic. Metacognition is a skill set that you work at developing.

Empathy

The core of caring behavior in the pharmacist patient relationship is empathy. Empathy is a reflexive understanding of patient and self.[8] In essence, the ability to empathize is to be able to put yourself in someone else's place, sometimes referred to as being able to "walk in someone else's shoes." Empathy is an important ability to draw upon at every stage of clinical reasoning. Without the use of empathic reasoning, you cannot identify what the patient views as a problem and how a patient feels about or accepts the possible solutions (or course of action) that you recommend. It is important to understand empathy as a skill set that is used to understand and learn what the patient is experiencing and needs. Empathy itself is not the emotional state of sympathizing, rather, it is understanding what exactly is being told to you through all forms of communication.

Empathy includes listening and responding skills. Listening involves hearing what is said and observing what is demonstrated in nonverbal behaviors. Listening involves interpreting the emotions of the patient. Responding involves determining what the most appropriate response to what your listening reveals in order to maximize what you learn from the patient about his or her concerns and needs.[9] Coulehan and Block have identified levels of responding to help describe what optimal responses to gain the full understanding of what the patient is trying to communicate. The first two levels are ignoring and minimizing. Ignoring is when you act like you didn't hear the patient and provide no acknowledgement about what the patient has told you. Minimizing is when you respond to what the patient has told you but you respond by indicating that things are less important or serious than what the patient has implied. Both forms of response result in the patient interpreting you as not listening—or being a poor listener, interpreting inaccurately what has just been communicated.

The two levels of response that are desired in empathic communication are known as interchangeable or additive. An interchangeable response is one that recognizes the feelings and symptoms expressed by the patient at an accurate level of intensity, and is provided back to the patient indicating that you have identified them and the intensity of the experience accurately. An additive response takes this skill one step further. You not only understand what the patient is expressing, but you can relate to what is being felt but not expressed in any way. Your response articulates these feelings back to the patient in words that indicate you understand. Additive responses become possible as you gain experiences over time with patients who have had similar problems. As their stories unfold, you assimilate a body of experiential knowledge that allows you to substitute words for the unspoken. This is an expert skill. We will examine empathic communication and levels of responding in the patient cases in this chapter.

The ways in which you use verbal and nonverbal language will influence your ability to be empathic. Patients do not use medical terminology to express the presence of or degree of intensity of their symptoms. Patients use words that express how they feel about their symptoms as well as what symptoms they are having. It becomes your job to translate what the patient is saying in patient language into the professional language you use.[10] **Table 8-1** shows a listing of words that describe levels of feelings to help you interpret both the quantity and intensity of what the patient is discussing with you.

Nonverbal communication involves the way a person uses his or her body—including personal and social space and paralinguistics—the "how" of speech. The body language of both you and your patient become important to empathic reasoning. You must act interested, make eye contact, and stay focused on the patient. Otherwise, the patient is likely to interpret your actions as disinterest and you will not learn what you need to know. The distance between you and the patient can also make a difference. For example, if you are trying to discuss a delicate and private aspect of the patient's condition, the patient is less likely to respond if he or she has to speak loudly in order for you to hear. Characteristics of the boundaries of space between you and the patient in any interaction are shown in **Table 8-2**. Consider using an appropriate distance from the patient for the type of interaction you expect to have.

The most subtle aspects of the communication exchange are probably the paralinguistic characteristics of the patient's speech. When we hear the words a patient is saying, we are also influenced by the rate of speech, pauses, tone or voice quality, pitch, volume, and word choice. These characteristics, combined with the words stated, tell us the patient's emotions, feelings, and sincerity. Learning the nuances of paralinguistics is a communication skill that develops through formal study and your accumulated experience in working with a wide range of patients. Overall, your main goal with the patient should be to assess the consistency between what is being said and the physical behavior. When there is consistency, the communication is likely to be accurate. When there is inconsistency, you should probe further to determine why.

Genuineness

Genuineness means being "you," both professionally and personally. It requires you to express your feelings within the boundaries of your professional relationships. This means that you must be able to distinguish

Table 8-1. Descriptive Words for Levels of Feelings

Intensity	Anger	Joy	Anxiety or Fear	Depression
Weak	Annoyed	Pleased	Uneasy	Sad
	Upset	Glad	Uncertain	Down
	Irritated	Happy	Apprehensive	Blue
Medium	Angry	Turned on	Worried	Gloomy
	Testy	Joyful	Troubled	Sorrowful
	Quarrelsome	Delighted	Afraid	Miserable
Strong	Infuriated	Marvelous	Tormented	Distraught
	Spiteful	Jubilant	Frantic	Overwhelmed
	Enraged	Ecstatic	Terrified	Devastated

Adapted from Coulehan JL, Block MR. The medical interview: a primer for students of the art. Philadelphia, PA: F.A. Davis Company.

Table 8-2. Space Boundaries in Patient Interactions

Interaction	Distance between You and Patient	Body Contact	Eye Contact	Vocalization
Intimate	0–1.5 feet	Expected (e.g., exam)	Not possible; restricted to small area	Low and frequent
Personal	1.5–4 feet	Close contact likely	May see whole face	Moderate
Social	4–12 feet	Out of reach	Eye contact important	Louder
Public	12–25 feet	No	Individuality lost	Louder; the pronounciation exaggerated

Adapted from Forsyth DM. Looking good to communicate better with patients. Nursing. 1983; July:34–7.

your personal self from your professional self. But this is where it gets more difficult for many people. You may have personal feelings in response to information provided or the behavior of a patient with whom you work; however, these feelings are inappropriate to act on. Your professional feelings must govern your response to these situations. The skill of being genuine requires that you restrict your responses to those that you think will help the patient therapeutically. It may be appropriate to confirm a patient's feelings through sharing a reflection of a personal nature, but only after you have evaluated it through a professional frame of reference and determined that it has therapeutic value to your relationship with the patient.

Respect for Others

Respect is about valuing the patient's traits and beliefs rather than considering your own feelings first. You must see the patient's attitudes, beliefs, and behaviors as a legitimate representation or extension of illness or problems. This means that you are personally nonjudgmental about the patient, and are able to serve the patient professionally with all of these factors taken into consideration. The skill of respect requires you to stay focused on what is needed to care for the patient and to help the patient improve. Follow the communication tips noted below to demonstrate your respect for the patient:

1. Introduce yourself and communicate specifically why you are there. You should address the patient by his or her proper last name when you first meet. The patient should be the one who invites you to use a first name in conversation.
2. Ask the patient how you might improve his or her comfort. Consider this response throughout your interaction.
3. Use proper communication skills for the specific situation.
4. Warn the patient when you are going to say something that may induce emotional harm or when you will do something that might be unexpectedly painful.
5. Always acknowledge through your response that you have heard what the patient has said.

ASSESSING MEANING FROM INFORMATION USING EVIDENCE-BASED CLINICAL REASONING

The subjective and objective data gathered through various sources must be interpreted for its significance to the patient's case. As you gain skills in clinical reasoning, it becomes clear that interpreting the language of the patient is a critical aspect of selecting relevant subjective information. As you gain technical knowledge about the conditions, effective treatments, and methods of management, it becomes clear that you must integrate this information with what you know to be significant to the patient. Both forms of knowledge are critical to expert clinical care. Use of these combined forms of knowledge as the framework for applying the components of clinical reasoning is evidence-based clinical reasoning. Research has been conducted on this subject with family physicians. The findings revealed that family physicians think about evidence during patient interactions but do so in the context of their patients and their communities. They appreciated evidence that had been appraised, summarized, and published as a guideline by an independent national organization. Evidence is an important part of clinical practice, and was considered along with many other factors in their practices. This work accurately summarized the place for evidence in clinical reasoning.[11]

IDENTIFYING THE PATIENT'S HEALTH CARE NEEDS

Why is the patient's care provider seeking help? To identify the patient's health care needs, you must evaluate the information in the patient database. Anticipating the most common problems before beginning your detailed evaluation is a proactive approach to patient assessment—and one that is strongly tied to the concept of pharmaceutical care. This approach is preferred to a reactive technique where you only perform an assessment and provide advice for existing problems noted by other people or for problems recognized by scanning the patient data only after they occur. The proactive approach evaluates the overall patient and his or her needs. You will likely identify therapeutic issues not recognized by others. You are able to identify and document "significant negatives" (i.e., the absence of problems) and "significant positives" (i.e., the presence of problems), improving the ability for yourself and others to monitor and assist the patient with his or her progress. Screening for problems that may not yet have manifested or been recognized increases your opportunity to prevent problems or serious sequelae. Your personal method for conducting the assessment should suit your personal style and experience level. However, the method should incorporate the following characteristics:

1. Anticipate and discuss if the most common potential problems encountered with patients are present or absent with *this* patient.
2. Be consistent between patients about the basic evaluation you conduct.
3. Individualize the depth and scope of the evaluation beyond the basic assessment provided to all.
4. Document the complete assessment (i.e., both significant positives and significant negatives).

The more effective your clinical reasoning process, the better you will be at identifying all of the potential problems.

IDENTIFYING THE PATIENT'S MEDICAL NEEDS

Once you have established an initial impression of the patient's overall health care needs, you narrow your assessment to determining the patient's actual medical needs. Specifically, the patient has some history to share with you and an accompanying list of medical problems or active conditions. Other sources of information (e.g., medical chart, pharmacy profile) may be accessible to you to provide this detail.

IDENTIFYING THE PATIENT'S MEDICATION-RELATED NEEDS

This level identifies all of the patient's medication-related needs. This list of needs must be prioritized by the most important or significant problems to be addressed to meet the patient's goals. The development of this list requires your clinical reasoning skills. For many of these needs, identifying those that must be addressed also requires the shared decisionmaking of the patient. Upon completion of your initial assessment of the patient, you will have a "picture" of the patient—the patient's story. This story leads you to an initial problem list that both you and the patient share. You must further discern the pharmaceutical care aspects of this problem list that require your attention. To identify the patient's drug therapy problems and needs, you should use a systematic process that meets your personal style but addresses the core practice and care considerations of the patient and his or her drug therapy care. The problem list contains everything that you should consider when setting pharmacotherapeutic goals. One approach is to use a systematic method to evaluate the patient's therapeutic plan by using a routine evaluation as a basis to start. The types of concerns about drug therapy are categorized and the questions to assess them are also included.

CORRELATION BETWEEN MEDICAL NEEDS AND MEDICATION-RELATED NEEDS

As you conduct your assessment, you must correlate the medical problems and needs with the medication-related needs that you uncover. This effort requires you to determine the drugs being used to treat each condition identified, conditions that are not being treated with any identifiable drug, and drugs being used with no identifiable indication. There may be more than one indication for a particular medication or, alternatively, more than one medication for an indication. In some situations, a patient may be taking unidentified medications. The patient may have unlabeled tablets—drug samples that were given during a clinic visit or tablets that were removed from the original prescription vials and put into another container. Additionally, the patient may have nonprescription medications with unknown contents, like those purchased through health food supplies. Or, the patient may be unable to provide the names and dosage regimens of medications taken prior to admission or a clinic visit. When you encounter these situations, you should draw upon your drug information skills. You may use your skills of inquiry to develop the patient database through patient interviewing strategies, contacting other health care providers who have needed information, or interviewing family or friends who care for the patient.

After all drugs have been accounted for in the matching process, consider if any drugs are being used that have no identified medical indication for the patient. This situation sometimes occurs when a condition is cured but the patient continues to take the medication or when the patient self-medicates and has no true medical need for the drug.

The patient may also have an untreated medical condition that requires drug therapy, but no medications are being given. You must identify these "missing" medications because untreated medical conditions may worsen.

Basic Medication-Use Assessment

To conduct a basic medication-use assessment, you should first identify all of the medications that a patient is actively taking. This process is done in different ways depending on the care environment. In the hospital setting, you may be the professional conducting a medication history on admission. On the other hand, this process may routinely be handled by the nurse and you may need to supplement or augment it. In many settings, you will be able to ask the patient to show you all of the medications that are being taken. Some pharmacists conduct "brown bag" medication reviews. This review occurs when the patient brings a bag containing all of the medication containers he or she is using. The pharmacist then interviews the patient based upon this information as an initial starting point.

Patients and their caretakers may also maintain written lists of active medications. This source is often the one that reflects what the patient is supposed to be doing presently with the medications. However, you may need to use your drug information inquiry skills. For example, you may need to check information resources for tablet or capsule identification based upon a physical description of a drug you are shown. You might also have to contact the patient's pharmacy(ies) or other providers to reconstruct what the patient is supposed to be doing. After the medications are identified, then you should assess the patient's current use of them.

The assessment of medications currently being used involves remembering the patients' health needs and medical problems as you evaluate their medication use. Several routine questions should be asked of every patient in order to understand what he or she is presently doing. As you are assessing the medications used, incorporate your technical knowledge of evidence. Knowledge of best clinical practices, evidence-based evaluations, and other methods of scientific support for optimal therapeutic management become critical to serving your patient. Key questions suggested for the basic medication-use assessment are shown here:

1. *Appropriateness of medication selection*
   Are the medications chosen for this patient optimal efficacy option(s)?
   Do these medications have the greatest relative safety option(s)?
   Have the medications selected been tailored to this individual patient's health and medical needs?
2. *Appropriateness of drug regimen*
   Are the prescribed dose and dosing frequency appropriate—within the usual therapeutic range and/or modified for patient factors?

Is p.r.n. use appropriate for those medications either prescribed or taken that way?

Is the route/dosage form/mode of administration appropriate, considering efficacy, safety, convenience, patient limitations, and cost?

Are doses scheduled to maximize therapeutic effect and compliance and to minimize adverse effects, drug interactions, and regimen complexity?

Is the length or course of therapy appropriate?

3. *Presence of therapeutic omission*

Have any conditions or problems gone untreated?

4. *Presence of therapeutic duplication*

Are there any therapeutic duplications?

5. *Existence of allergy or intolerance to medications*

Is the patient allergic to or intolerant of any treatments currently being taken or considered?

If the patient has an allergy or intolerance, is he or she using any method to alert health care providers of the allergy/intolerance (emergency bracelet, wallet card)?

6. *Potential for or actual adverse drug event*

Are any symptoms or medical problems possibly drug induced? What is the likelihood that the problem is drug related?

7. *Presence of clinically important interactions: drug, disease, nutrient, or laboratory*

Are there drug–drug interactions? Are they clinically significant?

Are any medications contraindicated (relatively or absolutely) given patient characteristics and current/past disease states?

Are there drug–nutrient interactions? Are they clinically significant?

Are there drug–laboratory test interactions? Are they clinically significant?

8. *Relationship of social or recreational drug use to medical management with drug therapy*

Is the patient's current use of social drugs problematic?

What is the patient's usual consumption of alcohol as a social or recreational drug?

Could the sudden decrease or discontinuation of social drugs be related to patient symptoms (e.g., withdrawal)?

By answering these basic questions, you are able to identify areas that require further individualized attention in your care planning.

Individualized Medication-Use Assessment

1. *Unique individual patient cultural, ethnic, and personal beliefs affecting determination of problems and goals*

Are there ethnic, cultural, or personal beliefs that are affecting the patient's behaviors related to medication use?

2. *Patient values related to goals of treatment and medication use*

Does the patient believe that using the medication is valuable and worthwhile?

3. *Patient adherence to treatment*

Is the patient taking the medications as prescribed?

4. *Financial barriers*

Is the chosen medication(s) cost effective?

Does the cost of medication pose a financial barrier to the patient adhering to use?

5. *Inadequate patient knowledge*

Does the patient understand the purpose of his or her medication(s), how to take it, and the potential side effects of therapy?

Would the patient benefit from educational tools (e.g., written patient education sheets, wallet cards, and reminder packaging)?

6. *Clinical outcomes, economic, and humanistic outcomes*

What are the clinical outcomes from the medication-use plan?

What are the economic outcomes associated with the medication-use plan?

What are the quality-of-life outcomes experienced by the patient that are directly related to the medication-use plan?

7. *Other factors affecting medication use*

SYSTEM OF CARE ISSUES RELATED TO MEDICATION USE

Your role as a clinician is to optimize the patient's care experience using evidence-based clinical reasoning to problem solve and determine appropriate care, and to implement that care with the patient. Sometimes, aspects of the larger systems of health care influence this beyond your control. For example, payers may not cover the costs associated with medications determined to be optimal for this patient's use. Or errors are made and the patient does not receive the intended medication in the way you have intended. These barriers will confront you and your patient. It is essential that you identify these obstacles in the reasoning process and work through possible solutions with the patient.

SYSTEM OF CARE—MODIFYING THE PATIENT'S REGIMEN

One barrier that may prevent a patient from modifying the drug regimen after your evaluation and assessment is the practical issue of having prescribed medications modified to reflect the recommendations you have determined optimal for the patient. In the inpatient setting, a medication order may be rewritten by a pharmacist as a verbal order and countersigned by the physician. The pharmacist may also participate in a practice guideline that indicates the authority that the pharmacist has to make medication regimen changes without the physician's countersignature. In many states, it is possible for the pharmacist to initiate or modify prescription medications in the outpatient setting by being delegated this authority by a physician. This authority is recognized through the establishment of a collaborative practice agreement. In some states, these agreements are not recognized as a legal vehicle to accomplish this goal. In these states, the pharmacist must contact the prescriber ahead of time and recommend a change. The prescriber will then initiate a prescription change and either fax the prescription to the pharmacist or require that the patient pick up the new prescription and have the changes made by the pharmacist.

HEURISTICS FOR CLINICAL REASONING

Occasionally, you may encounter a very difficult problem with a patient that is not solvable using your systematic methods. How does one clinically reason through these complex or messy problems? Heuristics are techniques we use as people to solve such problems. We each adopt different heuristic approaches to solving them. Here is a summary of some possible approaches:[9]

- Consider the most common problems first.
- Consider more seriously those problems for which effective therapeutic options are available; if you failed to initiate treatment, it would be harmful to the patient.
- Make sure that history taking and the physical examination are branching procedures.

- Strive for the degree of precision or reliability at hand.
- Form a reasoned plan to test your hypotheses, because there should be a reason for every piece of data you intend to gather.
- Seek out and evaluate evidence that tends to rule out any hypothesis or alternative.
- Consider the possibility that a patient with multiple symptoms or complaints may have more than one problem.

SUMMARY

Clinical reasoning is applied throughout the care process with the patient. As we progress through the care steps, clinical reasoning is used to determine the problems and the therapeutic options, design the care plan (including the goals and therapeutic regimen), design the monitoring plan, and determine the care behaviors supportive of achieving the goals. You will continue to use clinical reasoning as you implement the plan, assess a patient's response, and use this skill to redesign the plan.

CASES

See pages 173–191 for cases.

Case 1: *Nasir answers Lauren's question and establishes a collaborative drug therapy management service with her and her physician.*

Nasir and Lauren continue with the visit—refer back to Chapter 7.

Nasir (responds to her question): "The best thing for you to do will depend upon what is most important to you, and what you believe you can change about your own behaviors. Your health choices depend on it."

(Lauren looks somewhat troubled.)

Nasir: "You look troubled Lauren. What can I do to help you?"

Lauren: "You mentioned before that you offer a smoking cessation program."

Nasir: "Yes, and also blood pressure management."

Lauren (expressing herself with lack of confidence): "Is it possible for me to consider this as an option? You know…having this service?"

Nasir (detects her lack of confidence): "Yes it is. It would be my pleasure to provide this care for you. You are an excellent candidate for benefiting from these services. However, I would like to inform you of a few things before we both agree that this is the best choice for you."

Lauren (looks somewhat relieved): "Okay. I would like to hear more."

Nasir: "These services are not independent of your physician. By this, I mean that your physician must refer you to me for these services, and your physician and I have agreed to the range of decisions I will make to your drug therapy without approving it ahead of time. Your physician is doing what is called 'delegating her authority' to me to do certain tasks, like write prescriptions for medications. In other aspects of the service, I have 'independent authority.' With these services, such as smoking cessation counseling, I have earned a certificate that is recognized by health care payers as making me a qualified care provider."

Lauren (interrupts): "You mean that you are doing something that isn't legal?"

Nasir (acknowledging her concerns): "Not at all. This is the legal way in which you, your physician, and I will handle helping you with your care. This is also a method of assuring that you will receive quality services from me, and that your physician will be informed of our progress so that everyone involved in your care can be supportive. How does this sound so far?"

Lauren: "I think I understand. It sounds okay. Is there a charge for this service?"

Nasir: "Yes there is. The charges are established based upon the community standard; if you have insurance, I will bill them with your permission."

Lauren (looking depressed): "I do not have insurance, my parents have been paying for everything."

Nasir (sensing her reaction): "I have worked with many patients who do not have insurance. I have permission from the pharmacy to work out special payment programs and options for individuals in your situation. Joe (pharmacy technician) has a written explanation of how we can do this. If you think you would still like to pursue this, I will transfer the financial parts of this over to Joe. I will work on your care, and he will work with you to achieve a financial arrangement that meets your situation. I have not encountered a patient situation that Joe hasn't been able to work with yet."

Lauren (relieved): "That sounds good, Nasir. How do we proceed?"

Nasir: "I would like to share my collaborative practice agreement with you that Dr. Miller and I have prepared (**Appendix 8-1**, page 186). I also have to send a document to the state that indicates I have this arrangement. It is yours to keep and review. You will need to contact Dr. Miller and indicate that I have offered these services and that you would like to receive them. Her office will follow up with me after that. In the meantime, we will need to set up an evaluation and assessment appointment to establish your overall care plan and how we will go about implementing it. Joe will set this up for you too."

Lauren (looking grateful): "Thank you so much, Nasir. I will call Dr. Miller's office."

Nasir: "Great. Joe can facilitate that if you like. Just let him know if you want his help."

[Nasir updates Lauren's patient profile (**Figure 8-1**).]

Pharmacy Profile for:

| Patient: | Smith, Lauren | | **New Patient** | **Print** | **Close Record** |

| Demographic | OTC / Allergy | | Insurance | Diagnosis | Contacts |

| General Health | Care Plans | Surveys | Account Status | | Current Therapy |

| General Information | Illnesses | Systems Review | Vital Signs | | Lab Values |

Pharmacist's Progress Note: Date: 02-02

LS referred to Dr. Miller by NJ on 02-01 for evaluation of probable UTI. LS presented today with co-trimoxazole prescription. Upon brief history and examination the following was noted:
S: LS reports BP at physician's 148/100; using birth control patch after 2 year history of Lo-Ovral; 3-4 Advil 200 mg tablets 3-4 x per week for headaches – characterized by frontal discomfort and occasional periorbital pain; 1-2 ppd cigarettes. Denies allergy to medications.
O: BP 150/102 seated (repeated here)
A: UTI, probable essential HTN worsened by NSAID use and nicotine addiction - increased risk of thromboembolic events and elevated BP and , headaches – symptoms consistent with sinus headache – likely in need of a decongestant rather than Advil.
P: Dispensed co-trimoxazole and counseled to consume water, take to completion. Offered smoking cessation and hypertension management service. Research her question, "Does birth control patch affect BP also?" Asked her to visit in one week for follow-up.
                                    Nasir Jabr, Pharm.D.

Drug Information Search   Date: 02-03

LS inquiry: Does use of birth control patch carry similar cardiovascular risks when a patient smokes as the oral contraceptives do?
Risk is same with oral contraceptives or patch for those who smoke. (see Drug Information Worksheet)

Collaborative practice agreement   Date: 02-10

LS requested collaborative care for smoking cessation and hypertension management. Joe will make arrangements for referral, appointments, financial management of services. Nasir Jabr, Pharm.D.

Figure 8-1. Pharmacy profile for Lauren Smith updated by pharmacist Nasir Jabr.

Case 1: Specific Questions

1. What were some examples of nonverbal communication demonstrated by Lauren?
2. Describe some examples of empathic responses observed in Nasir. At what level of response would you categorize them?
3. Did Nasir demonstrate any moral reasoning skills? If so, identify them in this case.
4. What questions did Lauren ask that suggests she has a trusting relationship with Nasir?

Case 2: *Christine Johnston evaluates the sources of information she has available to help Mr. Montanez.*

After learning that there is a clinical hypoglycemic effect with cactus flowers when prepared as Mr. Montanez's family prepares them, Christine reevaluates the challenge she faces. She reviews the clinic chart, laboratory data, progress notes, information and impressions from the patient interview, and the biomedical literature-based evidence about alternative product use. In addition, she reviews the biomedical literature for evidence and clinical guidelines for dyslipidemia management, diabetes management, and hypertension management. She prepares a priority list of problems that she thinks require attention. She takes notes to prepare herself for her next meeting with Mr. Montanez and Maria to discuss his perceptions of the problems that need to be addressed (**Figure 8-2**). She will work with him and Maria to establish these issues.

Christine then reprioritizes her notes based upon the priorities she anticipates from Mr. Montanez. These priorities are different than her own, but she thinks that she will make more progress in their relationship by demonstrating this respect for Mr. Montanez's beliefs. She knows that she is at a disadvantage by not understanding the alternative care of his family. But she wants him to know that this is a limitation but that she will learn more and work with him in both areas.

Case 2: Specific Questions

1. How does Christine show genuineness in this description of her clinical reasoning?

Case 3: *Luisa Rodriquez evaluates and prioritizes Huong Tran's health, medical, and medication-related needs.*

Luisa reviews Huong Tran's admission progress note to pediatrics 5W, the Admitting Physician's Orders by Dr. Morris, her own medication history notes, and the drug information documentation she has collected thus far. She identifies all of Huong's health, medical, and medication-related needs, then prioritizes them. Since several other health professionals would benefit from knowing Luisa's analysis of Huong's case, she decides to write a Pharmacist's Progress Note identifying Huong's needs. Her personal notes are as follows:

Problems

#1 – Medically indigent patient with no personal resources for health care.
#2 – Without English speaking parents or caretakers—no translator.
#3 – Without a primary physician to advocate/provide care.
#4 – Uncontrolled asthma—moderate to severe.
#5 – Alternative medical treatment—acupuncturist, gingko (Bai Guo Ye).
#6 – Uses albuterol to control asthma; school nurse provides sample supply—not dependable or continuous.
#7 – Without spacer device for albuterol.
#8 – Needs resources to support discharge medications and followup.

Luisa prepares a Pharmacist's Progress Note to communicate her findings (**Figure 8-3**).

2. How does Christine demonstrate respect for Mr. Montanez in this situation?
3. Identify two examples in this case where Christine uses evidence-based clinical reasoning.

Case 3: Specific Questions

1. Which of the clinical reasoning skills dominates Luisa's prioritization of Huong's problems in this case? Explain why you identified this particular one.
2. What piece of technical knowledge did Luisa have that improved Huong's ability to respond to medication during his acute asthma exacerbation?

Christine's personal notes in preparation for next visit:

General health problems:
1. Poor vision needs correction.
2. Daily alcohol consumption is excessive.
3. Has beliefs about the cause of his diabetes that may not facilitate traditional care. Need to further evaluate the concept of susto with his daughter Maria.
4. Are his immunizations up to date? Recommendations of the American Diabetes Association "Standards of Medical Care in Diabetes", Diabetes Care 2004;27(1):S15-35.
5. Why isn't he on preventive aspirin therapy? He meets the criteria recommended in "Aspirin Therapy in Diabetes", Diabetes Care 2004;27(1):S72.

Medical problems:
1. Diabetes mellitus not controlled based upon blood glucose, HgbA$_1$c, urinary protein and signs and symptoms.
2. Neurologic pain in legs secondary to diabetes of 15 years
3. Dyslipidemia borderline – total cholesterol 220; LDL cholesterol not evaluated – need to determine this – will order LDL for next visit. Recommendations of the Third Report of the National Cholesterol Education Program Expert Panel on Detection, Evaluation, and Treatment of High Blood Cholesterol in Adults (Adult Treatment Panel III) NIH publication no. 01-3670.
4. May have stage 1 hypertension based upon last progress note in chart – needs evaluation. Recommendations of the Seventh Report of the Joint National Committee on Prevention, Detection, Evaluation and Treatment of High Blood Pressure (JNC 7) NIH publication no. 03-5233.
5. Evaluate for retinopathy secondary to diabetes based upon guidelines, "Retinopathy in Diabetes", Diabetes Care 2004;27(1):S84-87.

Medication related problems:
1. His use of oral diabetes agents is unclear to me. I will discuss with him further the use of these medicines. Confirm that he uses 1 tablet per day of Diabinese® 125 mgs and 1 tablet per day of tolinase 250 mgs.
2. His use of cactus flowers and yucca are sporadic. We need to decide if he will continue to use these. There is a drug interaction between his use of the cactus flowers and his oral hypoglycemics. However, difficult to assess if this is a manageable interaction for which he can continue both types of treatment. If so, then we need to agree on how this will be done. This may be difficult to work out with him.
3. He uses 1 tablet per day of Mevacor® 20 mgs. Does he take this with an evening meal or at bedtime to maximize its effect?
4. Need to evaluate use of Tylox® and drinking. Concerned about dizziness and falls related to this combination, as much as the diabetes. Need to sort this out.
5. Mr. Montanez does not have a contraindication to codeine use - he needs to be reeducated. This is based upon the opioid decision tree departmental guideline.
6. Not sure if Mr. Montanez relates his poor vision, leg pain, frequency of urination, thirst and hunger to his diabetes – need to discuss and assess.
7. Not sure if Mr. Montanez's beliefs will be compatible with educational effort and adherence to plan recommendations.

Figure 8-2. A summary of pharmacist Christine Johnston's notes used to prepare for Mr. Montanez's next visit.

Memorial Hospital and Health System

PROGRESS NOTES

VITAL SIGNS:

Age: 8 years old   Sex: Male

Weight: 40 kg   Height: 5'   B/P: 109/72   Temp: 98.6°

Pulse: 82   Resp.: 16

Date: 04/02/04

PHARMACIST'S PROGRESS NOTE:

HT is an 8 yo male admitted to 5W Pediatrics from the ER with 3rd exacerbation of asthma in 2 weeks. Admitting pharmacist history reveals the following problems:
#1 Medically indigent patient
#2 Non-English speaking Vietnamese parents - no other caretakers
#3 No primary provider
#4 Uncontrolled asthma – exacerbations are moderate to severe
#5 Alternative medical treatment pursued by family – acupuncture and Bai Guo Ye (gingko) – no evidence of effectiveness of gingko in asthma.
#6 Albuterol samples only medication source – provided sporadically by the school nurse.
#7 Benefits from spacer-device albuterol administration – does not have one.
#8 Needs resources/support for discharge medications and follow up.

A: Child will continue to have uncontrolled asthma episodes without resource support, primary provider, and continuous medication supply with pharmacist's care. Will discuss acceptable solutions with family and social work. Need the interpreter to make progress with parents! I will wait to discuss solutions with family until interpreter is made available.

Signature *Luisa Rodriguez*

Patient Identification (Stamp)

Name: Huong Tran
Reg.No. 2364590
Location: 5W Pediatrics
Date: 04-02-04

Figure 8-3. Pharmacist Luisa Rodriguez prepares a progress note to update everyone on the health care team about the patient's medication-related problems and assessments.

Case 4: *Michael Jones analyzes his data sources and determined Mr. Robinson's health, medical, and medication-related needs.*

Michael stops to reflect on the information he now knows from his various data sources. It becomes a bit overwhelming, so he decides to extract the meaningful findings he has learned and update Samuel Robinson's Patient History Form—Pharmacist's Recommendations/Plans (**Figure 8-4**). While he is updating this form, Charlotte (the nurse) conducts an Instrumental Activities of Daily Living (IADL) (**Figure 8-5**) on Mr. Robinson. Just then, Mr. Robinson's two lady friends, Althea Jones and Dorothy Roberts, stop by to see him. Charlotte briefly interviews them and documents their responses in the IADL. She brings this form to show Michael. Michael assesses Mr. Robinson's health, medical, and medication-related problems (**Figure 8-6**). His overall problem list includes:

#1   Essential need for inhome assistance with ADLs, including medication administration.
#2   Anticoagulation management
#3   CHF management
#4   A Fib management
#5   Thyroid management
#6   Evaluate drug drug interactions:
        warfarin—vitamin E
        warfarin—NSAID and aspirin
#7   Evaluate drug disease interactions:
        warfarin thyroid disease/synthroid
#8   Evaluate possible clonidine-induced hypotensive episodes
#9   Evaluate duplication in drug therapy: aspirin

Michael decides to wait for laboratory data before making a dosing recommendation about warfarin.

CASE 4: SPECIFIC QUESTIONS

1. How are Michael's metacognitive skills observed in this case?
2. Which of the problems identified by Michael are solved predominantly with evidence-based clinical reasoning?

GENERAL ASSESSMENT QUESTIONS

1. Can someone have sound clinical reasoning skills without having content expertise in the subject matter of concern? Explain the rationale for your answer.
2. Differentiate the characteristics of empathy from sympathy.

ASSIGNMENT

1. Identify a family member or friend to interview about his or her general health, medical needs, and medication-related needs. During the interview, practice the skills of empathy, genuineness, respect for others, and clinical reasoning. List this person's health needs, medical needs, and medication-related needs. Prioritize them based upon your own opinion of priority. Then reprioritize them based upon the priorities of the individual. How do they compare? How do you account for the differences?

REFERENCES

1. Bezold C, Halperin HA, Ashbaugh RR et al. Pharmacy for the 21st century—planning for an uncertain future; 1984.

2. Latif DA. The link between moral reasoning scores, social desirability, and patient care performance scores: empirical evidence from the retail pharmacy setting. *Journal of Business Ethics.* 2000; 25:255–69.

3. Benor DE, Notzer N, Sheehan TJ et al. Moral reasoning as a criterion for admission to medical school. *Med Educ.* 1984; Nov 18(6):423–8.

4. Newell KJ, Young LJ, Yamoor CM. Moral reasoning in dental hygiene students. *J Dent Educ.* 1985; Feb 49(2):79–84.

5. Sheehan TJ, Husted SD, Candee D et al. Moral judgment as a predictor of clinical performance. *Evaluation and the Health Professions.* 1980; 8:379–400.

6. Baldwin DC, Adamson E, Self DJ et al. Moral reasoning and malpractice: a study of orthopedic surgeons. *American Journal of Orthopedics.* 1996; 25(7):481–4.

7. Schon DA. Educating the reflective practitioner. San Francisco, CA: Josey-Bass, Inc.; 1990.

8. More ES. Empathy as hermeneutic practice. *Theoretical Medicine.* 1996; 17(3):243–54.

9. Coulehan JL, Block MR. The medical interview: a primer for students of the art. Philadelphia, PA: F.A. Davis Company; 1987.

10. Brennan PF, Strombom I. Improving health care by understanding patient preferences: the role of computer technology. *J Am Med Inform Assoc.* 1998; May Jun 5(3):257–62.

11. Putnam W, Twohig PL, Burge FI et al. A qualitative study of evidence in primary care: what the practitioners are saying. *CMAJ*. 2002; Jun 11 166(12):1525–30.

Patient's History Form – Pharmacist's Recommendations/Plan

Demographic and Administrative Information:		Room No.	ID No. 02946372	
Date: 09-25-04		Gender: M	Primary Language: English	
Name: Samuel Robinson		DOB: 11-23-28	Height:	Weight:
Street Address: 1362 Mockingdale Lane		BP: 156/102	Temp:	Pulse: 110R
City, State, Zip Biloxi, Mississippi 78023		Race/Ethnicity: AF-		Religion: Baptist
Home Phone #: (901) 468-4832		MD/Phone No. Dr. Rangert/Dr. Friedland		
Work Phone #: N/A		Pharmacist/Phone No. Joe Daly		
Occupation: Retired - farmer		Insurance: Medicare		
Family Members/Care Givers: Wife deceased – friends: Dorothy Roberts, Althea Jones				

Problem List:	Pharmacist's Recommendations/Plan:
1.	
2.	
3.	
4.	
5.	
6.	
7.	
8.	
9.	
10.	

Pharmacist's Name: Michael Jones   Date: _____   Phone/Pager #: _____

Chief Complaint/History of Present Illness: "Hard time breathing – was going to suffocate." Became dizzy – started to faint – called 911.
Past Medical History/Surgery/Genetics: S/P myocardial infarction
Family and Social History (significant relationship/co-habitants): wife died 1 yr ago. Friends visit almost daily; however, medication use is not properly managed.
Physical Examination/Review of Systems: (-) S + Sx of bleeding and bruising; (-) bleeding gums; (-) blood In urine or stool. Sleeps 2 pillow orthopnea.
ADL: see evaluation
Lifestyle/Diet/Exercise:

Acute and Chronic Medical Problems/Associated Symptoms:	
1. Congestive heart failure	6. Poorly managed drug regimen
2. Hypertension (type unknown)	7.
3. Atrial fibrillation	8.
4. Hypothyroidism	9.
5. Status post myocardial infarction	10.
Describe Patient's Health Beliefs and Values:	

Figure 8-4. Samuel Robinson's patient history form. (cont'd)

Does Patient Receive Assistance in Medication Administration? **Describe:** No – friends pick up and take him to Daly's pharmacy

Allergies/Intolerances: (*) No Known Drug Allergies

Allergen:	Reaction:	Treatment:
Allergen:	Reaction:	Treatment:
Allergen:	Reaction:	Treatment:

Social Drug Use: Alcohol: 0   Caffeine: ---   Tobacco: 1 ppd-3 ppd   Other:

Current Drug Therapy (prescription and over the counter, vitamins, remedies, alternative treatment):

Drug Name Strength/Route	Problem Number	Usual Schedule	Describe PRN Use	Does Med Work?	Side Effects or Concerns	Compliance Issues
1. Blood thinner/warfarin 5 mg		qd			(pt. Interview)	He can't remember -
2. Heart pills x3/Digoxin 0.25 mg		qd				Problems -
3. Clonidine 0.5 mg		qd				reports
4. Hydrochlorothiazide 25 mg		qd				using
5. Synthroid 120 mcgs		qd				warfarin
6. Multivitamin		qd				and Vitamin
7. Advil			1-2x/wk			E qd
8. Vitamin E 1,000 I.U.'s		qd				
9. Dofetilide 250 mcgs		2x/day				
10. Aspirin (baby) 81 mgs		qd			(bottle label)	
11. Warfarin 5 mgs		qod			(nurse admit)	
12. Warfarin		Mon-Sat			(bottle label)	
13. Aspirin tab 1 tab		qd			(nurse admit)	
14.						
15.						

Past Drug Therapy:

Time Line: Circle administration times and record appropriate medications and meals below:

Patient's Actual Use:

6 7 8 9 (10 11 12 1) 2 3 4 5 6 7 8 9 (10 11 12 1) 2 3 4 5
am   noon   pm   midnight   am

Prescribed Schedule:

6 7 8 9 (10 11 12 1) 2 3 4 5 6 7 8 9 (10 11 12 1) 2 3 4 5
am   noon   pm   midnight   am

Costs of Meds/Month: $ Insurance: ( ) Yes   ( ) No
     Co-pay: Medicaid: Annual Income:

Completed by: _____   **Date:** _____

Figure 8-4. Samuel Robinson's patient history form.

Instrumental Activities of Daily Living (IADL)

Patient's Name: S. Robinson   **Date:**

I = Independent   A = Assistance Required   D = Dependent

Obtained from Patient	Obtained from Informant	Activity	Guidelines for Assessment
(I) A D	I (A) D	**Using Telephone**	I = Able to look up numbers, dial, receive and make calls without help A = Unable to use telephone D = Able to answer phone or dial operator in an emergency but needs special phone or help in getting number, dialing
I (A) D	I A (D) *"We take him everywhere"*	**Traveling**	I = Able to drive own car or travel alone on buses, taxis A = Able to travel but needs someone to travel with D = Unable to travel
(I) A D	I (A) D	**Shopping**	I = Able to take care of all food/clothes A = Able to shop but needs someone to shop with D = Unable to shop
I (A) D	I (A) D	**Preparing Meals**	I = Able to plan and cook full meals A = Able to prepare light foods but unable to cook full meals alone D = Unable to prepare any meals
I (A) D	I (A) D	**Housework**	I = Able to do heavy housework, i.e., scrub floors A = Able to do light housework, but needs help with heavy tasks D = Unable to do any housework
I (A) D	I A *"If we don't do it for him, it doesn't get done."* (D)	**Taking Medicine**	I = Able to prepare/take medications in the right dose at the right time A = Able to take medications, but needs reminding or someone to prepare them D = Unable to take medications
(I) A D	I A D	**Managing Money**	I = Able to manage buying needs, i.e., write checks, pay bills A = Able to manage daily buying needs but needs help managing checkbook, paying bills D = Unable to handle money

Adapted from Lawton M.P. and Brody E.M. Assessment of older people: self-maintaining and instrumental activities of daily living. Gerontologist 1969; 9: 179-186.

Figure 8-5. Instrumental Activities of Daily Living (IADL) for Mr. Robinson.

ANTICOAGULATION ASSESSMENT RECORD

Patient's Name Samuel Robinson   **Age** 76   **Date of Birth** 11-23-28   **Race** B

Home Telephone (901) 468-4832   **Alternate Telephone** (   )   **Doctor/Emergency Contact Person** None

Habits (describe pattern of use): Smoking 1-3 ppd   Alcohol ⊘   **Drugs** ⊘

Indication for Anticoagulation	Check One	INR Goal
Prophylaxis of DVT		2-3
Treatment of Venous Thrombosis		2-3
Treatment of PE		2-3
Prevention of systemic embolism		2-3
Tissue heart valves		2-3
Acute MI		2-3
Valvular heart disease		2-3
Bileaflet mechanical valve/aortic position		2-3
Mechanical prosthetic valve		2.5-3.5
Antiphospholipid syndrome		2.5-3.5
Acute MI (prevent recurrence)	√	2.5-3.5

Bleeding History/Risk Factors for Bleeding

Factor	Check if present
Hosp. Admission for bleed	
Falls	
Oral bleed	
Vaginal bleed	
Lower GI bleed	
Upper GI Bleed	
Rectal bleed	
Guaiac + - / / ND	
hemorrhoids Ulcer	
Seizure	
Urinary bleed	
Hct <30%	
Hematuria	

Conditions Requiring Dose Adjustment

Condition	Dose Change
ETOH Acute	No change
ETOH Chronic	Inc dose
Advanced renal disease	Dec dose
> 65 years old	(Dec dose)
Liver disease	Dec dose
Congestive heart failure	(Dec dose)
Thyroid disease	(Dec dose)

Baseline Hematology

Hemoglobin	
Hematocrit	
Platelets	
WBC's	

Figure 8-6. Anticoagulation assessment record for Samuel Robinson prepared by pharmacist Michael Jones. (cont'd)

Considerations for dosage determination:

Indication for anticoagulation   Concurrent conditions requiring dosage adjustment   Drug Interactions

Target INR   Bleeding history/risk factors for bleeding   Dietary/alternative sources of Vitamin K

Initial dose recommendation taking into consideration all factors:

Date	Dose	INR	RP Initials	Comments	Date	Dose	INR	RP Initials	Comments

Vitamin K Food Intake History (Foods High in Vitamin K)

Food Source	Amount	Consumption Qty	Food Source	Amount	Consumption Qty
Fats and Dressings			Green Scallion - raw	2/3 cup	
Mayonnaise	7 tbsp		Kale - raw	3/4 cup	
Oils: Cannola, Salad, Soybean	7 tbsp		Lettuce - raw bib, red leaf	1-3/4 cup	
Vegetables			Mustard greens - raw	1-1/2 cup	
Broccoli	1/2 cup		Parsley - chopped	1-1/2 cups	
Brussel Sprouts	5 sprouts		Spinach - raw leaf	1-1/2 cups	
Cabbage	1-1/2 cups		Turnip greens - raw	1-1/2 cups	
Collard greens	1/2 cup		Watercress - raw chopped	3 cups	
Endive - raw	2 cups				

Concurrent Medications Known to Interact with Warfarin (Prescriptions and OTC -name, dose, frequency):

Drug	Using	Action to be Taken	Drug	Using	Action to be Taken
Acetaminophen - large dose>1week (OTC)	Yes	None	Dicloxacillin		Inc W dose
Alcohol - acute ingestion	No	Redraw INR in 24 hrs	Diflunisal		DecW dose

Figure 8-6. Anticoagulation assessment record for Samuel Robinson prepared by pharmacist Michael Jones. (cont'd)

Drug	Y/N	Effect	Drug	Y/N	Effect
Alcohol - chronic ingestion	No	Inc W dose-stop ETOH	Disulfiram		DecW dose
Allopurinol		?Inc W dose	Fluconazole		DecW dose
Aminoglutethimide		Inc W dose	Griseofulvin		Inc W dose
Aminoglycosides		?DecW dose	Isoniazid		DecW dose
Amiodarone		DecW dose - delayed effect	Ketoconazole		DecW dose
>500 mgs/day ascorbic acid		?Inc W dose	Lovastatin		DecW dose
Azathioprine		?Inc W dose	Metronidazole		DecW dose
Azithromycin		?DecW dose	Miconazole		DecW dose
Barbiturates		Inc W dose	Multivitamin with Vit K	Yes	
Carbamazepine		Inc W dose	NSAIDS-varies with each agent (OTC)	Yes	Inc/DecW dose
Cephalosporins		?DecW dose	Omeprazole- slight increase in INR		DecW dose
Cholestyramine		Inc W dose/displace time of administration	Phenytoin		Inc/Dec W dose
Chloramphenicol		DecW dose	Quinidine		DecW dose
Cimetidine (OTC)		?DecW dose	Simvastatin		DecW dose
Ciprofloxacin		?DecW dose	Sulfinpyrazone		DecW dose
Clofibrate/Gemfibrozil		DecW dose	Tamoxifen		DecW dose
Colestipol		Inc W dose/displace time of administration	Thyroid hormones		DecW dose
Corticosteroids		Unpredictable	Tricyclic Antidepressants		?DecW dose
Cyclophosphamide		Inc W dose	TMP-SMX		DecW dose by 1/3
Cyclosporine		IncW dose	Vitamin E (OTC)	Yes	DecW dose
Danazol		DecW dose	Valproic Acid		DecW dose
			Zafirleukast		DecW dose

Figure 8-6. Anticoagulation assessment record for Samuel Robinson prepared by pharmacist Michael Jones.

Appendix 8-1.

Application
STATE OF <u>MICHIGAN</u>
DIVISION OF LICENSING
BOARD OF PHARMACY

PHARMACIST COLLABORATIVE PRACTICE APPLICATION

Instructions: Complete this application form and submit, along with the written protocol, to the above address for approval by the board. For hospitals with protocols approved by the hospital pharmacy and therapeutics committee, an "umbrella protocol" may be accepted by the board.

Title of Protocol:____<u>Therapeutic Drug Management Services</u>____

Principal Pharmacist:

____<u>Nasir Jabr</u>____   License #____<u>16492</u>____
Name

For protocols involving multiple pharmacists, list participating pharmacists and license numbers, or identify by description those participating (i.e.; all pharmacists employed by XYZ Pharmacy):

____<u>All pharmacists employed by Werbert's Pharmacy</u>____

Practice Site:

<u>Werbert's Pharmacy</u>   License #____<u>9001</u>____
Pharmacy Name

<u>6907 Detroit Avenue</u>
Street Address

<u>Detroit, MI 48169</u>   Telephone Number: <u>(712) 501-4279</u>
City/State/Zip Code

Principal Authorizing Prescriber:

                                          Type of License:<u>Doctor of Medicine</u>

<u>Joyce Miller, M.D.</u>   License #____<u>1269478</u>____
Name

For protocols involving multiple prescribing practitioners, list participating practitioners and license numbers, or identify by description those participating (i.e.; all staff physicians at XYZ Hospital):____

<u>All physicians participating at Metropolitan General Family Medicine Clinic</u>

Practice Site:__<u>Metropolitan General Family Medicine Clinic</u>

<u>1234 Detroit Ave.</u>
Street Address
<u>Detroit, MI 48169</u>   Telephone Number: <u>(712) 493-8560</u>
City/State/Zip Code

CONTINUED ON NEXT PAGE

Required in accordance with Pharmacy practice rules and regulations

	Yes	No
(1) Does the protocol contain an agreement in which practitioners authorized to prescribe legend drugs in this state authorize pharmacists licenses in this state to administer or dispense in accordance with that written protocol?..	☒	☐
(2) Does the protocol contain a statement identifying the practitioners authorized to prescribe and the pharmacists who are party to the agreement?...	☒	☐
(3) Is a time period for the protocol specified (May not exceed two years)........................	☒	☐
(4) Does the protocol include the types of collaborative authority decisions that the pharmacists are authorized to make, including (A) types of diseases, drugs, or drug categories involved and the type of collaborative authority authorized in each case?..	☒	☐
(B) Procedures, decision criteria, or plans the pharmacists are to follow when making therapeutic decisions, particularly when modification or initiation of drug therapy is involved?..	☒	☐
(5) Does the protocol include the activities that pharmacists are to follow in the course of exercising collaborative authority, including documentation of decisions made, and a plan for communication and feedback to the authorizing practitioners concerning the specific decisions made?..	☒	☐
(6) Does the protocol contain a list o the specific types of patients eligible to receive services under the written protocol?..	☒	☐
(7) Does the protocol include a plan for the authorizing practitioners to review the decisions made by he pharmacist at least once every three months?......................................	☒	☐
(8) Does the protocol include a plan for providing the authorizing practitioners with each patient record created under the written protocol?...	☒	☐
(9) Are the authorizing practitioners in active practice, and is the prescriptive authority within the scope of the practitioners' practice?...	☒	☐
(10) Does the protocol specify and require completion of additional training, if required for the procedures authorized under the protocol?...	☒	☐

Also please note:
- Documentation related to the written protocol must be maintained for at least two years.
- The written protocol may be terminated upon written notice by the authorizing practitioners or pharmacists. The pharmacists shall notify the board in writing within 30 days after a written protocol is terminated.
- Any modification to the written protocol must be approved by the board as required by this section for a new written protocol.

Nasin Jahn
_____
Signature of Principal Pharmacist

Joyce Miller
_____
Signature of Principal Prescriber

2/10
_____
Date

2/10
_____
Date

CONTINUED ON NEXT PAGE
Page 2 of 6

COLLABORATIVE PRACTICE REGULATIONS

PHARMACIST COLLABORATIVE PRACTICE AUTHORITY. (a) A pharmacist planning to exercise collaborative practice authority in the pharmacist's practice by initiating or modifying drug therapy in accordance with a written protocol established and approved for the pharmacist's practice by a practitioner authorized to prescribe drugs must submit the completed written protocol to the board and be approved by the board before implementation.

(b) A written protocol must include

(1) an agreement in which practitioners authorized to prescribe legend drugs in this state authorize pharmacists licensed in this state to administer or dispense in accordance with that written protocol;

(2) a statement identifying the practitioners authorized to prescribe and the pharmacists who are party to the agreement;

(3) the time period during which the written protocol will be in effect, not to exceed two years;

(4) the types of collaborative authority decisions that the pharmacists are authorized to make, including

(A) types of diseases, drugs, or drug categories involved and the type of collaborative authorized in each case;

(B) procedures, decision criteria, or plans the pharmacists are to follow when making therapeutic decisions, particularly when modification or initiation of drug therapy is involved;

(5) activities the pharmacists are to follow in the course of exercising collaborative authority, including documentation of decisions made, and a plan for communication and feedback to the authorizing practitioners concerning specific decisions made;

(6) a list of the specific types of patients eligible to receive services under the written protocol;

(7) a plan for the authorizing practitioners to review the decisions made by the pharmacists at least once every three months; and

(8) a plan for providing the authorizing practitioners with each patient record created under the written protocol

(c) To enter into a written protocol under this section, practitioners authorized to prescribe must be in active practice, and the authority granted must be within the scope of the practitioners' practice.

(d) Unless the board is satisfied that the pharmacist has been adequately trained in the procedures outlined in the written protocol, the board will specify and require completion of additional training that covers those procedures before issuing approval of the protocol.

(e) Documentation related to the written protocol must be maintained for at least two years.

(f) The written protocol may be terminated upon written notice by the authorizing practitioners or pharmacists. The pharmacists shall notify the board in writing within 30 days after a written protocol is terminated.

(g) Any modification to the written protocol must be approved by the board as required by this section for a new written protocol.

DEFINITIONS

(c) "monitoring of drug therapy" means a review of the drug therapy regimen of patients by a pharmacist for the purpose of evaluating and rendering advice to the prescribing practitioner regarding adjustment of the regimen. "Monitoring of drug therapy" includes

(1) collecting and reviewing records of patient drug use histories;

(2) measuring and reviewing routine patient vital signs, including pulse, temperature, blood pressure, and respiration; and

(3) ordering and evaluating the results of laboratory tests relating to drug therapy, including blood chemistries and cell counts, drug levels in blood, urine, tissue, or other body fluids, and culture and sensitivity tests that are performed in accordance with a written protocol.

CONTINUED ON NEXT PAGE

COLLABORATIVE PRACTICE AGREEMENT

DEFINITIONS

Collaborative Practice Agreement refers to the written agreement identifying the collaborating professionals and delineating jointly agreed upon parameters for the delivery of health care services, by which the collaborating individuals agree to function in practice.

Collaborating Professionals refers to ___ Dr. Joyce Miller ___ and ___ Nasir Jabr, RPh, Pharm.D. ___ respectively physician and pharmacist, which have entered into collaborative practice.

Clinical Practice Guidelines refers to written documents, jointly agreed upon by the collaborating professionals that describe a specific plan, arrangement, or sequence of orders, steps, or procedures to be followed or carried out in providing patient care in various clinical situations.

HIERARCHY

Nasir Jabr is a pharmacist employed at ___ Werbert's Pharmacy ___. Dr. Joyce Miller is employed at ___ Metropolitan General Family Medicine Clinic ___.

1. **Methods of Patient Care** – Nasir Jabr is authorized to provide professional services within the scope of a general pharmacist practitioner within collaborative practice guidelines agreed upon by the collaborative parties.

   The parameters of this practice include initial or follow-up assessment, history taking, physical examination of patients, utilization of differential diagnosis, appropriate interventions, consultation and referral as indicated. Emergency treatment and stabilization are also authorized.

2. **Clinical Practice Guidelines** agreed upon within this collaborative arrangement are meant to provide guidelines for safe and effective care and will:

   - Be mutually agreed upon by the decision of the collaborating professionals.
   - Be specific to a variety of clinical situations, and to the practice setting.
   - Describe a general plan, arrangement, or sequence of orders, steps, or procedures to be followed in providing patient care in various clinical situations, including medications and referral procedures.
   - Be adjusted on an on-going basis to fulfill individual patient's needs/situations and to accommodate ongoing research and changing standards.
   - Be maintained on site and readily available in the clinic to the collaborating professionals.
   - Be reviewed and signed yearly or more frequently, as appropriately by both parties.

   Responsibilities of the pharmacist are to see patients in a timely manner, follow practice guidelines and consult collaborating physician as needed. All documentation is to be completed within 48 hours.

CONTINUED ON NEXT PAGE

Responsibilities of the collaborating physician are to be available for collaboration during clinic hours, review selected charts weekly, and provide call coverage for all patients.

3. **Chart Notes and Co-Signatures** – documentation of active medical records, such as the SOAP format will be utilized. Medical documentation will include subjective data, objective data, assessment, and recommendations for treatment, referral, and/or follow-up. Documentation will indicate cases discussed in the clinical setting. In the instances of cases not discussed in the clinical setting, a selection of those charts will be reviewed periodically, as agreed upon between collaborating practitioners.

4. **Diagnostic/Lab Requests** – Diagnostic tests and/or laboratory tests, will be ordered by the pharmacist according to mutually agreed upon office evaluation and management practice guidelines. If results are abnormal, the pharmacist will follow practice guidelines utilizing appropriate consultation, treatment, and/or referral as indicated.

5. **Medications/Prescriptions** – The distribution or administration of medications by the pharmacist within the collaborative practice agreement shall comply with current state and federal law. The physician will initiate pharmacological intervention not addressed by current practice guidelines only after appropriate consultation with the collaborating physician or directly.

6. **Radiology Requests** – Ordering of all radiological exams will be guided by practice guidelines. Radiological testing not addressed by current practice guidelines will be initiated only after appropriate consultation with the collaborating physician or by the physician directly. The radiologist will do final evaluation of all radiological examinations.

7. **Specialty Consults** – Specialty consultations/referrals will be completed according to practice guidelines. If need falls outside of practice guidelines, consultation with the physician will be completed prior to specialty consultation or referral.

8. **Hospital Admissions and Privileges** – All patients who need hospital admission will be registered under the collaborating physician. The pharmacist will cooperate with the hospital pharmacists in continuing to provide information relevant to the care for the patients admitted.

9. **Emergency Absences** – One of the collaborating physicians will manage the pharmacist's patients if the pharmacist is absent. Back-up physician and pharmacist to manage MD's patients if MD absent.

10. **After Clinic Hours Coverage** – The collaborating physician, or designee, covers all hospitalized patients, and manages "on call" coverage. In the event that a patient contacts the pharmacist outside of pharmacy hours, that patient will be referred to the on-call physician or the emergency center, as deemed appropriate for the circumstance.

11. **Cancellation of Collaborative Arrangement** – collaborating parties individually retain the right to terminate the collaborative arrangement with written notification of both parties with a timeline of sixty (60) days.

CONTINUED ON NEXT PAGE
Page 5 of 6

12. **Availability of the collaborating Physician** – Be available for immediate consultation to the pharmacist at all times, either personally or via telecommunications. The collaborating physician will visit the practice site periodically to:

   A. Review patient histories with the pharmacist.
   B. Verify that treatment and acts of limited prescriptive authority are in accordance with the clinical practice guidelines.

13. **Pharmacist's professional Liability Insurance** - $1,000,000.00 each claim up to $5,000,000.00 aggregate professional liability coverage renewed yearly.

Signature: _*Nasir Jabr*_____   _16492____
           PLEASE TYPE NAME UNDER SIGNATURE   License Number
           Nasir Jabr, RPh,Pharm.D.
           Collaborating Pharmacist

Signature: _*Dr. Joyce Miller*_____   _1269478___
           PLEASE TYPE NAME UNDER SIGNATURE   License Number
           Dr. Joyce Miller

Signature: _*Dr. Mark Campos*_____   _1279326___
           PLEASE TYPE NAME UNDER SIGNATURE   License Number
           Dr. Mark Campos

CHAPTER 9

Designing the Patient Care Plan

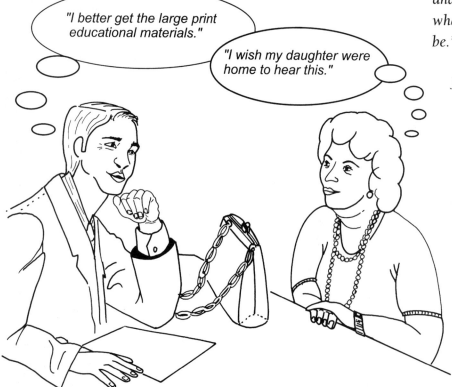

"*If you treat an individual as if he were what he ought to be and could be, he will become what he ought to be and could be.*"

Johann Wolfgang von Goethe

Chapter Outline:

- **Specify Patient Care Goals**
  Determine the Patient's Health, Medical, and
  Medication-Related Goals
  Prioritize the Patient's Health Care Goals
  Determine the Role of Your Care in Addressing
  Patient Needs
- **Design the Pharmacotherapeutic Regimen**
  Determine Therapeutic Regimen Options
  Select the Optimal Pharmacotherapeutic Regimen
  Based upon Drug Regimen Characteristics
  and Patient Characteristics
  *Drug Regimen Characteristics: Dose, Frequency,
  Form, Method, Route, and Duration of
  Administration*
  Comparative Efficacy and Safety of Drug Regimens
  Patient-Related Characteristics
  Age
  Gender
  Pregnancy and Lactation
  Religion and Occupation
  Ethnic Background
  Cognitive Impairments

  Sensory and Physical Limitations
  Patient Preference and Behavior
  Factors Influencing Drug Therapy Adherence
  Simplicity and Cost
- **Design the Monitoring Plan**
  Determine Proxy Outcome Indicators to Maximize
  Efficacy and Minimize Toxicity of Drug Therapy
  Determine Frequency of Monitoring
  Establish Desired Endpoints of Indicators
  Determine a Followup Plan to Evaluate Findings with
  the Patient, Family, and/or Other Health Care
  Providers
- **Determine the Pharmacists' Care Behaviors
  Supportive of Achieving Care Goals for
  the Patient**
  Advocacy Behaviors Required to Achieve Optimal
  Therapeutic Regimen
  Educational Needs to Be Addressed and Appropriate
  Audiences to Target
- **Document the Patient Care Plan**

Objectives / To be able to understand:

1. a patient's drug therapy problem list;
2. pharmacotherapeutic goals based on a patient's health care needs;
3. how disease characteristics influence pharmacotherapeutic goals;
4. pharmacotherapeutic goals requiring immediate solutions;
5. the effects of various drug products, dosage forms, routes of administration, dosage schedules, lengths of treatment, and modes of administration on achieving your desired pharmacotherapeutic goals;

6. a drug therapy plan for achieving desired pharmacotherapeutic goals;
7. the pharmacist's relationship to other health care professionals in the patient's care plan;
8. pharmacotherapeutic parameters and endpoints for a patient's drug therapy for maximizing efficacy and minimizing toxicity;
9. a monitoring plan measuring the achievement of the desired pharmacotherapeutic endpoints; and
10. an efficient format for recording a pharmacist's care plan.

Purpose: This chapter integrates the knowledge and skills developed in the previous chapters to show you how to design and document a patient care plan that is individualized for each patient.

A patient care plan is the roadmap you create to achieve the desired outcomes agreeable to both you and the patient. It is an action plan, and it is dynamic. This means that once you and the patient have established an initial starting point, you implement the plan and monitor progress. If the results (outcomes) do not meet expectations, you modify the plan of action and re-monitor. If you think about delivering your care from this perspective, the need for a relationship with the patient built upon trust and ongoing communication becomes apparent. However, one of the most common problems in pharmaceutical care is the lack of a starting plan. Your ability to assist the patient is compromised without it. This chapter focuses on the design of the initial care plan and the documentation to support your actions. Let's look at the initial care plan in greater depth.

SPECIFY PATIENT CARE GOALS

You will design a care plan that synthesizes all of the data you have gathered using your expertise as a pharmacist. You must first define the patient's health care needs and then specify care goals. After these goals are established, you can design a therapeutic regimen and develop a monitoring plan. Your design of the care plan should take both the initial care plan as well as the monitoring and redesign of the care plan, based upon patient progress, into consideration. Application of your clinical reasoning skills will guide you through a constant reevaluation and updating of the plan based upon the patient's progress.

Determine the Patient's Health, Medical, and Medication-Related Goals

You are now ready to begin the first phase of a pharmacist's care plan: identifying the patient's health care needs. Pharmaceutical care emphasizes that you are dealing with a "whole" person whose care is entrusted to a team of health professionals, including you as the pharmacist. *A patient's health care needs are elements of care required to improve or prevent deterioration of health and well being.* Each health care need focuses on the *elements of care required to improve or prevent deterioration of health and well being.* At this point, you should understand how these health care needs relate to the pharmaceutical care concept. Therefore, your plan of action must also include both the patient's medication-related and total health concerns and the goals of other team members who serve the patient when relevant.

Probably the most important influence on successful care is the personal relationship between you and the patient. Your relationship provides the way to learn from the patient what he or she believes those needs to be. It is *this* relationship that facilitates a genuine exchange between you both.

The second phase of a pharmacist's care plan is to establish pharmacotherapeutic goals. You must set goals to meet each health care need. To determine these goals, you must integrate various influences: disease characteristics, goals of other health professionals, drug therapy problems, and nondisease factors. Patients may possess characteristics that interfere with the achievement of desired therapeutic outcomes. Patients may be noncompliant with prescribed medication use regimens, or there may be unpredictable variations in a patient's biological responses. Thus, in an imperfect world, intended outcomes from medication-related therapy are not always achievable. Again, your relationship with the patient will dictate the degree and amount of information that he or she will share with you. Your ability to help is related to the extent to which the patient is open to sharing and disclosing information, including values and beliefs.

Concurrent disease characteristics. The patient's disease dictates the drug therapy regimen and monitoring plan. When you identify pharmacotherapeutic goals for treating a disease, you must understand both the normal physiology of the system involved and the pathophysiology of the disease. The goal of treatment is to approach normal physiology as much as possible. By understanding where you are and where you would like to be, the pharmacotherapeutic goals for a given disease become clear. Your expert knowledge about conditions and their management provides the patient with the greatest number of care management options.

Previously identified health care goals by other health professionals. The advantage of the team approach is that many people with different expertise levels and viewpoints contribute to a patient's care. You can ultimately develop a plan that will take the priorities of the team into consideration in order to provide optimal patient care.

Previously identified health care goals by patient. Patients have often formed their own concepts about what is possible to achieve with their health. You must know this so that you can incorporate goals that are healthy and realistic, providing you with the information needed to establish a care plan with a greater chance of success. It also allows you to work with the patient to establish new goals or modify those that are not realistic or appropriate.

Current drug therapy problems. Most of your work begins after the patient has had care initiated by another provider. You often inherit patients and drug therapy problems that they are already experiencing. Frequently, patients do not understand that they are experiencing problems *because* of their drug therapy plan, rather than solving their health problems *with* their drug therapy plan. Trust must be established in order for the patient to be receptive to the primary care provider not optimizing this aspect of care, and to allow you to work on it on his or her behalf. Patients also develop many drug therapy problems by self-diagnosis, self-treatment practices, and the solicitations of multiple advisors to their health who may not have adequate expertise in the management of drug therapy. (A detailed discussion of how to identify drug therapy problems was presented in Chapter 8.)

Social, financial, cultural, and system factors. Many nondisease factors can influence pharmacotherapeutic goals. If a patient is elderly or has diminished renal or hepatic function, for example, the pharmacokinetics of drugs may be altered. Drug dosing, then, will need to be adjusted or an alternative drug chosen. Or, if penicillin is the drug of choice for treating an infection but the patient is allergic to it, a second-line agent is indicated. Likewise, if you would select a calcium channel-blocker for the treatment of hypertension but the patient cannot afford it, you must recommend a less expensive agent. Such nondisease factors will influence your pharmacotherapeutic goals and your clinical decisionmaking.

Prioritize the Patient's Health Care Goals

After identifying the care problems and goals that need to be addressed, your next step is to determine what to address first. Your clinical reasoning skills should guide you through these decisions. In matters of urgency, you are expected to take action immediately. In less urgent situations, you must express to the patient and other team members (when appropriate) what you believe are the foremost concerns. Evaluate the disease characteristics and/or drug therapy problems related to the pharmacotherapeutic goals. Consider both the possible risks and onset of toxicity. Rank your corresponding pharmacotherapeutic goals by their importance. Then the prioritized list of problems and goals will guide you and your patient in care.

Determine the Role of Your Care in Addressing Patient Needs

The pharmacist's care plan documents a strategy to provide care that helps the patient achieve goals. Based on patient-, disease-, and drug-specific data, your plan states pharmacotherapeutic goals, a strategy to achieve them, and a means to measure or evaluate their achievement. This plan also serves as a reference when you recommend therapy to the patient, the patient's family, and other health care providers. Although all patients are different, they should all be evaluated in the same way.

DESIGN THE PHARMACOTHERAPEUTIC REGIMEN

Determine Therapeutic Regimen Options

The first step in the development of your drug therapy plan involves optimizing drug selection. Three factors to consider in your choice are 1) comparative efficacy, 2) comparative safety, and 3) patient-related characteristics. You should combine information on appropriate therapy with patient-specific data. Remember the three primary factors noted above that are used to select optimal appropriate drug. Based upon the patient's prioritized problems, you may be recommending discontinuation of therapy, modifications in existing therapy, or new therapies to consider.

Select the Optimal Pharmacotherapeutic Regimen Based upon Drug Regimen Characteristics and Patient Characteristics

Drug Regimen Characteristics: Dose, Frequency, Form, Method, Route, and Duration of Administration

For each medication to be ordered, you should know the usual dosing regimen for both dose and frequency and then determine the most appropriate dose based upon patient characteristics. Medications with multiple therapeutic indications may be dosed differently for each indication. For example, the maximum daily dose for propranolol is 240 mg for vascular headaches, 320 mg for angina, or 640 mg for hypertension. Other factors such as age, height, weight, and concomitant disease states or drug therapy may affect the usual dosing regimen. Renal or liver function impairments are especially important when selecting a dose. For example, a digoxin dose should be modified for age, reduced renal function, and concomitant quinidine or verapamil therapy. In addition, medications with narrow therapeutic indices should be dosed pharmacokinetically when feasible to optimize efficacy and reduce toxicity.

Various dosage forms also may present safety considerations. While both oral and inhaled steroids can often improve asthma, a patient should use the oral product *only if* symptoms cannot be controlled with the inhaled medication. Finally, you should consider the length of therapy when evaluating a medication's safety. For example, buspirone may be acceptable for a patient needing long-term anxiolytic therapy, while a benzodiazepine such as diazepam may be better for short-term therapy needs.

Many medications can be administered by multiple routes. For example, nitroglycerin can be administered orally, topically (either via patch or ointment), sublingually, or intravenously. The advantages and disadvantages of administration routes should be considered for a particular medication and medical symptom/problem. The mode of drug administration is important for reasons of safety and/or patient tolerance. Some drugs cause serious adverse effects when administered by rapid IV push and must be given more slowly; phenytoin, for example, can cause hypotension when administered rapidly. The use of patient-controlled analgesia may be more appropriate than intramuscular injection in patients with decreased muscle mass. For example, both oral and topical tetracycline are effective for acne. The severity of the condition and the likelihood of toxicity, along with patient preference, may determine the best route for treatment.

Standard references provide information about preferred routes for a particular drug. Some drugs can be administered intravenously but cause tissue damage when given intramuscularly. Other drugs are designed to be administered intramuscularly because rapid administration causes adverse effects. Alternative routes of administration often are chosen for patients who cannot tolerate oral therapy or for enhanced efficacy and delivery. For example, IV antibiotics are used to treat serious infections because higher doses can be administered and drug delivery to the bloodstream is certain. However, parenteral therapy is almost always more expensive than oral. In these situations, it is common for the pharmacist to recommend switching from an IV to a PO dosage form to reduce the cost impact of long-term parenteral therapy. In some cases, side effects may be more prevalent with one dosage form than another (e.g., clonidine patch is often better tolerated than the oral form).

Dosage form considerations are similar to those for administration route. In contrast to older patients, liquids and chewable tablets often are selected for pediatric patients. Furthermore, various dosage forms of a medication may have different advantages and disadvantages. Either Cortisporin suspension or solution can be used to treat external otitis. Although the solution may cause stinging (due to propylene glycol), it allows reexamination of the ear canal that would be obscured by the suspension.

Scheduling of medication doses throughout the day can be a concern for both inpatients and outpatients. The goal is to select dosing times that optimize therapeutic benefits and compliance and minimize the potential for adverse effects, drug interactions, and regimen complexity. For example, antiarrhythmics should be administered at equally spaced intervals for optimal efficacy, whereas nonsteroidal anti-inflammatory drugs (NSAIDs) (e.g., ibuprofen and acetaminophen) should be given with meals to minimize GI intolerance. To increase outpatient compliance, you should link drug administrations with the patient's regular daily schedule and try to reduce total dosing times per day.

Finally, you must determine the length of therapy for each drug. Appropriate length of therapy can vary from a single dose to lifelong administration, depending on the condition. One problem is drug use exceeding the course of therapy (e.g., ranitidine treatment exceeding the recommended 6 weeks for duodenal ulcer). Conversely, length of treatment could be shorter than recommended (e.g., for a patient with thrombosis, beginning concomitant warfarin/heparin therapy may allow the heparin to be stopped several days earlier).

Comparative Efficacy and Safety of Drug Regimens

To determine comparative efficacy, you should consider the severity of the patient's problem. For example, although many medications have analgesic properties, product selection should depend on the severity of pain. Acetaminophen or a NSAID may be acceptable for moderate chronic pain, while a narcotic analgesic is better for acute postsurgical pain.

Safety is usually evaluated in terms of potential adverse effects. When you assess a drug, consider both the likely side effects and the uncommon but serious adverse effects. Serious adverse effects can obviously threaten a patient's health. Common side effects, regarded as nuisance events, also may have more serious sequelae–therapeutic failure if compliance is compromised. If additional therapy is prescribed to manage these side effects, the patient may be at risk for adverse drug reactions, drug–drug interactions, and even increased therapy costs. In certain situations, you may want to consider the safety of a drug with an overdosage and/or in an unsupervised situation (e.g., patient with suicidal ideas or elderly patient with mild dementia).

Patient-Related Characteristics

Age

You should consider a patient's age primarily in the *dosing* of drugs and occasionally as it influences *selection*. For example, tetracyclines and the sulfa antibiotics are contraindicated for some pediatric *age* groups. Age also may be a factor that indicates the potential for adverse effects. For example, with some drugs such as digoxin and antipsychotics, doses for elderly patients are lower than the usual adult dosage due to the likelihood for adverse reactions. This "sensitivity" to certain medications may be linked to physiologic changes associated with aging (e.g., decreased renal clearance). Age also may determine the route or dosage form used for a medication. Both young and elderly patients, for example, may have difficulty with dexterity, being unable to properly use a metered-dose inhaler. Therefore, you may need to treat these patients with either another drug or another form of the same medication.

Gender

Gender, as a factor in drug selection, is important for dosing certain drug classes (e.g., hormonal drugs) where some adverse effects are gender specific. Gender also is important in dosing if the illness presents differently in men than women. For example, men are not treated with a single dose of antibiotic for an uncomplicated urinary tract infection, but women may be. Gender also might be considered in prescribing for women of childbearing age. Gender also plays a role in dosing drugs that are cleared renally or when dosing is based on the calculation of the creatinine clearance. In some cases, the most efficacious therapy for women is not clearly defined, given the lack of clinical trial data.

Pregnancy and Lactation

Pregnancy and lactation are two special health states that you should consider when selecting drug therapy. During pregnancy and lactation, the welfare of two individuals is at stake. For example, while warfarin therapy—if indicated—would be safe for a pregnant woman, heparin is universally prescribed because of warfarin's potential to harm the fetus. Standard references often are not useful for answering questions about fetal/child safety or maternal drug use. Therefore, you should consult specialty references when selecting either prescription or nonprescription medications for a pregnant or lactating patient. Excellent professional sources for this information need are listed in Chapter 7.

Religion and Occupation

Religion and occupation are other demographic characteristics that may occasionally influence drug selection (e.g., avoiding blood products for Jehovah Witnesses or avoiding sedative medications for airline pilots).

Ethnic Background

Although ethnic background is rarely considered in drug selection, studies suggest some differences in both efficacy and toxicity of medications in various ethnic groups. As more data become available, pharmacists can select appropriate therapy depending on a patient's genetic background. For example, ethnic differences in response to therapy have been noted with hypertension. The different hemodynamic profiles of Caucasian and African-American patients may influence the selection and/or dosing of antihypertensive medications used for them. Therapy decisions must be modified to initiate dosing regimens appropriately. Evidence from published studies should be sought and applied clinically in each patient case. Ethnic background plays an important role in the types of products that individuals may use to self-treat as well as their beliefs about illness and what will actually work in their treatment.

Cognitive Impairments

Cognitive impairments may influence dosing frequency or route/dosage form in your therapy recommendation. For example, a transdermal patch (e.g., nitroglycerin or Clonidine) or medication requiring infrequent administration (e.g., piroxicam versus ibuprofen) is better for an elderly or incapacitated patient who relies on a working adult caregiver. This caregiver could then administer the medication during time at home.

Sensory and Physical Limitations

Sensory and physical limitations also may affect drug selection. For example, insulin is a commonly used medication. For a visually impaired patient, special education or devices to assist visually impaired patients may be incorporated into the pharmacist's counseling practice. Without these aids, it may be inappropriate to use this medication because of the increased risk for clinically significant errors in a visually impaired patient. Similarly, a physical limitation such as poor grip strength may eliminate the selection of an inhaler for an asthma patient.

Patient Preference and Behavior

Finally, you should consider a patient's preference and behavior when selecting therapy. Some preferences are assumed and, therefore, selected—once-a-day dosing is preferred to multiple daily doses and oral medication is preferred to a parenteral drug. At other times, you should ask the patient about a preference.

Patients may also be asked for their preference about the mode of drug administration. For example, a patient admitted for elective surgery may be asked to decide between scheduled and patient-controlled administration of a narcotic analgesic for postsurgical pain. Occasionally, the patient will prefer a certain dosage form based on convenience (e.g., lozenges versus cough syrup for a working adult).

Factors Influencing Drug Therapy Adherence

You should use your knowledge of the patient's medication adherence to evaluate the suitability of a drug. A patient who cannot remember to take a NSAID three or four times daily should be prescribed a once-a-day product. A patient's ability to manage a certain regimen may influence its suitability. For capable patients, a combination of long-acting insulin with variable doses of regular insulin (depending on blood glucose) is appropriate. But for a less capable or motivated patient, a once-a-day combination of long- and short-acting insulins may be better.

Simplicity and Cost

The simplicity and cost of the drug therapy regimen influence medication adherence. It is well established that a patient's adherence to a drug regimen improves when there are fewer drug treatment episodes a day. Patients on once- or twice-a-day treatment adhere to a greater degree than patients who need to take medications three or more times a day.

DESIGN THE MONITORING PLAN

The starting point in a monitoring plan is the selection of parameters, both quantitative and qualitative, that help to determine whether the desired pharmacotherapeutic goals or drug therapy outcomes are met. *Quantitative* parameters include measurements such as blood pressure, pulse, temperature, weight, and serum glucose. Relief of pain, decrease in swelling, and resolution of nausea are examples of *qualitative* parameters.

When selecting parameters, you should consider the following:

- Drug characteristics.
- Therapeutic efficacy and adverse effects of regimen.
- Physiological changes in the patient.
- Practicality, availability, and cost of monitoring.
- Patient's willingness to participate.

Determine Proxy Outcome Indicators to Maximize Efficacy and Minimize Toxicity of Drug Therapy

Many conditions for which you manage drug treatments can only be monitored using proxy outcome indicators. They are indicators of the likelihood of the patient's outcome based upon his or her response to therapy. To illustrate this, we can examine the condition of hypertension. If a patient continued to live with essential hypertension for many years and it went untreated, the patient would likely experience a stroke, renal failure, or blindness; all are undesirable outcomes. The indicator that

predicts the likelihood of these outcomes is the patient's blood pressure, both systolic and diastolic, at rest. When the patient is treated with antihypertensive therapy, you monitor the blood pressure. The blood pressure is a proxy indicator for actual clinical outcomes. If it is well controlled, the likelihood of blindness, stroke, or renal failure is low. If it is not well controlled, the likelihood of these outcomes increases. Other examples of proxy indicators include $HgbA_1c$ for blood glucose control in diabetes mellitus, FEV_1 for asthma management, or pulse and rhythm for management of atrial fibrillation ($HgbA_1c$ is a laboratory measure of blood glucose control over time; FEV1 is the forced expiratory volume over 1 second—a measure of lung capacity).

Determine Frequency of Monitoring

In the design of your monitoring plan, the final step is determining the frequency of monitoring. Factors that will influence monitoring frequency include

- Specific needs and willingness of the patient to participate.
- Details of the drug therapy.
- Specific physiologic effects of the drug therapy (drug characteristics).
- Cost and practicality of monitoring.
- Desires of other health professionals.

Your first consideration should be patient-specific needs, such as a person's disease state or socioeconomic state. Patients may require more frequent monitoring early in the course of therapy (or, conversely, later in therapy). You should also consider cost and practicality when determining the frequency of monitoring. Measurement of serum drug concentrations can be useful if performed correctly, but various studies have shown that many serum drug levels are poorly utilized. If a serum drug concentration is measured too soon after the dose or prior to steady state, the information is probably not useful. Also, serum drug concentrations that are not obtained at the correct times may result in remeasurements or incorrect therapeutic decisions. In both cases, resources are wasted and patients may be exposed to toxicity or ineffectiveness. Hospitalized patients can be monitored frequently, but they may have to be monitored less frequently as outpatients. When developing your monitoring plan, review the monitoring parameters, desired endpoints, and monitoring frequency for each pharmacotherapeutic goal *before* you obtain measurements. In this way, you can minimize unnecessary monitoring.

Establish Desired Endpoints of Indicators

An endpoint signifies the achievement of a goal or completion of a process. The next step in your monitoring plan is the determination of desired endpoints—either measurable or observable—for each parameter.

A *measurable* endpoint for a patient receiving quinidine for atrial fibrillation is a serum quinidine concentration of 2–5 mcg/ml. Another measurable endpoint might be the heart rate, heart rhythm, or the pulse. Other examples might include a 10% weight loss for a patient with both hypercholesterolemia and hypertension and an absolute neutrophil count less than 1,200/mm^3 for a patient receiving ticlopidine. Examples of *observable* endpoints include elimination of pain in a cancer patient receiving opioids and elimination of dyspnea in an asthma patient.

When determining desired endpoints, you should consider

- Patient-specific factors
- Drug characteristics
- Efficacy and toxicity

Factors such as age and concurrent illness will influence your desired endpoints of therapy. Drug characteristics will also impact your therapeutic endpoints. You must consider the medication's ability to affect the disease being treated. The availability of various dosage forms, routes of administration, and modes of administration will also influence your desired endpoints. Finally, when setting endpoints, you must consider the drug's efficacy and toxicity.

Determine a Followup Plan to Evaluate Findings with the Patient, Family, and/or Other Health Care Providers

Monitoring plans are designed to measure the achievement of pharmacotherapeutic goals established with the patient. You should begin by determining what parameters can be measured (either quantitatively or qualitatively) as valid indicators that a given goal has or has not been achieved. Next, you should establish desired endpoints for these parameters to indicate that the goal has actually been achieved. These endpoints can be observable or measurable. Finally, you must determine how frequently to monitor each parameter.

Some factors that will influence your monitoring plan include the needs of the patient and other professionals caring for the patient, characteristics of the drug, and policies of the health care setting. Additionally, your assessment process requires documentation that conveys your thought process to other health professionals caring for the patient.

DETERMINE THE PHARMACISTS' CARE BEHAVIORS SUPPORTIVE OF ACHIEVING CARE GOALS FOR THE PATIENT

Your care behaviors influence the success that a patient experiences in attaining positive outcomes as a result of therapy. You can use empathy skills to relate to how a patient is feeling, and your expertise to know what the best options are for treatment. However, what you do with this set of skills is what will make a difference for the patient.

Advocacy Behaviors Required to Achieve Optimal Therapeutic Regimen

The pharmacist–patient relationship requires you to sometimes serve as an advocate for the patient. An advocate, in this context, is someone who helps the patient obtain information to make decisions about health care. The advocate discusses with the patient and the family/caregivers the patient's preferences and represents his or her views to other members of the health care team. Working with other team members who agree with you most of the time is less challenging than when they don't agree with you. If you know a patient's preferences and they differ from those of other health care team members, it is your obligation to advocate on behalf of the patient. Your expertise, experience, and confidence in your recommendations is needed to feel assertive about the care plan to be adopted. As a health professional yourself, it is reasonable to expect other health professionals to listen and respect your recommendations. As you practice, you will gain comfort in displaying advocacy behaviors for your patient.

Educational Needs to Be Addressed and Appropriate Audiences to Target

Patients vary greatly in their educational needs to achieve the desired outcomes. You should not assume that the most highly educated patient has adequate and appropriate knowledge to participate effectively in achieving desired care outcomes. Patients require health-focused education to achieve desired outcomes. The term defining a patient's level of health knowledge is *health literacy*. Health literacy is a comprehensive concept, which means having the knowledge, values, and attitudes required to become and stay healthy. As you work with patients, you are assisting them with their health literacy. As you gain more experience, you come to realize how uncomfortable many patients are in the health care setting. This further blunts their response to your efforts to educate and inform. It is worsened when we encounter cultures alternative to our own or language barriers. Your training as a health professional centers your thinking about the health concerns and needs of the patient, often without adequate consideration for the context of the world in which patients live.

Many patient education resources are available to improve a patient's health literacy related to medication use. **Table 9-1** provides several key consumer or patient-centered web sites that can be recommended to patients who have access to and aptitude for using computer-based resources. However, many patients do not have

Table 9-1. Databases for Patient Education and Consumer Health

Reading Level	Database Name and Developer or Sponsor/Website/and Description	Languages English	Spanish
4th – 6th grade	**Micromedex Care Notes System™ - Micromedex, Inc.** **Web site: www.micromedex.com** **Description: Patient education and drug leaflet documents provide a patient-oriented overview of common conditions and frequently prescribed drugs. This is a system accessible by health care providers whose organizations have purchased it. It is not designed for direct use by patients.**	•	•
Varies	**Consumers and Patients – Agency for Healthcare Research and Quality** **Web site: www.ahcpr.gov/consumer** **Description: A comprehensive web access site about a wide range of health topics. The site provides information about helping patients choose providers wisely, health conditions/risks, consumer versions of clinical practice guidelines, health plans, prescriptions, prevention and wellness, quality of care, surgery, and specific conditions—such as cardiac rehabilitation, pressure sores, and smoking cessation.**	•	•
Varies	**Consumer and Patient Health Information Section (CAPHIS) Top 100 List – Medical Library Association** **Web site: www.caphis.mlanet.org/consumer/index.html** **Description: This site links consumers to over 100 evaluated consumer health sites. The Medical Library Association and CAPHIS endorse the criteria for assessing the Quality of Health Information on the Internet of the Health Summit Working Group. Their symbol denotes consumer web sites that have met their quality standards based upon the following criteria: credibility, sponsorship, authorship, controls, authors, currency, disclosure, purpose, links, design, interactivity, and disclaimers.**	•	•
Varies	**MedlinePlus™ - National Library of Medicine** **Web site: www.medlineplus.gov** **Description: MedlinePlus provides over 650 English and 600 Spanish health topic pages representing information from 850 organizations. There are over 15,000 links to authoritative health information.** **Drug information is provided from two sources: Medmaster—a product of the American Society of Health-System Pharmacists and Drug Information—Advice for the Patient, published by the United States Pharmacopoeia.**	•	•

computers available to them and are not able to assist themselves with these resources. Part of your care plan should address this need.

DOCUMENT THE PATIENT CARE PLAN

Chapter 4 provides an overview about the elements of documenting your care plan and its progress. Maintaining a sound documentation system is integral to your ability

to deliver, monitor, and modify care based upon the patient's outcomes. Documentation in a permanent record provides you with the history to assess patient progress. If you share care of a patient with other colleagues, it creates a vehicle for all of you to access the history and keep each other informed. Documentation offers other advantages. It is a legal record showing the evidence of care provided and the resultant outcomes for the patient. It may be important to payors as you develop a billing system for providing care to patients. But the heart of it all is the ongoing tracking tool that documentation provides to facilitate your quality of care.

This chapter emphasizes the skills for documenting care using traditional paper and pencil methods. Integrated computerized clinical record systems are emerging to support pharmacist's documentation of clinical care. As billing for cognitive services becomes a common practice in pharmacy, the computerized systems will improve, become less costly, and be more readily available. The skills you acquire about what to record and how to record will remain important, no matter what media is used in the future.

Figure 9-1 provides a worksheet to think through plan development for each problem or patient priority. It is only intended to be helpful for focusing your thoughts on plan development. **Figure 9-2** provides a template for documenting the pharmacists' comprehensive initial care plan. It is representative of a chart note format commonly used in the inpatient or clinic setting. However, the elements for inclusion are universal for any patient care setting. **Figure 9-3** provides guidance about how to prepare an excellent progress note. You will focus your skill development on creating and documenting patient care plans in the patient case section of this chapter.

SUMMARY

Designing the patient care plan requires a systematic approach. An initial assessment of care goals, followed by designing the specific therapeutic regimen and monitoring plan, require you to synthesize all of the patient-specific information with your clinical knowledge. Once the plan is developed, you further determine what care behaviors you should employ to accomplish the care plan. Documentation is essential to ensure continuity of care and progress assessment.

CASES

See pages 205–214 for cases.

Health Care Need: _____

Pharmacotherapeutic Goal: _____

Recommendations for Therapy: _____

Monitoring Parameter(s) and Frequency: _____

Expected Outcomes: _____

When to Reassess: _____

Health Care Need: _____

Pharmacotherapeutic Goal: _____

Recommendations for Therapy: _____

Monitoring Parameter(s) and Frequency: _____

Expected Outcomes: _____

When to Reassess: _____

Health Care Need: _____

Pharmacotherapeutic Goal: _____

Recommendations for Therapy: _____

Monitoring Parameter(s) and Frequency: _____

Expected Outcomes: _____

When to Reassess: _____

Health Care Need: _____

Pharmacotherapeutic Goal: _____

Recommendations for Therapy: _____

Monitoring Parameter(s) and Frequency: _____

Expected Outcomes: _____

When to Reassess: _____

Health Care Need: _____

Pharmacotherapeutic Goal: _____

Recommendations for Therapy: _____

Monitoring Parameter(s) and Frequency: _____

Expected Outcomes: _____

When to Reassess: _____

Health Care Need: _____

Pharmacotherapeutic Goal: _____

Recommendations for Therapy: _____

Monitoring Parameter(s) and Frequency: _____

Expected Outcomes: _____

When to Reassess: _____

Figure 9-1. Worksheet to identify core elements to patient care plan.

PROGRESS NOTES

PHARMACIST CONSULTATION NOTE

Time: [patient's initials] _____ is a [years] _____ yo [gender] _____ who presents to clinic today with:

[patient's initials] _____ history includes:

chief complaint (CC)

history of present illness (hpi)

past medical history (pmh)

review of systems (ros)

physical examination (pe)

laboratory values (labs)

social history (sh)

past/present medications

over-the-counter medication use (otc)

other treatments (vitamins, natural products, home remedies)

After interviewing the patient, the following problems were identified:

PROBLEM #1 [problem label or diagnosis]

Subjective (S): Interval history, subjective complaints, adherence to program/care plan, ability to adhere.

Objective (O): Physical findings, labs, x-ray, other tests, mini-mental status exam (MMSE) results, cognitive assessment.

Assessment (A): Appraisal of progress, interpretation of new findings, determine likelihood of progress.
Assessment of severity/status and relevant etiologies/risk factors of active **problems.**
Assessment of current non drug and drug **therapy** & patient **compliance.**
Rationale for changes/additions in drug therapy/health maintenance.

Plan (P):
<u>Key patient specific,</u> **goals and endpoints** (i.e. needed to titrate or discontinue therapy):

Diagnostic (either referral to physician or pharmacy based diagnostics which need to be done).

Non-drug therapy:

Therapeutic (any recommendations modifying the drug therapy-related care plan).

New / current drug therapy and **health maintenance** (continue/discontinue, drug/dose/route/frequency/duration):

Patient education/adherence: Document what's done during visit. Document what is long-term educational plan.

Monitoring parameters for <u>efficacy and toxicity</u> (include monitor(s) and interval/frequency):

Follow-up: Describe plans for follow-up, e.g., telephone follow-up, return to clinic (when), contact physician or other providers, etc.

Pharmacist Name/Signature _____ Date/Pager No. _____

Figure 9-2. Format for pharmacist consultation note: initial care plan development.

General guidelines for a properly prepared patient chart note include:

- *Write in ink, not in pencil. Notes are permanent.*
- *If a correction is needed, cross through the statement with a single line and place your initials next to it.*
- *Black ink is conventional. It is a requirement of some research-related agencies that records be kept in black ink.*
- *The note should be written in brief, straightforward, concise sentences or statements.*
- *The note should be complete.*
- *Dates, times, content, spelling must be accurate.*
- *The note must be legible. Practice handwriting to eliminate interpretation errors.*
- *You should print your name and then place your signature next to or below this.*
- *Some method to communicate back to you should be identified by your name (e.g. Pharmacy department phone extension 1234, or pager number 1234).*
- *Abbreviations of any kind should not be used.*
- *The patient should be identifiable by at least two demographic characteristics on the note, e.g., name and age, or name and birth date.*

The following might serve useful in self- or peer-quality assessment of a pharmacy chart note:

Meets criteria	Criteria
	Consistent with SOAP format/accepted medical conventions.
	Includes **key data** necessary to support assessment.
	Identifies **complete problem list** and **health maintenance/compliance** issues.
	Assesses each **problem** and current **therapy.**
	Assessment of disease and therapy is **complete, specific, correct, and clear.**
	Provides correct, specific rationale for **all changes/additions** in therapy.
	Plan is complete, clear, correct, and specific & can be carried out by another professional.
	Is **neat, legible,** concise, and correctly **spelled.**
	Wording is **appropriate** for health care professionals & for medical record.

Figure 9-3. Characteristics of proper documentation—criteria for quality of patient chart notes.

Case 1: *Lauren Smith has her first formal pharmacist's consultation and care visit at Werbert's Pharmacy.*

One week later, Lauren returns for her first appointment with Nasir. Nasir has already contacted Dr. Miller and had her most recent outpatient records (patient information/clinic admission form) (**Figure 9-4**) faxed over to the pharmacy to establish written support for his pharmacy profile information.

Nasir: "Welcome Lauren. Let's go to the private counseling area. I am going to gather the needed materials for this initial visit. While I am doing this, please complete the history form in front of you." (There is a self-administered medical history questionnaire on the desk surface where Lauren sits.)

Lauren: "What is it you will need?"

Nasir: "Today, we will be checking your baseline blood pressure, so I will need a cuff. I will also be performing a quick ophthalmic check to make sure that there are no signs of advancing hypertension. And I will be using the Clinical Practice Guidelines for Hypertension Management and Smoking Cessation."

(Lauren completes the self-administered history form. Nasir reviews Lauren's history form for any new information or inconsistencies. He determines there is no additional followup required.)

Nasir: "Thank you, Lauren. I don't see any new or additional complaints or concerns based upon this history form. Is there anything you would like to mention that is not here?"

Lauren: "No Nasir. I think we have discussed most things in passing."

Nasir: "Good. Let's establish your care plan together then. What I see based upon the records I keep in the pharmacy, the copy of records I requested from Dr. Miller's office, and our conversations suggests that there are five health care needs to address: a recent urinary tract infection, headaches, hypertension, smoking, and your method of birth control as it relates to cardiovascular risk."

Lauren: "I would agree. However, I think the urinary tract infection is gone."

Nasir: "Have you taken the antibiotic that was in the prescription bottle until it was completely gone?"

Lauren: "Yes, and I have not had any burning or discomfort for several days now."

Nasir: "Terrific. Let's work on the other issues then. First, I will take your blood pressure and check your pulse. (Lauren is seated. Nasir places the cuff around her upper arm and rests her arm on the table while inviting her to relax.) Your blood pressure at rest is 148/98. A little high (he records it on a note). Lauren, do you find it difficult not to smoke in situations where you would normally do so?[1]"

Lauren: "Yes, I do find it difficult."

Nasir: "Have you tried quitting smoking for good in the past but found that you could not?"

Lauren: "Yes, again. I need help."

Nasir: "Do you want to stop smoking for good?"

Lauren: "Yes, that would be wonderful. I really hate this habit."

Nasir: "Are you interested in making a serious attempt to stop in the near future?"

Lauren: "Yes, I want to start now."

Nasir: "Are you interested in receiving help with your attempt to quit?"

Lauren: "Well yes, I am here, aren't I?" (Lauren becomes a little impatient.)

Nasir: "Yes you are. I would like you to complete the following questionnaire. It will only take a minute. This is called the Fagerstrom Test (**Figure 9-5**)."

Nasir: [He evaluates the results realizing that she is at the "attempting to stop" phase of her effort to stop smoking (**Figure 9-6**)]. "This test helps you and I understand the depth of your dependence on nicotine, Lauren. As it turns out, your score of 5 out of 10 indicates you are moderately dependent upon nicotine. This means that you are likely to fail at quitting a few times before finally achieving it. It also means that you may do better with medication or focused counseling, as opposed to trying on your own without either of these approaches.[1,2]"

Lauren: "What do you recommend?"

Nasir: "Have you ever tried the nicotine gum programs?"

Lauren: "No."

Nasir: "Why don't we start with this approach? There are other alternatives to consider if this does not achieve success."

Lauren: "Okay. I would like to try that."

continued

Case 1: *Lauren Smith has her first formal pharmacist's consultation and care visit at Werbert's Pharmacy. (cont'd)*

Nasir: "If you can quit smoking, your hypertension is likely to resolve. However, it is not appropriate to let this go without treatment. Your blood pressure readings suggest that you are in stage I hypertension. The national guidelines for managing stage I hypertension suggest that we should start you on a medication—a thiazide-type diuretic. I believe this is appropriate for now, until we have a better understanding of how successful you will be with smoking cessation in the short term."

Lauren: "What if I can quit right away? Will being on the medicine be a problem for me?"

Nasir: "No. A person of your age is not likely to develop hypotension in response to a low-dose thiazide diuretic. And as we monitor your blood pressure, we will be able to determine if you need to continue drug treatment. I believe this is a relatively short-term need; hopefully, it will resolve when you quit smoking."

Lauren: "We haven't talked about Advil or birth control."

Nasir: "Well, we have spoken about the concerns before now. Advil, if used frequently, will cause additional fluid retention that may lead to an elevation of your blood pressure. This makes it more difficult for you to control your blood pressure. And when it is more difficult to control this, then it is more difficult to control your hypertension. Since your headaches may be related to smoking, getting control over the smoking is likely to be the solution. But in the meantime, why not use acetaminophen, for example, Tylenol?" (Lauren nods her head affirmatively.)

"The birth control is a bigger issue. Although uncommon, you are definitely at a greater risk for a stroke by taking birth control pills while smoking and having hypertension. I would urge you to consider switching to barrier birth control protection until we get this resolved. This is a choice that you will have to make. If there was a better alternative, I would suggest it. But there is not. (Lauren looks thoughtful with a resigned expression on her face.) Is there more you want to discuss about this?"

Lauren: "Well, not today. I understand what you are telling me."

CASE 1: SPECIFIC QUESTIONS

1. Evaluate the pharmacotherapeutic regimen that was designed for Lauren by Nasir. Was the clinical reasoning applied to develop the pharmacotherapeutic regimen appropriate based upon Lauren's characteristics as a patient? Describe why you believe it is.

2. Was Nasir patient centered in his approach to Lauren? What is the evidence that supports your opinion about this?

3. How likely is Lauren to follow Nasir's recommendations? Describe why or why not (support your answer).

Metropolitan General Family Medicine Clinic
1234 Detroit Avenue
Detroit, Michigan 48169
PATIENT INFORMATION/CLINIC ADMISSION FORM

Allergies, Adverse Drug Reactions

Prob. No.	Entry Date	Problems/Diagnosis	Medications	Renew	Start Date	Stop Date
1		Urinary Tract Infection	Co-trimoxazole		02-02	02-10
2		Headaches	Over the counter NSAIDs			
3		Essential Hypertension	Pharmacist collaborative practice referral			
4		Smoking	No treatment at this time. Pharmacist smoking cessation program under evaluation by patient			
5		Birth Control/ CV Risk	Patch with 2 years Lo Ovral			

Risk Factors: family illnesses, occupation, alcohol, drug and tobacco use, lifestyle, etc.				Patient Information	
Entry date		Entry date			
	Smokes 2ppd			**Patient Name**	Smith, Lauren
				Birthdate	10/13/81
				Sex	F
				Chart Number	13614

Figure 9-4. Faxed copy of Lauren Smith's clinic admission form.

Fagerstrom Test   **Name: Lauren Smith**

Q1. How many cigarettes per day do you usually smoke? (Write a number in the box and circle one response)	10 or less / (11 to 20) / 21 to 30 / 31 or more	0 / 1 / 2 / 3
Q2. How soon after you wake up do you smoke your first cigarette? (Circle one response)	Within 5 minutes / (6-30 minutes) / 31 or more	3 / 2 / 0
Q3. Do you find it difficult to stop smoking in non-smoking areas? (Circle one response)	(No) / Yes	0 / 1
Q4. Which cigarette would you most hate to give up? (Circle one response)	First of the morning / (Other)	0 / 1
Q5. Do you smoke more frequently in the first hours after waking than the rest of the day? (Circle one response)	No / (Yes)	0 / 1
Q6. Do you smoke if you are so ill that you are in bed most of the day? (Circle one response)	(No) / Yes	0 / 1
	SCORE	5

Figure 9-5. Lauren's responses to the Fagerstrom test. The Fagerstrom test for nicotine dependence: a quantitative index of dependence. The numbers in the gray shaded column corresponding to the smoker's responses are added together to produce a single score on scale of 0 (low dependence) to 10 (high dependence). (Adapted from Heatherton et al. Br J Addict. 1991; 86:1119–27.)

Smoking

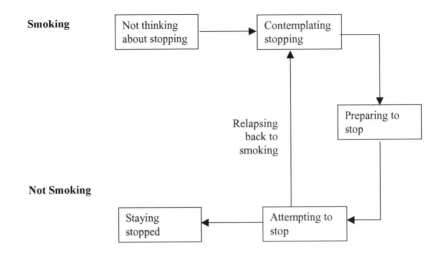

Figure 9-6. *Stages of change in the process of stopping smoking. (Adapted from Prochaska et al. Clin Chest Med. 1991; 12:727–35.)*

Case 2: *Christine Johnston visits with Mr. Montanez and Maria to develop a care plan.*[3,4]

Christine: "Bueños dias Señor Montanez and Maria. It is nice to see you once again. Thank you for returning to discuss your medicine needs with me."

Mr Montanez and Maria (simultaneously): "Bueños dias, Señora Johnson."

Christine: "Well Mr. Montanez, overall you are doing pretty well. What do you think?"

Mr. Montanez: "Si, yes, overall I think so. But sometimes I just don't feel so good."

Christine: "Yes…I can understand that. I think there are few things that are starting to show up in you because you have had diabetes for a long time. But you know, diabetes does not have to be a problem like it has been. There is no shame in having it. This is a medical problem that you can manage very well. And if you manage it well, those leg pains are not likely to worsen and may improve, and it is possible that your eyesight will not worsen as well. You may notice that you feel quite a bit better. What I would like to do is decide with you what we think is important to do…and to also agree on what is realistic for you. Can we discuss this and come to a decision together?"

Mr. Montanez: "Yes Señora, Johnston. This would be a good thing to do."

Christine: "Okay. Let's start with what you think is your most important need."

Mr. Montanez: "Well…I don't like my blurry vision. I feel so dependent on Maria and others sometimes. They are great, but I should be able to read myself."

Christine (writes down poor vision in her progress note): "Okay, what is next?"

Mr. Montanez: "Well…my leg pains keep me awake in the afternoon when I want to siesta and sometimes at night."

Christine: "Does having to use the bathroom at night bother you too?"

Mr. Montanez: "Well yes, but not as much as the leg pains. I have gotten used to getting up to use the bathroom."

Christine: "We can work on all of these issues at once by working on managing the diabetes. Are you interested in discussing how to do this in more detail?"

Mr. Montanez: "Yes, I am very much interested." (Maria looks a little surprised at her father-in-law's reaction, then smiles and nods her head yes in agreement.)

Christine: "Good! Let's start with the Cactus Flowers and Yucca Plant. If I told you that the Cactus Flower makes the other diabetes medicine not work as well, would that surprise you?"

Case 2: *Christine Johnston visits with Mr. Montanez and Maria to develop a care plan.*[3,4] *(cont'd)*

Mr. Montanez: "Yes! Really? That is what my family has always done."

Christine: "I understand…and it is not a bad thing to do by itself. But, the medicine that is more powerful and more effective that we are giving you does not work as well when it is put together. So, I want to know if you think you can accept stopping the use of the Cactus Flowers?"

Mr. Montanez (looks at Maria who nods her head affirmatively): "I will try this…wouldn't that be something else."

Christine: "Yes it would. I think we are off to a good start, Mr. Montanez. Let's work through the other concerns and get a good plan set up. Okay?"

Mr. Montanez: "Yes. Okay. I want you to know how much I appreciate you taking this time."

(Christine continues the discussion with Mr. Montanez and Maria, and she develops a care plan and progress note as shown in **Figure 9-7**.)

CASE 2: SPECIFIC QUESTIONS

1. Was Christine patient centered in her approach to Mr. Montanez? What is the evidence that supports your opinion about this?

2. Was Christine correct to focus her attention toward Mr. Montanez, and not to both Maria and Mr. Montanez? Why?

3. Do you agree with the problems and priorities that are displayed in the Progress Note prepared about Mr. Montanez's care? Do you have any suggestions or alternative approaches you might consider using in his case that was not demonstrated by Christine?

HEART OF TEXAS SYSTEM CLINICS		Patient Identification (Stamp)

HEART OF TEXAS SYSTEM CLINICS

PROGRESS NOTES

Name: **Eduardo Montanez**

Reg.No. **16254**

Location: **Main Clinic**

Date: **06/19/04**

	Age	**Sex**	Leukocytes _____
V S	Weight _____	Height _____	Nitrite _____ ph _____
I I			Protein _____ Glucose _____
T G	B/P _____	Temp _____	
A N			Ketones _____ Urobilinogen _____
L S	Pulse _____	Resp. _____	Bilirubin _____ Blood

Hct _____ Preg. __ __ Hemocult _____ Strep _____ Other _____

UA Micro: WBC _____ RCB _____ WBC _____ Epis _____ Bacteria _____

Appt. _____ _____ Call/Walk In _____ Primary Physician ___ _____ /Staff _____

Date: _96-19-04____

3:30 p.m.

EM is a 68 year old Hispanic male who presents to clinic today upon referral of Dr. Mattis. EM's history is well described in Dr. Mattis's clinical progress note of 9/15/03. I discussed and confirmed the accuracy of EM's history in the note. Discussed the problems identified with EM and prioritized plan of care. EM indicates that his vision, leg pain, and nocturia are most troublesome to his comfort.

#1 vision

S: does not like blurriness

O: possible retinopathy secondary to diabetes (as noted in Dr. Mattis's note)

A: vision impairment likely secondary to diabetes. Needs evaluation for retinopathy.

P: refer for visual assessment, evaluation of retinopathy, visual correction

#2 diabetes neuropathy in legs

S: EM dislikes leg pain

A: likely 2ndary to diabetes.

P: Control diabetes.

#3 Nocturia

S: has had nocturia so long is 'used to it'.

O: HgbA$_1$c = increased from 12 to 12.5 mg%, Fasting Blood Sugar = 220 mg%

A: 2ndary to poor blood sugar control

P: Control diabetes

#4 Diabetes poorly controlled

S: problems 1-3. Self treats with cactus flowers and yucca plant. Has alternative health belief of 'susto'. Confirmed that he uses 1 tablet a day each of Diabinese 125 mgs and Tolinase 250 mgs. Uses alcohol socially and frequently. Also uses Tylox.

O: slightly cloudy urine - proteinuria consistent with Diabetes Mellitus. HgbA$_1$c = increased from 12 to 12.5 mg% in past 6 months, Fasting Blood Sugar = 220 mg%.

A: EM is non-compliant with his diabetes care plan. He self treats and uses alcohol excessively. Evaluation is complicated by possible drug interaction with cactus flower plant consumption.

P: Educate EM about: a) the relationship between controlling blood sugar and his symptoms, b) the interaction with cactus flowers and his diabetes medication, c) educate to stop using the cactus flower treatment, d) educate to stop alcohol consumption, e) reinforce once a day consumption of both Diabinese and Tolinase, f) schedule follow up for blood sugar and urine protein in two weeks.

#5 Other problems

A: May have hypertension and dyslipidemia, not sure if immunizations up to date. Not on preventive aspirin. Has an incorrect belief that he is allergic to opioids.

P: Although these all need to be corrected, will plan to work on these at next visit, if progress made on problems of primary concern to EM. Take resting blood pressure and obtain Total Cholesterol and Low Density Lipoprotein at end of visit.

Pharmacist's Signature/Pager: *Christine Johnston, PharmD* Date: _6/19/04_

Figure 9-7. Progress note documenting care plan for Mr. Montanez prepared by pharmacist Christine Johnston.

Case 3: *Luisa Rodriguez develops a care plan with Huong Tran.*

Luisa visits with Huong and his family after developing her Progress Note and placing it in the chart. She knows that she needs to implement the social service aspects of care that Huong needs and also educate his family about basic asthma care before Huong goes home. She is concerned that there is no continuity of care plan but believes she can ask the social worker to be an ongoing advocate to interface Huong with a regular care provider or service. One thought is to interface Huong with a community health center in his vicinity. However, a problem to overcome is that no interpreter is available who speaks Huong's language. The hospital is willing to contract with someone in the community; however, they make one visit, and that visit must be well planned to accomplish the goals of the meeting. Luisa decides to try to make more progress on her own, considering use of the interpreter as a last step in the process (if necessary).

Luisa: "Hello Huong, Mr. and Mrs. Tran. You are looking much better, Huong. Your breathing seems to have returned to normal and your facial skin color looks very good. How are you feeling?"

Huong: "I am feeling much better, thank you."

Luisa: "Huong, I would like to speak with you about having a social worker check on you at home periodically. I know this is not something that you or your family has experienced previously, but I think that it would be a good way to get the medical help you need so that you are less likely to have asthma attacks requiring hospitalization. Could you communicate our conversation to your parents, while we are speaking, so that I might understand their concerns and wishes and answer any questions they have?"

Huong (turns to his parents and explains Luisa's request; they nod their heads affirmatively): "I would be most happy to do this. Please go on."

Luisa: "To keep you from coming to the hospital, we need to make sure that you see someone at least once a month or so about your asthma and that you always have medicine available to take regularly. This means that you should have enough so you do not run out." (Huong translates to his parents—they nod affirmatively.)

Luisa: "I think one way to do this will be to ask if a social worker could be assigned to assist you and your family with this once you leave the hospital."

(Huong translates for his parents who in turn ask: What is a social worker?)

Luisa: "This is a person who is paid by our community government to assist families, especially those who have children or elderly parents to care for. These people know about the programs and services available in the community. They would make sure Huong had a doctor that would accept him as a patient, and make sure that he received his medicines without interruption."

(Huong translates for his parents, who in turn ask: How do they do this?)

Luisa: "They come to your home by making an appointment with you. In your family's case, we will need to make sure that Huong is home with you to speak comfortably with the social worker."

[Huong and his parents briefly discuss this issue. His parents accept it and indicate that they are willing to try this, although they do not yet understand how this will work. Luisa records another care note to detail this discussion and request a social work consult (**Figure 9-8**).]

CASE 3: SPECIFIC QUESTIONS

1. Was Luisa patient centered in her approach to Huong and his parents? What is the evidence that supports your opinion?
2. Was Luisa correct to focus her attention toward all of the family members? Why?
3. Do you agree with the problems and priorities that are displayed in the Progress Note prepared about Huong's care? Do you have any suggestions or alternative approaches you might consider using in his case that was not demonstrated by Luisa?

Memorial Hospital and Health System **PROGRESS NOTES**	Patient Identification (Stamp) Name: **Huong Tran** Reg.No. **2364590**

Age: 8 years old Sex: Male VITAL SIGNS:	Location: **5W Pediatrics** Date: **04-02-04 1500 hrs**

Weight 40 kg   Height 5'   B/P 109/72   Temp 98.6°

Pulse 82   Resp. 16

Date: 04/02/04

Pharmacist's Progress Note:

HT is an 8 year old male admitted to 5W Pediatrics from the Emergency Room secondary to 3rd exacerbation of asthma in 2 weeks.

Could not obtain an interpreter for regular participation in communication because there is no interpreter available for regular and repeated interaction in the hospital who can speak Huong's language. Will be able to arrange for an interpreter on contract for one visit that summarizes overall care plan and how to implement it when discharge plan prepared.

Discussed the problem of asthma management requiring regular care visits and use of medication without interruption. (Huong interpreted for his parents). I presented the possible solution of having a social worker assigned to Huong after he is discharged to the community. The family did not know what a social work was. I provided an explanation of their roles and responsibilities in the community and what the value would be to Huong.

A: Family was supportive of the idea of participating with a social worker, however the family has limited knowledge and does not know what is involved.

P: 1) Will request the hospital social worker for the unit to come and provide an explanation of services and how the social worker participates with the family in the community.
2) Will request an interpreter be contracted for discharge consultation meeting.

Luisa Rodriquez, PharmD.
Signature

Figure 9-8. Progress note documenting care plan for Huong Tran prepared by pharmacist Luisa Rodriquez.

Case 4: *Michael Jones develops a care plan for Mr. Robinson.*

Michael Jones knows that as soon as Mr. Robinson is determined to be medically stable, he will be discharged from the hospital. This usually means that the anticoagulation therapy is not stabilized to the ideal dose before the patient is discharged. He decides to speak with his physician about problem areas he sees to determine if there is support for some care plan actions he will recommend.

Michael: "Dr. Rangert, I had a chance to review Mr. Robinson's coagulation needs as well as how they relate to his other medications and health care needs. You may not have had a chance to see this yet, but Charlotte administered the IADL and found that Mr. Robinson needs in-home assistance in order to use his medications safely. I think that his hospitalization is a direct result of his inability to safely self-medicate."

Dr. Rangert: "I appreciate what you are doing Michael, but I didn't ask for a comprehensive evaluation about him…I need him stabilized and out (looking a little frustrated)."

Michael: "I understand. Actually Charlotte and I are doing what we always do in response to a request for anticoagulation consultation and management. The evidence is clear that if we don't address his needs comprehensively, he is much more likely to be re-hospitalized within the next 30 days because of anticoagulation failure or toxicity. I would like to adjust his anticoagulant dose in response to how he answers my questions about use of vitamin E (doses greater than 300 IUs per day interfere with vitamin K dependent factors leading to increased risk of bleeding), his use of thyroid replacement (increases effect of anticoagulant if used regularly), and his use of NSAIDs and aspirin. I would also like to participate in the discharge planning process with the unit and make sure that in-home medication assistance is planned for him in some way. If you countersign a consult that I write, including these recommendations, I will then be authorized to handle these specific actions. I know you are very busy—I am qualified to do these things and just need your countersignature. It should not cause you more work at all."

Dr. Rangert: "All right."

Michael: "Thanks, Dr. Rangert. I will place the progress note in the chart after I speak with Mr. Robinson."

(Now that Michael has a better sense of what Dr. Rangert is thinking and will support, he discusses his thoughts and recommendations with Mr. Robinson. He picks up the home medication bag so he can clarify Mr. Robinson's medication-taking behavior.)

Michael: "Hi, Mr. Robinson."

Mr. Robinson: Hi, Michael. How ya' doin'?

Michael: "Okay sir, thanks for asking. I just spoke with Dr. Rangert, and we discussed a few ideas about your care that I want to talk with you about further. Can I take a few minutes?"

Mr. Robinson: "Sure, I'm not going anywhere!"

Michael: "Okay. I want you to tell me about this medicine (he holds up vitamin E). How much of this do you take, sir?"

Mr. Robinson: "I take one of those a day. I don't miss those because my wife told me these were most important for my heart. So I do it."

Michael: "Okay. And how about these (holds up his Synthroid)?"

Mr. Robinson: "Well, I haven't been taking too much of those."

Michael: "Why not?"

Mr. Robinson: "I haven't known what they're for, really. Just decided they probably weren't that important."

Michael: "Now tell me about these pills, Mr. Robinson (he holds up the warfarin)."

Mr. Robinson: "Oh those…well I take one of those every day."

Michael: "Do you skip Sundays, or do you skip every other day?"

Mr. Robinson: "Well, not usually. Only if I forget."

Michael: "Okay. Thanks Mr. Robinson."

[Michael Jones prepares a progress note summarizing his impressions and plan based upon his discussion with Mr. Robinson (**Figure 9-9**).]

	Patient Identification (Stamp)
Madison Hospitals and Health Systems	Name: **Samuel Robinson**
	Reg. No. **02946372**
	Location: **INPT 347-1**
PROGRESS NOTES	Date: **09-2-04**

Anticoagulation Care Consult by Pharmacist

1:45 p.m. SR is a 76 year old African American male who was referred to this service to initiate warfarin therapy for prophylaxis for atrial fibrillation Dr. Rangert has determined the target INR (International Normalized Ratio) goal range to be **2.0 – 3.0**.   Upon initial assessment of the patient, the following is noted:

#1 Atrial fibrillation – poorly controlled
#2 congestive heart failure
#3 hypothyroidism
#4 hypertension
#5 s/p myocardial infarction
#6 unable to self-manage drug therapy regimen
#7 poorly controlled anticoagulation therapy

S: After a brief interview, the patient does not report any bleeding history. Risk factors include dizziness and falling at home. Patient reports symptoms concurrent with congestive heart failure and hypothyroidism, reports use of over the counter use of acetaminophen, Advil (NSAIDs) and vitamin E (1,000 IU's) at home.
O: There are no signs or symptoms observed in the patient to suggest a greater bleeding risk. Baseline hematology (Hemoglobin, Hematocrit, platelets, prothrombin time) and stool guaiac have not been done.
A: The patient is an acceptable candidate for warfarin therapy, pending acceptable baseline hematology results and a care plan at home that includes assistance with medication use from a regular care provider. Dose modification likely needed based upon age > 65 years, concurrent congestive heart failure and hypothyroidism, over the counter use of acetaminophen, Advil (NSAIDs) and vitamin E (1,000 IU's).
P: Order hemoglobin, hematocrit, platelets, prothrombin time and INR from laboratory as soon as possible. Perform stool guaiac test. Will review results and recommend initial dose and monitoring plan. If acceptable, plan to dose warfarin at 4 mgs po qd at 5 p.m. on 9/02/04. Obtain Prothromin Time/INR at 9 a.m.

Michael Jones, RPh x4269
Pharmacist's Signature/phone extension or pager

Figure 9-9. Progress note documenting care plan for Samuel Robinson prepared by pharmacist Michael Jones.

CASE 4: SPECIFIC QUESTIONS

1. Did Michael take the best approach in establishing Mr. Robinson's care plan by speaking with Dr. Rangert first? Why do you think so?
2. What additional questions would you ask of Mr. Robinson to further refine his care plan?

GENERAL ASSESSMENT QUESTIONS

1. Why is it important to write a care plan and document it?
2. What is the name of the section of the care plan that describes your evaluation of the patient's condition and the rationale for this evaluation?
3. Describe how to prioritize the patient's problems.

ASSIGNMENT

1. Identify a neighborhood health clinic or community health center that is in a cultural community different than your own. Alternatively, attend a church and the social time surrounding worship that is different from your own religious practice. Use this experience to understand what it is like for someone from a different background to navigate his or her health care. To facilitate this assignment, do the following:
   a. Introduce yourself to some individuals.
   b. Ask the following questions after explaining your purpose of understanding the difficulties encountered in the health system:
   c. Tell me how you feel about going to the doctor's office? The pharmacist? The hospital?
   d. Do you believe the health professionals that care for you understand your needs and preferences?
   e. What would you like to see done in the pharmacy service area to improve your experience in receiving care?

Reflect upon the answers.

REFERENCES

1. West R. ABC of smoking cessation. Assessment of dependence and motivation to stop smoking. *BMJ.* 2004; 328:338–9.
2. Heatherton TF, Kozlowski LT, Frecker RC et al. The Fagerstrom Test for Nicotine Dependence: a revision of the Fagerstrom Tolerance Questionnaire. *British Journal of Addiction.* 1991; 86:1119–27.
3. Lawson KL, Horneffer KJ. Roots and wings: a pilot of a mind-body-spirit program. *Journal of Holistic Nursing.* 2002 Sep; 20(3):250–63.
4. Bradley C. Health beliefs and knowledge of patients and doctors in clinical practice and research. *Patient-Educ-Couns.* 1995 Sep; 26(1-3):99–106.

CHAPTER 10

Implementing the Patient Care Plan

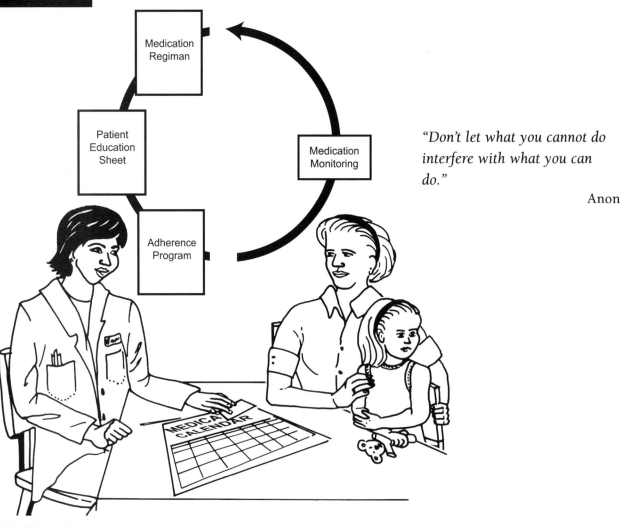

"Don't let what you cannot do interfere with what you can do."

Anon

Chapter Outline:

Objectives / To be able to:

1. recommend a pharmacist's care plan to the prescriber clearly, persuasively, and appropriately;

2. confirm the care plan for the patient with pertinent members of the patient care team;

3. use appropriate procedures to implement a care plan;

4. understand how to implement all aspects of the patient's care plan;

5. use evidence-based literature to support patient care decisions and communicate them whenever possible;

6. maintain responsibility for the patient care outcomes by advocating for the patient's health and well-being;

7. use effective patient education techniques to provide counseling to both patients and caregivers; and

8. document your recommendations in the patient's health record.

Purpose: In this unit, you will learn to how to implement the different aspects of the patient's care plan based upon your role as a care provider.

Implementing the care plan for the patient is one of the most challenging aspects of providing clinical care. To be successful, you must have a clear plan to implement, use a variety of communication approaches, and follow through for completion of the plan. Sometimes you are advocating for the patient's needs in addition to the challenge of designing the optimal plan. You must be prepared to modify the plan in response to rejection of your recommendations. All in all, this step requires you to keep the patient as the central focus of your efforts.

DELIVER CARE TO THE PATIENT

In advocating for the care plan you are implementing, you must identify your role in order to know what actions you must take and with whom. There are three likely roles: 1) recommending a care plan to the patient's primary medical care provider that you initiate; 2) recommending a care plan to the patient's primary medical care provider or other health professional in response to a formal consult request; or 3) recommending a care plan directly to the patient. When you are in the first role—recommending a care plan to another provider that you initiate, then you will also follow up with the patient—taking on the third role.

Recommending the Care Plan

In all three roles, you must select the components from the pharmacist's care plan that should be included in your recommendation. Once you know what they are, consider alternative approaches to communicating those recommendations. Communication can take place by several methods: 1) face-to-face conversation, 2) telephone communication, and 3) written documentation left in the patient's health record, faxed, or e-mailed to the relevant care provider. Finally, you will learn about two formats for recording your recommendation to health care providers: the formal consult and the progress note.

Recommendations require selecting the appropriate information to convey. You should consider including four components in any recommendation: 1) the patient's health care need, 2) pharmacotherapeutic goals, 3) recommended therapy, and 4) a monitoring plan.

Remember that the health care needs you identified for your patient are based primarily on subjective data. The second integral component of your recommendation, pharmacotherapeutic goals, can be viewed as objective in some ways. Since these goals are developed from issues such as drug response and disease process, you can make clear, measurable observations (objective

information). However, your pharmacotherapeutic goals also have some relationship to your assessment of the patient. The third component of your recommendation should be your treatment suggestions, both an assessment and a plan of action. You will assess the potential for the therapies that you are recommending to achieve the pharmacotherapeutic goals and discuss plans to reach them. Your recommendation should include clear instructions for other members of the health care team about how to follow this plan. Here, you will outline your monitoring parameters, desired endpoints, and monitoring frequency.

Practice-Setting Considerations, Site-Specific Policies, Professionalism, and Practice Standards

Although you can follow a general systematic approach to recommending your care plan, four factors may influence your approach: 1) practice setting considerations, 2) site-specific policies, 3) practice standards, and 4) professionalism.

You should first consider your practice setting (e.g., home care, outpatient clinic, inpatient unit, or skilled nursing facility). Your approach to relaying a recommendation in the inpatient unit of a hospital, where the patient is examined many times daily, may differ from your approach in a home care setting. You may have many opportunities for face-to-face communication. You may also write your recommendations in the chart, having a reasonable degree of confidence that your recommendations will be reviewed by all relevant health professionals who, in turn, can respond and follow up. In contrast, the home care setting does not provide you the privilege of high-frequency communication opportunities. You may not see a patient's chart for several days nor see another care provider involved with that patient, possibly ever. Therefore, verbal communication over the telephone and written recommendations transmitted via facsimile or e-mail may be more appropriate.

Next, you must consider site-specific policies when making recommendations. A written recommendation in the patient chart may be preferable, but some sites have restrictions on who is allowed to do it. If restrictions exist, it is usually because of concerns about the volume of entries into the medical chart (hospitals are typically most concerned with this) or litigation fears (organizational philosophy driven). Even though some settings or site-specific policies may influence your approach, the accepted standards of practice developed by the pharmacy profession should guide your behavior. If your practice setting does not allow pharmacists to record information in the chart, you should advocate for updating the hospital's policies.

Professionals display the concepts of mutual respect when communicating about their work. To achieve acceptance of your recommendations, it is important that you adopt this approach. Many professionals appreciate being contacted prior to any written documentation taking place no matter what the circumstances. Being considerate of the other professionals' viewpoint will go a long way in having your recommendations accepted. Failure to achieve getting your recommendations accepted by other providers may result in failure to deliver some pharmaceutical care you know will improve the patient care. Therefore, use proper judgment when selecting an approach to deliver your recommendation initially.

Pharmacist-Initiated Recommendations to the Primary Care Provider

When your primary role is to make recommendations to improve a patient's care that were *not solicited* by the primary care provider, you should speak directly to the primary care provider on behalf of the patient. Your success at accomplishing this will depend upon practical issues. If you are working in a community pharmacy, you may not be able to implement a change via telephone at the point of care with the patient. Other providers are in the same situation. They have ongoing work and may not be able to interrupt it in order to resolve the situation. You may have to schedule a return time with the patient to initiate the changes needed. On the other hand, in the hospital setting, you may be using an informal chart note system requesting the prescriber make the changes you are recommending. The prescriber can rewrite orders to meet the request. Alternatively, you may page the care provider and take a verbal order via the telephone, transcribing the order to an order sheet for prescriber countersignature at a later time.

Recommendations for drug therapy regimens, by their nature, allow the prescriber the option of rejecting the recommendation. However, phrases such as "I would consider" or "I would recommend" allow the prescriber to contemplate the recommendation. Being too forceful can result in failure to have your recommendations accepted. The exception is when your recommendation can offset a life-threatening or substantially harmful situation. You may have to choose to be more aggressive about your communication to effect the change necessary. The prescriber may have other information to consider that you do not have. However, your communication should include an evidence-based approach to your recommendation, including risks to the patient should the recommendations not be accepted and the benefits to the patient if they are accepted. If you are helping the prescriber to make the best decision, it is highly unlikely that your recommendation will be rejected. You are advocating for the patient in this role in the most challenging situation you can encounter—

uninvited. This is a unique privilege when caring for a patient, and it requires an understanding of the communication challenges.

Your clinical reasoning should guide you as to whether you should inform the patient about your intention to contact the prescriber beforehand. Discussing the options and your intention with the patient is generally the right thing to do. However, in the event of a life-threatening, or very high-risk situation, you have a responsibility to protect the patient. Therefore, you cannot ask for permission to contact a prescriber because it gives the patient an option to say "no." You have a duty to contact the prescriber. It is appropriate to take charge and contact the prescriber, offer the recommended solution to the problem, and inform the patient about it once completed.

Pharmacist Recommendations in Response to a Formal Consult

When a request for your services has been initiated formally, the need to make your recommendations through conversation first is less apparent. It is typical in this form of care to prepare your written consultation and send it directly to the requesting provider or place it in the chart (setting appropriate). If practical, you should briefly meet the patient if you have not done so already, and inform him or her that you have been requested to provide this consultation. It provides the patient with an opportunity to give you information, ask questions, and realize that your expertise is valuable. It is also important to tell the professional who requested your consult that you intend to communicate directly with the patient. Anything you learn that is relevant to the consultation for this patient should be included in the written summary.

Pharmacist Recommendations Provided Directly to the Patient

In many practice settings (particularly outpatient and community), it is most common for you to provide recommendations directly to the patient. A wide range of patient needs can be met through your direct consultation and advice. Direct consultation occurs less frequently in the inpatient setting, although the improved practices of both medication history taking on admission and discharge care planning involving medications has increased direct consultation with the patient during a hospitalization. It is also far more common to directly consult with the patient in decentralized pharmacist service models in the hospital setting. Your direct interaction with the patient will continue to be a substantially more important aspect of work with the models of care delivery moving to interprofessional approaches.

Implement the Care Plan

Successful implementation of the care plan is dependent upon followup with the recommendations so actions and changes are made promptly. Part of your role is to identify and eliminate barriers to implementation. The following areas of discussion emphasize what you should do as a pharmacist to eliminate or minimize barriers and optimize everyone's opportunity, especially the patient's, to successfully implement the plan.

Ensure that Medication Orders and/or Prescriptions Are Written to Facilitate Care and Monitoring of the Patient

Medication orders and prescriptions are the customary vehicles that initiate treatment for the patient by other providers. These are legal terms, with the word "prescription" indicating an outpatient dispensing act associated with the product. *Inpatient medication orders* are orders written within the hospital or institutional setting that are intended to have the medication administered to the patient there. Similarly, *outpatient medication orders* are orders written in a physician office or clinic setting that are intended to be administered within the office before the patient leaves. In neither case is there dispensing of a prescription to the patient that takes place—even though the patient is administered the drug. In contrast, *discharge or outpatient prescriptions* are written by individuals having legal authority to prescribe with the intention that the prescribed treatment or device will be used outside of the facility and generally under the control of the patient once it has been dispensed by the pharmacist. The reason for overtly discussing this terminology is to be accurate. However, the overarching concepts emphasized in this chapter do not depend upon the legal definitions of these terms. The important point is that the proper writing of medication orders and prescriptions is essential to facilitate optimal care and monitoring of a patient's response to therapy.

It is the pharmacist's responsibility to make sure a medication order is complete, including identification of the correct patient with both the patient's name and at least another identifier (age or birth date), drug name, dose, route, frequency and instructions for use, intended duration, and indication for use. The indication for the drug provides the pharmacist with knowledge of its intended use. This information is important for advising other health care providers involved in the medication management of the patient, for monitoring the drug's effectiveness toward its intended use, and for counseling patients optimally.[1] It is particularly important for medications that are ordered for nonscheduled, or "p.r.n." used to specify the indication so that correct patient instructions may be provided based upon intended use of the medication.

Whenever a treatment is being considered and eventually is either committed to a medication order or prescription, the natural thought processes of the prescriber move to monitoring the effectiveness. But most often, there is not a corollary order for monitoring that identifies key proxy outcomes or monitoring parameters and when they should be evaluated. If basic monitoring activities are required to assess a patient's response to treatment, you should take the initiative to contact the prescriber and have them ordered if the action of the prescriber is required (e.g., order laboratory monitoring test). If legal orders are not required, you may recommend a monitoring plan described in the patient's medical record or pharmacy profile that you can employ to assess the patient's response to therapy.

Transfer of Orders between Facilities or Settings

When patients transfer to different care environments, either within the hospital to different units or from one care facility to another, *transfer of medication orders* are written. This is a particularly error-prone time for patient care. Transfer orders typically must be rewritten as either required by standards in policy or by regulations in many states. The value of rewriting transfer orders is to ensure that the prescriber evaluates the need, safety, and effectiveness of the treatments ordered at the time of transfer (i.e., a natural time to evaluate effectiveness and safety). However, any time an order is rewritten, it creates the opportunity to omit or commit an error in transcription. Determining safety and effectiveness is your responsibility as a pharmacist prior to exposing the patient to a treatment. Evaluation of transfer orders is a "red flag" area for you.

Similarly, prescription transfers in the outpatient pharmacy setting are common. This often takes place between pharmacies, from hospital outpatient discharge pharmacies to community pharmacies, or from clinic pharmacies to outpatient community pharmacies. The same assessment issues that are discussed above in the order transfer considerations apply here too.

Ensure Patient Receives Medications and Supportive Technologies

Implementing a successful care plan with medications poses many challenges: 1) many prescriptions for medications are never turned in to a pharmacy to be filled by a pharmacist; 2) many are turned in but never picked up; and 3) many are initially filled, but subsequent refills are not requested by the patient. There are multiple reasons that this may occur. One study designed to evaluate why patients' chronic medication prescription refills were not picked up reveals the following reasons provided by patients:[2]

1. Patient went to a different pharmacy for refills than the original pharmacy that filled the prescription. The pharmacist thinks that the patient is not compliant, but the patient is using multiple pharmacy providers leading to lack of continuity in medication refill records.
2. Medication was discontinued by the prescriber before refill was needed.
3. Medication samples were provided by the physician, replacing the prescription.
4. The dosage was changed—prescription was no longer valid and a new prescription was issued.
5. Patient already had the medication at home—did not need more at the scheduled time. This often happens because patients are "partially compliant" (i.e., they take medication some of the time as they are supposed to).
6. Medication was used on an as-needed basis; didn't need the refill yet.
7. Self-reported noncompliance with medication—"I just don't take it."
8. Patient denies noncompliance—just didn't pick it up.
9. Patient had an adverse event from medication and no longer wanted to continue it.
10. Patient did not understand that he or she was supposed to continue medication.
11. Patient did not believe the medication works and decided not to continue.
12. Patient was unable to afford the medication prescribed.
13. Patient felt he or she had a self-limited need/short-term use despite the duration and refill status of the prescribed medication.
14. Patient was unable to pick up medication on time because of an illness or hospitalization.

Many causes require your advocacy to initially get the patient started on the medications. You must interact enough with the patient to know whether he or she has taken the first step—picked up and started the medication! A comprehensive list of factors associated with nonadherence to care is provided in **Table 10-1**.

Ensure Patient Takes Medication Once It Has Been Obtained

Even after obtaining the medication, many factors may cause a patient to not take it or take it incorrectly. There are social, economic, health, and other factors that contribute to this problem. Listed below are factors identified in prior research to consider when evaluating whether a patient is inclined to comply with proper medication use. If you can link the presence of one or more of these characteristics with the patient, you can then determine what to address if the patient's behavior is nonadherent to the medication regimens determined in the care plan.

To learn about the influence of these factors on your patient's behavior, you must communicate with him or her in order to follow up for clinical monitoring and provide encouragement and support. Three approaches to use are as follows:

- *Followup telephone calls that you initiate* within a specified time period after visiting with a patient when seen in a community pharmacy, outpatient clinic practice, or home care visit. These calls can be reassuring to the patient, further enhancing your relationship. Your genuine concern to assist the patient may result in offering solutions you might not have known about in your patient interactions.
- *Followup monitoring visits that you initiate at the time of care plan development and each subsequent visit* in order to assess your patient's response to therapy. At these visits, focus on communication about barriers and successes to care approaches in order to identify early on what might not be working and why.
- *Invitation and encouragement of patient to call you for assistance* when encountering any difficulties or barriers to implementing the care plan.

Conduct Counseling Relevant to the Care Plan

Effective counseling starts with involving the patient in treatment decisions. When you individualize the medication management plan by considering the patient's age, culture, gender, and attitudes, you eliminate many barriers that reduce the effectiveness of counseling.

Working with other health professionals and health care organizations to develop interdisciplinary compliance programs further improves the effectiveness of your counseling. The National Council for Patient Information and Education (NCPIE) has made several recommendations to health care organizations and hospitals that, when combined with the individual efforts of professionals such as the pharmacist, are likely to result in true improvement in patient adherence to care plans. These suggestions include

- Use existing databases to determine the extent of medicine noncompliance among patients.
- Develop and implement programs for patient compliance support (e.g., group support programs, educational interventions, monitoring clinics, compliance packaging aids, and multiple medicine reviews). Keep health care providers informed about these programs so they can refer appropriate patients as part of an individualized compliance regimen.
- Develop and implement innovative programs that teach patients responsibility for and involvement in their health care.
- Identify, implement, evaluate, and encourage successful compliance-promoting organizational practices and policies.
- Review drug use policies, such as formulary policy

Table 10-1. Published Evidence of Factors that Influence Nonadherence

Access - Economic
Able to purchase medications
Willing to purchase medications
Sample use
Lack of insurance[15]

Access - Transportation
Transportation available/dependable[2–6]
Distance for travel/convenience[4,5,7]

Social Support
General[5,8,9,11,12]
Live alone[5,12,13]
Assistance from people living with[5]
Married[5,12,14–16]
Care provider[17,18]
Church – active support
Home health assistance if needed
Assisted living

Complexity of Condition - Medication
General[11,19]
Number of medications[5,8,18–22,26–29]
Number of doses/day[8,18,21,22]

Complexity of Condition - Condition
Number of chronic conditions
Type of chronic condition:
   Diabetes
   Congestive heart failure
   High blood pressure
    Number of times BP taken[16]
   High cholesterol
   Stomach disorders
   Asthma
   Arthritis
   Depression[11,12,17,18,20,23,24,26]
   Alcoholism[15]
   Substance Abuse Problems[11,15]
   Tobacco use[15,16]

Perceived Effects of Medication
Past-current adverse event[2–5,10,11,18,20,24,25,30–34]
Past or current failure of therapy[2,3,18]
Desired reversal of symptoms
Patient perceives no impact on disease[8]

Health Effects
Belief that medication works[4,5,11,23,35]
Self efficacy accomplished with health[36]
Self efficacy accomplished with drugs[14,36–38]
Health beliefs support need[36]
Satisfied with health providers[3,4,11,36]

Lack of insight[11]
Denial of illness[11,42]
Low family value of med[11]
Stigma attached to illness[1]
Belief that MD orders improve health[42]
Use of home remedies[5]
Express concern about missed meds[5]

Coping Skills[26]

Other – Process steps
Physician–patient communication[8]
Formal education program[17]
Admin. of own medication[29,47]
Counseled by pharmacist[47]
Single dose pack of medication[47]
Receive medication in emergency room[15]

Other – General
Three or more meals per day[47]
Drug free holiday[5,31]
Self-care[14]
General practitioner prescribed[47]
Medication class effect adherence[5,22]
Inconvenient clinic hours[4]
Unable to pick up due to illness/hospitalization[2]
Self-limited need for med[2]
"As needed" use of scheduled med[2]

Health Cognition
Forgetfulness[3,5,7,11,32,39]
Knowledge of disease[3,4,5,11,18,36,40]
Knowledge of drug regimen[3,4,5,11,14,18,24,25,36,41]
Reading level
Grade level completed[5,12,13,14,16,42]
Functional health skills (psychomotor)
Physical impairment/accommodation status
Vision impairment/accommodation status
Hearing impairment/accommodation status
Ability to open medication containers[4,43]
Ability to self-administer medications
Language is a health communication barrier[35]

Other - Demographic
Age[5,12,14–18,20,22,26–29,44,45]
Sex[14,15,16,17,22,26–29,44]
Socioeconomic status[8,16,42]
Cost of medication[3,5,6,16,23,25,39]
Occupation[27,42]
Employed[5,15,26]
Number of drug allergies[5]

Other – Disease Specific

Seizure type[20,29]
Psychiatric disorder[46]
Transplantation stress[23]
Anxiety[11,17,18,24]
Dementia[4]
Anger hostility symptoms[17,20]
Severity of disease[11,18,27,43]
Duration of illness/need for med[5,9,19,20]
Duration of seizure control[29]
BP primarily checked in emergency room[15]
Poor cycle control[25]

Other – Patient Beliefs

Health locus of control[12,20,23,42]
Shouldn't have to take med[32]
Self-esteem[46]
Belief that patient did not need medication[3,33,34,39]

Other – Patient Characteristics

Family disorganization[18]
Medication cost to much/financial[3,5,16,23,25,39]
Low health care provider visits[15,16,22]
Use of avoidance behavior[3,17]
Recent hospitalization[28]
Poly pharmacy[28]
Lack of insight[11]
Race/ethnicity (influence side effect profile)[11,26]

---

* Spirituality as a determinant of health or healing – would like to include, however, no prior useful research in area to assist us with this.

---

guidelines, from a patient compliance perspective. Revise policies accordingly to facilitate compliance.

- Develop and implement computerized systems that allow departments to share clinical patient information electronically.

Methods of Counseling to Optimize Patient Adherence

Your patient needs to know why you think a treatment plan is most appropriate for him or her. However, to determine this, you must have an understanding of the patient's values—what is personally important. If you can link the value of taking the medication (because of expected outcomes) to what is important to the person, you are likely to achieve adherence.

You conduct counseling in an environment that enhances your chance of success with the patient. You are more likely to engage the patient and hold his or her attention by communicating in an atmosphere that protects patient privacy and confidentiality. If your facilities are inadequate, work with pharmacy management to redesign them to increase pharmacist/patient contact

and provide a private counseling area. Uninterrupted adjustments in operational flow may be necessary. Efficient use of supportive personnel to facilitate this important responsibility is needed.

Patients must also be advised to become an active participant in their own treatment decisions and work to overcome potential barriers that prevent proper medicine use. You should counsel your patients to ask questions and to offer information without being prompted by you as it relates to all of their medicine use. You should expect the patient to carry out his or her responsibilities that are required to succeed at the treatment regimen. Your expectation of the patient is held in high regard by patients and is likely to be taken seriously. This will reinforce your effectiveness.

Counseling should be provided orally. One approach is to ask the patient questions that stimulate a conversation. Engage the patient in a conversation about the care plans and have him or her tell you (back) what approach will be used to adhere to the plan.

You should also provide written support materials at the appropriate educational level and other media that provide additional information about the medications and their proper use or monitoring skills so the patient can comply with the care plan. Use written materials to reinforce oral counseling, not as a substitute or replacement for it. Use educational brochures, patient education leaflets, books, lists of web sites, videos and CDs, and access to specialized classes, if appropriate, for the patient and his or her needs.

Document Care Provided in the Patient's Record

Oral communication with a written followup is the usual and common way in which most documentation will occur. When you prepare the initial assessment and plan, you usually record it using a S.O.A.P. note. This format follows the development of a pharmacist's care plan discussed previously. Subjective information, what the patient relates to you, correlates to the health care need on your pharmacist's care plan. Objective data, which are quantitative, observable, or measurable, partially correlate to the information obtained from the pharmacist's patient database. The third part of the SOAP note, assessment, correlates to the information on your drug therapy problem list and/or the pharmacotherapeutic goals listed on your pharmacist's care plan. Finally, the recommendations for therapy and monitoring information on your pharmacist's care plan correlate to the fourth part of the SOAP note: the plan.

A narrative recommendation may not be labeled as clearly as the SOAP note. This format uses the same parts as the SOAP note but combines subjective and objective information into one paragraph. All information relayed by a patient, not just related to symptoms, could be documented in a "history" category. Sometimes, both subjective and objective information will come from a patient.

Either format can be used. The vast majority of physicians are accustomed to reading SOAP notes. Use the most effective and appropriate format for your practice setting. Remember to record the data and time when you write a patient's progress notes. Misinterpretation may arise if these items are missing.

Patient/Caregiver Response to Care Plan

The ways that both the patient and caregiver respond to a care plan are key subjective indicators of their intentions to support it. The reaction and responses of the patient and care provider should be captured and documented in the record. You will find it helpful to keep track of the responses that you perceive from the patient and caregiver in order to better understand why the plan is succeeding or failing. These impressions may be captured in the subjective and assessment areas of your notes.

Types of Notes Documented in the Patient Record

Several variations on the documentation notes used in charts are predominantly based on purpose. The *admission note* summarizes the data and initial assessment and plan as you prepare for the patient upon admission to the hospital. These notes usually follow a more formal format, using the chief complaint, history of present illness, past medical history, and other headings that provide a thorough representation of the impression on admission. The *progress note* is written to keep everyone up-to-date after each care provider has supplied some care and assessed the patient's response. *Medication history notes* are prepared specifically to communicate medications active on admission or to establish prior medication use history on the patient for the pharmacist in all practice settings. *Consultation notes* reflect your expert professional opinion, when requested by others, and communicate this opinion for their use. There are notes related to changes in the patient service location or provider. The *transfer note* is written to officially move a patient from one service to another and from one setting to another. A professional will leave a *sign-off note* when leaving the direct care of the patient. Sometimes professionals will write these notes at time of shift change for the benefit of the next group of professionals covering care in the hospital or long-term care setting. Finally, sometimes the notes summarize the *discharge* care plans for the patient.

Educate Patients about How to Contact You and Other Health Professionals

As you implement the patient's care plan, you will coordinate the medication regimens with other health professionals who provide services to the patient. In some cases, this coordination may require you to communicate with a visiting nurse representative, physician assistant or nurse practitioner, other pharmacists who are involved in caring for the patient, or family members or other caretakers. Use a business card that provides contact information for you and your backup contacts. Make sure to have 24-hour emergency contact information.

Ensure Patient Followup Is Scheduled

A key to successful care plan implementation is improving adherence by scheduling followup and monitoring with the patient. With chronic medications, you may be asking the patient to change the daily behaviors he or she has become accustomed to for a substantial time. Success with a patient adhering to a care plan at this point is largely education, assessment through monitoring, and feedback to the patient regarding his or her progress. The traditional model of care—development of a plan with no scheduled followup—is an ineffective model of care.

To complete each visit successfully, consider using a "checklist" to assure you have provided all of the care steps needed (**Figure 10-1**).

PATIENT RESOURCES

An increasing number of resources are available to facilitate the patients' shared responsibility for ensuring the most appropriate care is taking place. The National Council on Patient Information and Education (NCPIE) has some useful safe medication tips for distribution to your patients (**www.talkaboutrx.org**). The Agency for Healthcare Research and Quality has produced a Patient Fact Sheet entitled, "From the Source: 20 Tips to Help Prevent Medical Errors" (**Appendix 10-1**). Both the American Society of Health-System Pharmacists and the American Pharmacists Association have web site access to medication information for consumers and patients at **www.safemedication.org** and **www.pharmacyand you.org**, respectively.

CHECKLIST FOR PATIENT CARE PLAN IMPLEMENTATION

Check when Completed	Step in Care Plan Implementation
	Recommend the care plan to the appropriate individuals • Patient • Health care providers • Caretakers
	Ensure that medication orders and/or prescriptions are written to facilitate care and monitoring of the patient
	Ensure patient receives medications and supportive technologies
	Conduct counseling relevant to the care plan • Patient resources
	Use methods of counseling to optimize patient adherence
	Document care provided in the patients' record • Follow up with health care providers as appropriate
	Document patient/caregiver response to care plan
	Document appropriate type of note in the patient record
	Educate patients about how to contact you and other health professionals • Business card
	Ensure patient followup is scheduled

Figure 10-1. Checklist for patient care plan implementation.

SUMMARY

Implementing the care plan is one of the most challenging aspects of providing clinical care as a pharmacist. You must attend to the patient-centered approach by advocating for the patients' needs with others when recommending care. You must also directly monitor patient progress and needs by removing barriers to adherence. You will need to keep abreast of structural issues, such as workplace environment, and work flow and technical support, to allow you to focus uninterrupted time and attention on the patient. With these actions at the core of your efforts, you will be successful in supporting your patients with implementation of care plans.

GENERAL ASSESSMENT QUESTIONS

1. There are many reasons why a patient may be nonadherent to a medication plan. Interview a close friend, neighbor, relative, or another classmate who has had a need to take medications. Question this individual about the medication-taking behavior. What were challenges to adhering for this individual? How do they match what you have learned in this chapter?
2. What are tools you might use to assist the patient with carrying out the care plan you develop?

ASSIGNMENT

1. What do you do when there is a substantial mismatch between what you think is optimal treatment and what the patient tells you is optimal? This is a difficult situation that requires strength on your part to remain true to the relationship you have with the patient. Interview another pharmacist in your community about this subject to learn about the approach he or she uses in this situation.
2. There are different systems to document patient care. Visit a pharmacy to observe the system that the pharmacists use. Evaluate the system to determine what you are able to document and not document on that particular product. Discuss what you observe with the pharmacist.

CASES

See pages 226–235 for cases.

Case 1: *Lauren Smith continues her first formal pharmacist's consultation and care visit at Werbert's Pharmacy to implement the care plan with Nasir.*

Nasir: "It would seem we have a fairly clear idea of the care steps we should take. I would like to go over each one briefly so that you can tell me if we are on track."

(Nasir describes the following assessment from his progress note.)

Nasir: "I will send a summary of this visit to Dr. Miller's office so she is aware of our progress. If she has any questions, she will contact me for clarification. Here are two prescriptions to start out treatment (**Figure 10-2 A & B**). The first one is hydrochlorothiazide for managing your hypertension. The second one is nicorette gum to start decreasing your dependence upon nicotine.

You need to take one tablet of hydrochlorothiazide every day. You need to use the nicorette gum, tapering it according to the schedule I will discuss with you. These directions are also provided in the packages. After you receive the medications, you may have questions—just call me so I can answer them."

Nasir: "Let's concentrate on smoking cessation now. I would like to present you with material about smoking cessation to help you with this process, Lauren. I am providing written material that has questions you will need to answer. I would like you to return with the answers to these questions on our next visit. Today, I will concentrate on the correct way to use the chewing gum so that you can get the most benefit from it."

(Nasir counsels Lauren on the specifics of how to use the chewing gum and answers specific questions.)

Lauren: "Thanks so much, Nasir. I will make an appointment for followup with Joe at the check-out area."

Nasir: "Good. I will see you again in 3 weeks or so. I look forward to it."

[Nasir completes the documentation in the pharmacy profile for Lauren and also emails the summary to Dr. Miller's office (**Figure 10-3**).]

Nasir: "You are welcome, Lauren. I have included a return visit approximately 3 weeks from now. We can reassess your progress and determine if there are changes needed in the approach we have chosen here."

Lauren: "Sounds good. Nasir provides a business card with scheduled appointment." (**Figure 10-4**)

First Prescription:

Joyce Miller MD   DEA No. AC 1269478
Don Hancock, M.D.   DEA No. AD 3497682

Metropolitan General Family Medicine Clinic
1234 Detroit Avenue
Detroit, Michigan 48169

Rx: Hydrochlorothiazide 25 mgs tablets
Quantity: 30 tablets
Sig: Take one tablet by mouth every day in the morning.
Refills: 6

                       Nasir Jabr, Pharm.D./Joyce Miller, M.D.

_____   _____
Dispense as Written   May Substitute Generic/Therapeutic Equivalent

---

Second prescription:

Joyce Miller MD   DEA No. AC 1269478
Don Hancock, M.D.   DEA No. AD 3497682

Metropolitan General Family Medicine Clinic
1234 Detroit Avenue
Detroit, Michigan 48169

Rx: Nicorette gum 2 mg
Quantity: 108
Sig: Chew 1 piece q 1-2 hours or when you have the urge to smoke.
Follow plan of pharmacist after initiation.
Refills: 2

                       Nasir Jabr, Pharm.D./Joyce Miller, M.D.

_____   _____
Dispense as Written   May Substitute Generic/Therapeutic Equivalent

---

Figure 10-2 A&B. Prescriptions prepared by pharmacist under Collaborative Practice Authority Agreement.

Pharmacy Profile for:

Patient:	Smith, Lauren		New Patient	Print	Close Record

Demographic	OTC / Allergy		Insurance	Diagnosis	Contacts
General Health	Care Plans	Surveys	Account Status	Current Therapy	
General Information	Illnesses	Systems Review	Vital Signs	Lab Values	

Pharmacist's Progress Note - continued: Date: 02-10

S: Compliant with antibiotic and signs and symptoms resolved no burning or discomfort for several days. Headaches continue.

O: BP #1 150/102 seated, BP #2 148/99 seated. Scored 5 of 10 on Fagerstrom test – moderate dependence upon nicotine and classified at the "attempting to stop" in stages of change phases.

A: UTI resolved – patient complied with antibiotic and took until gone. Mild, intermittent headaches responsive to Advil. Advil may worse fluid/sodium retention – contributing to hypertension. Headaches probably secondary to sinus discomfort or possibly allergies; worsened by smoking. Stage I hypertension. Both headaches and hypertension may improve if eliminate Advil use and smoking. Patient is ready to quit smoking. Patient is not comfortable with use of barrier method of birth control despite the risk benefit discussion that has taken place.

P:

#1 – Urinary Tract Infection

P: Counseled patient to drink 8 – 10 glasses water/day and contact immediately if symptoms return. Patient confirms understanding.

#2 – Headaches

P: Use acetaminophen instead of Advil to decrease risk of fluid retention and worsening of hypertension. Patient agrees to use acetaminophen instead of Advil.

#3 – Hypertension

 P: Initiate hydrochlorothiazide 25mgs, 1 tablet every morning per hypertension protocol with Dr. Joyce Miller. Reassess in 3 weeks. Patient given a prescription and instructed BP will be rechecked in 3 weeks.

#4 - Smoking

P: Initiate smoking cessation program. Provide counseling materials and prescription for chewing gum. Follow up at next visit regarding medication compliance.

#5 – Method of birth control

 P: Patient considering options. Will follow up at next visit to determine choices that patient has made.

Figure 10-3. Pharmacist's progress note prepared about patient visit with pharmacist in community pharmacy.

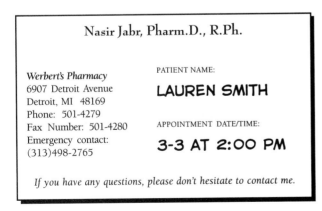

Figure 10-4. Business card used as patient reminder for next scheduled appointment.

CASE 1: COUNSELING MATERIALS

1. You Can Quit Smoking. Information kit for consumers. November 2003. U.S. Public Health Service. www.ahrq.gov/consumer/tobacco/
2. Help for Smokers: Ideas to Help you Quit*

Ideas to Help You Quit

Do you smoke? Do you want to quit? Here are some ideas to help you kick the habit. Check with your family physician on the best way for you to stop smoking.

Want to Quit?

You promised yourself that you would finally quit smoking.

It isn't easy giving up something that is so much a part of what you do every day.

But you are not alone. Over 1 million people each year decide to quit and are successful.

Tried Quitting Before?

Maybe once, maybe more...

You started out feeling the time was right but, for whatever reason, you're smoking again. Now, you're asking whether it's worth it to try quitting again. You bet it is!

Quitting is Hard, but Don't Give Up!

Some smokers try a number of times before they quit for good. Studies show that each time you try to quit, the more likely you will be to eventually succeed. With each try, you are better able to know what helps and what hurts. Any attempt to quit is a step in a healthier direction.

Pregnant?

There's no better time to quit.

And for two very good reasons:
- You.
- Your baby.

Even if someone you know smoked during pregnancy and had a problem-free delivery, smoking puts your baby's health at risk. Quitting at any time during pregnancy is still the best chance for you and your baby to get a fresh start.

It is also important to remember that infants and children exposed to second-hand smoke are more likely to develop health problems such as chronic ear infections and asthma. Helping to eliminate these health risks is another good reason to quit.

How Do I Start?

Make a Plan
- You may want to consult a health care professional to choose a quit smoking plan that is best for you.
- Set a quit date and stick to it.
- Get the support and understanding of your family, friends, and co-workers.
- Get rid of all tobacco products and ashtrays.

Get Support and Encouragement

U.S. Public Health Service (PHS)-funded research shows the more support you have, the greater your chance for success.

Join a quit smoking program or start your own quit smoking group. Check with your health care professional, local hospitals, the American Cancer Society, American Lung Association, or American Heart Association for schedules for existing groups.

Learn How to Handle the Urge to Smoke

Be aware of the things that may cause you to smoke, such as:
- Other smokers.
- Stress.
- Depression.
- Alcohol.

What Works?

Current Treatments

There are no magic solutions for quitting smoking. But, if you are ready to quit, effective treatments are available that can help reduce the urge to smoke.

Studies show that almost everyone can benefit from these nicotine and non-nicotine replacement therapies.

Nicotine Replacement Therapy
- Nicotine patch.
- Nicotine gum.
- Nicotine nasal spray.*
- Nicotine inhaler.*

Non-Nicotine Therapy
- Bupropion.*
  *Available only by prescription.

You can get these therapies through your pharmacy or health care provider.

More Resources

Additional free materials on quitting smoking from the U.S. Public Health Service may be requested:

Publications Clearinghouse
P.O. Box 8547
Silver Spring, MD 20907-8547

Or call toll-free in the United States at 800-358-9295

(outside the United States, please call 410-381-3150). Electronic requests may be made to: ahrqpubs @ahrq.gov.

Also, you can access and download materials from the Surgeon General's web site at: www.surgeongeneral.gov/ tobacco/default.htm

These materials include the consumer guide: *You Can Quit Smoking* (PDF File, 280 KB).

The Surgeon General's Report for Kids about Smoking is an excellent resource for children, parents, and teachers to discourage tobacco use and encourage youth to quit smoking.

Internet Citation:
*Help for Smokers: Ideas to Help You Quit. Based on the U.S. Public Health Service Tobacco Cessation Guideline, June 2000. Agency for Healthcare Research and Quality, Rockville, MD. www.ahrq.gov/consumer/helpsmok.htm Current as of June 2000

3. You Can Quit Smoking

5-Day Countdown

FOLLOW THIS 5-DAY COUNTDOWN TO YOUR QUIT DATE

5 Days Before Your Quit Date
- Think about your reasons for quitting.
- Tell your friends and family you are planning to quit.
- Stop buying cigarettes.

4 Days Before Your Quit Date
- Pay attention to when and why you smoke.
- Think of other things to hold in your hand instead of a cigarette.
- Think of habits or routines to change.

3 Days Before Your Quit Date
- What will you do with the extra money when you stop buying cigarettes?
- Think of who to reach out to when you need help.

2 Days Before Your Quit Date
- Buy the nicotine patch or nicotine gum.
- Or see your doctor to get the nicotine inhaler, nasal spray, or the non-nicotine pill.

1 Day Before Your Quit Date
- Put away lighters and ashtrays.
- Throw away all cigarettes and matches.
- Clean your clothes to get rid of the smell of cigarette smoke.

Quit Day
- Keep very busy.
- Remind family and friends that this is your quit day.

- Stay away from alcohol.
- Give yourself a treat, or do something special.

Smoke Free

CONGRATULATIONS!!!

If you "slip" and smoke, don't give up. Set a new date to get back on track.
- Call a friend or "quit smoking" support group.
- Eat healthy food and get exercise.

For More Help

For help in quitting smoking, call the National Cancer Institute's Smoking Quitline.
Toll-free: 1-877-44U-QUIT.
U.S. Department of Health and Human Services
Public Health Service
Current as of May 2003

Internet Citation:
You Can Quit Smoking. Follow this 5-Day Countdown to Your Quit Day. Consumer booklet, May 2003. U.S. Public Health Service. Agency for Healthcare Research and Quality. www.ahrq.gov/consumer/tobacco/5daybook.htm

CASE 1: SPECIFIC QUESTIONS

1. What are the specific points that Lauren needs to be counseled about in order for her to maximize use of the nicotine polycrilex gum (Nicorette gum)?
2. What aspects of implementing a care plan were demonstrated well by Nasir? What aspects need improvement? Support your opinion using the methods described in the chapter.

Case 2: *Christine Johnston implements the care plan with Mr. Montanez and Maria.*

Christine describes the plan that she, Mr. Montanez, and Maria have produced through the conversations in the visit.

Christine: "Now that we have discussed these areas, do you have any additional questions?"

Mr. Montanez: "No, I understand."

Maria: "I do, too, Christine. However, I am concerned that our memories will not keep up with so much. There is a great deal of information that we have covered."

Christine: "Yes, you are both right. I have some written materials to help us all remember and review. There is a great deal to learn. It is possible to do so if you have information to read. However, the most important things to do immediately are to

- Make the appointment with the eye doctor.
- Cut down on alcohol to no more than 1 drink a day.
- Take the two medicines for diabetes each morning (diabinese, tolinase).
- Read the materials I give you so that we can talk next time.
- Start to change your diet to improve diabetes control."

Mr. Montanez: "I will. Thank you." (He looks at Maria who nods her head affirmatively.)

Christine: "There are many things we should do to help you take care of yourself. We have covered a great deal of information today. We will need to visit several times to understand how to best approach these needs. Please plan on another visit in 4 weeks, and we will see how you are progressing." [She prepares the progress note (**Figure 10-5**).]

Mr. Montanez: "Si…Maria and I will visit again. Gracias."

[Christine provides both Mr. Montanez and Maria with her business card (**Figure 10-6**).]

CASE 2: SPECIFIC QUESTIONS

1. What approach did Christine adopt with Mr. Montanez to improve her chances of successful implementation?
2. Prioritize the problems that need to be addressed. What would be the next logical focus of the subsequent visit? How would you organize the tasks and responsibilities within each of the visits?

HEART OF TEXAS SYSTEM CLINICS PROGRESS NOTES	Patient Identification (Stamp) Name: **Eduardo Montanez**
Leukocytes _____	Reg.No. **16254**

Appt. _____ Call/Walk In _____ Primary Physician _____ /Staff _____ Date: 06-19-04

Progress Note

S: Does not like blurriness; leg pain continues; nocturia continues.
O: Possible retinopathy. Fasting Blood Sugar = 220 mg%. Patient has total cholesterol = 410 mg/dL; and High Density Lipoprotein=130 mg/dL.
A: EM is non-compliant with his diabetes care plan. He self treats and uses alcohol excessively. Evaluation is complicated by possible drug interaction with cactus flower plant consumption. Needs ophthalmologic evaluation now by someone who specializes in diabetes. Follow-up retinopathy status. Leg pain likely secondary to diabetes. Nocturia continues secondary to poor blood sugar control. :Newly diagnosed hypertension needs management.

#1 vision
P: Please initiate referral to Dr. Jones; an ophthalmologist, for evaluation of retinopathy status and need for visual correction.
#2 diabetes neuropathy in legs
P: Control Diabetes
#3 Nocturia
P: Control diabetes
#4 Diabetes poorly controlled
P: Patient education provided about:
 1. the relationship between controlling blood sugar and his symptoms,
 2. the interaction with cactus flowers and his diabetes medication,
 3. educate to stop using the cactus flower treatment,
 4. educate to stop alcohol consumption,
 5. reinforce once a day consumption of both Diabinese 125 mg po qd and Tolinase 250 mg po qd,
 6. schedule follow up for blood sugar and urine protein in two weeks.
#5 Hypertension
 1. Patients blood pressure at 146/96 – needs treatment.
 2. Educate patient about relationship between diabetes and hypertension.
 3. Discuss dietary control
 4. Discuss need for treatment. Risks and benefits of treatment vs. no treatment- consult primary care provider.
#6 Immunization status
Check immunization status – next visit.
#7 Dyslipidemia
 1. Recommend dyslipidemia therapy to primary care MD
 2. Initiate dietary counseling and establish goals.
 3. Reduce cardiovascular risk. Start on once a day 325 mg aspirin.
#8 Allergy status education
      Reeducated the patient that he does not have an opioid allergy.

Pharmacists Signature/Pager: ___*Christine Johnston*___ Date: _6/19/04_

Figure 10-5. *Pharmacist's progress note for patient clinic visit with pharmacist.*

Christine Johnston, Pharm.D., R.Ph.

*Heart of Texas
System Clinics*
(address)
San Antonio, TX
Phone: 332-689-7123
Fax: 332-689-7100

PATIENT NAME:

MR. E. MONTANEZ

APPOINTMENT DATE/TIME:

7/20/04 AT 9 AM

Please contact me if you have any needs or questions.

Figure 10-6. *Business card used as patient reminder for next scheduled appointment.*

Case 3: *Luisa implements the care plan for Huong Tran.*

Luisa contacts Dr. Morris to have him order the contracted service interpreter for Huong's family. She also discusses it with the social worker Ms. Sheri Turner.

Luisa: "Sheri, I think this family is going to have a hard time if we don't engage someone to translate the medical information and instructions."

Sheri: "I agree. And I can see this really deteriorating as a problem in the community for Huong as soon as he arrives home. I work with a colleague who is in Huong's area. I wonder if he couldn't take the medication plan and orders intended and have one of the residents in the community translate this until we get a better solution?" (This started Luisa thinking.)

Luisa: "You know, Sheri, if your colleague were able to take Huong as the case, I could contact the local pharmacies in the area to see if there was someone who could provide support and feedback to the family. Ideally, a pharmacist who speaks Vietnamese may be a large part of the solution for them."

Sheri: "You are right. Let's work on that."

[Luisa goes back to the floor and reviews the Medication Administration Record (**Figure 10-7**), determines the discharge medication plan for the patient, and prepares the discharge prescriptions for Huong Tran to be countersigned by Dr. Morris (**Figure 10-8**).]

(Luisa contacts several pharmacies and discovers one pharmacist who is willing to help Huong Tran. She prepares a discharge counseling note for Mr. Tran with the pharmacy information and has it ready when the interpreter and social worker Sheri are present with her and the family.)

Luisa: "It is a pleasure for me to introduce you to Xi Chang, our interpreter." (Xi repeats the introductory remarks.)

Luisa: "I have the medication prescriptions for you, Huong. These medications must be taken to a pharmacy in order for them to be dispensed. I have contacted a pharmacy that is able to provide these and also speak Vietnamese. I have written down the name and address of the pharmacist who will help you. I would also like to visit with you in a month or so. To accommodate this, Sheri, our social worker, has made arrangements with another social worker in your area to visit and assess how you are doing. She will bring you back here for an educational visit with me in the pharmacy within 4 weeks or so. Here is my business card so that you have the information. I am so pleased to work this out with you" (**Figure 10-9**).

CASE 3: SPECIFIC QUESTIONS

1. Was Luisa successful in the implementation of the care plan for Huong? Why or why not?
2. Why should Luisa take the responsibility to ensure continuity of Huong's medication management care after he is discharged?

Memorial Hospital and Health System

MEDICATION ADMINISTRATION RECORD

Name: Huong Tran
Reg.No. 2364590

INJECTION SITE CODE

A (R)Deltoid	H (L) Upper Quad
B (L)Deltoid	I (R) Lower Quad
C (L)Lat. Thigh	J (L) Lower Quad
D (R)Lat. Thigh	K (L) Glutial
E (R)Ant. Thigh	L (R) Glutial
F (L)Ant. Thigh	M(L) Ventro-Glutial
G (R)Upper Quad	O (R) Ventro-Glutial

DIAGNOSIS:
ACUTE ASTHMA
EXACERBATION

GENERATED:
FOR PERIOD:
THROUGH:

ALLERGIES:

START	STOP	MEDICATION	ORDER#	07:01-15:00	15:01-23:00	23:01-07:00
		ALBUTEROL 2 PUFFS Q 6 HRS	1246987	0600 1200	1800	2400
		FLUTICASONE 50 MCG Q 12 HRS	1246989	0900	2100	

INITIALS	NAME & PROFESSIONAL DESIGNATION	INITIALS	NAME & PROFESSIONAL DESIGNATION	INITIALS	NAME & PROFESSIONAL DESIGNATION	INITIALS	NAME & PROFESSIONAL DESIGNATION

Figure 10-7. Medication administration record for Huong Tran's hospitalization.

Dr. Morris   DEA No. AC 1269478

Memorial Hospital and Health System
Patient: Huong Tran   Date: April 4, 2004

Rx   Fluticasone 50 mcgs twice daily -inhaled
Disp: 1 inhaler

Refills: 11

_____   *Luisa Rodriguez /Dr. Morris*
Dispense as Written   May Substitute Generic/Therapeutic Equiv

---

Dr. Morris   DEA No. AC 1269478

Memorial Hospital and Health System

Patient: Huong Tran   Date: April 4, 2004
Rx: Albuterol two puffs every 6 hours
Disp: 1 inhaler

Refills: 11

_____   *Luisa Rodriguez /Dr. Morris*
Dispense as Written   May Substitute Generic/Therapeutic Equiv

---

Dr. Morris   DEA No. AC 1269478

Memorial Hospital and Health System

Patient: Huong Tran   Date: April 4, 2004
Rx: Spacer Device for hand held inhaler
Disp: 1

Refills: 1

_____   *Luisa Rodriguez /Dr. Morris*
Dispense as Written   May Substitute Generic/Therapeutic Equiv

---

Figure 10-8. Discharge prescriptions for Huong Tran.

Luisa Rodriguez, Pharm.D., R.Ph.
Memorial Hospital and Health System
Omaha, NE

Phone: (409)678-2345 Fax: (409)678-2320

If you have any questions, please don't hesitate to contact me.

Figure 10-9. Business card for pharmacist Luisa Rodriguez.

Case 4: *Michael Jones implements a care plan for Mr. Robinson.*

[Michael Jones follows up on interpreting the laboratory tests ordered so that he may confirm the appropriateness of the anticoagulation dose and begin the education process needed with this drug. His therapeutic monitoring of Mr. Robinson is described in the progress note (**Figure 10-10**).]

Michael Jones is reviewing another patient's chart when Dr. Rangert shows up on the patient floor.

Michael: "Good morning, Dr. Rangert."

Dr. Rangert: "Morning Michael. How is Mr. Robinson doing?"

Michael: "He appears to be doing well. His laboratory parameters indicate that the use of warfarin is appropriate. We are evaluating his response to using a 4-mg per day dose."

Dr. Rangert: "I am looking at discharge 2 days from now or so if all goes well. Will that be enough time to stabilize his warfarin?"

Michael: "If no dosage change is indicated tomorrow based upon his INR, this will be appropriate. I will contact you in the morning if there is an unexpected result. Otherwise, I will begin the anticoagulation education of Mr. Jones and, if possible, his acquaintances Althea Jones and Dorothy Roberts."

Dr. Rangert: "Sounds like a good plan. Thanks so much. I will countersign the orders."

CASE 4: SPECIFIC QUESTIONS

1. Was Michael Jones effective at communicating his care plan for Mr. Robinson to Dr. Rangert? If yes, what did he specifically do to accomplish this?
2. Under what circumstances would it be appropriate for Michael Jones to also educate Mr. Robinson's friends Althea Jones and Dorothy Roberts? What should he do to ensure that this is appropriate?

GENERAL ASSESSMENT QUESTIONS

1. There are many reasons why a patient may be nonadherent to a medication plan. Interview a close friend, neighbor, relative, or another classmate who has had the need to take medications. Question this individual about his or her medication-taking behavior. What were challenges to adherence for this individual? How do these match what you have learned in this chapter?

2. What are tools you might use with a patient to assist the individual with carrying out the care plan you develop?

ASSIGNMENT

1. What do you do when there is a substantial mismatch between what you think is optimal treatment and care and what the patient tells you is optimal? This is a difficult situation that requires strength on your part to remain true to the relationship you have with the patient. Interview another pharmacist in your community about this subject to learn about the approach he or she uses in this situation.

2. There are different systems to document patient care. Visit a pharmacy to observe the system that the pharmacists use. Evaluate the system to determine what you are able to document and not document on that particular product. Discuss what you observe with the pharmacist.

REFERENCES

1. Kuyper AR. Patient counseling detects prescription errors. *Hosp Pharm*. 1993; 28(Dec):1180–1, 1184–9.

2. Galt KA, Backes JB, Sondag LD. Indentifying noncompliance by combining refill audits with telephone follow-up. *Am J Health-Syst Pharm*. 2000; 57:219–20.

3. Pozsik CJ. Compliance with tuberculosis therapy. *Tuberculosis*. 1993; 77(6):1289–1301.

4. Galloway R, McGuire J. Determinants of compliance with iron supplementation: supplies, side effects, or psychology? *Soc Sci Med*. 1994; 39(3)381–90.

5. Shaw E, Anderson JG, Maloney M et al. Factors associated with noncompliance of patients taking antihypertensive medications. *Hosp Pharm*. 1995; 30(3):201–7.

6. Happ MB, Naylor MD, Roe-Prior P. Factors contributing to rehospitalization of elderly patients with heart failure. *J Cardiovasc Nurs*. 1997; 11(4):75–84.

7. McCaffrey DJ, Smith MC, Benahan BF. Why prescriptions go unclaimed. *US Pharmacist*. 1993; Aug:58–65.

8. Matesui ME. Drug compliance in pediatrics: clinical and research issues. *Pediatric Clinics of North America*. 1997; 44(1):1–14.

9. Kern Rm, Penick JM, Hamby RD. Prediction of diabetic adherence using the BASIS-A Inventory. *The Diabetes Educator*. 1996; 22(4):367–73.

10. Bittar AE, Keitel E, Garcia CD, et al. Patient noncompliance as a cause of late kidney graft failure. *Transplantation Proceedings*. 1992; 24(6):2720–1.

11. Marder SR. Facilitating compliance with antipsychotic medication. *J Clin Psychiatry*. 1998:59 (suppl 3) 21–5.

12. Safdar N, Baakza H, Kumar H et al. Non-compliance to diet and fluid restrictions in haemodialysis patients. *JPMA*. 1995; 45(11):293–5.

13. Eisen SA, Miller DK, Woodward RS et al. The effect of prescribed daily dose frequency on patient medication compliance. *Arch Intern Med*. 1990; 150:1881–4.

14. Geest SD, Borgermans L, Germoets H et al. Incidence, determinants, and consequences of subclinical noncompliance with immunosuppressive therapy in renal transplant recipients. *Transplantation*. 1995; 59(3):340–7.

15. Shea S, Misra D, Martin H. Correlates of non-adherence to hypertension treatment in an inner-city minority population. *Am J Public Health*. 1992; 82(12):1607.

Madison Hospitals and Health Systems	Patient Identification (Stamp)
	Name: **Samuel Robinson**
	Reg. No. **02946372**
	Location: **INPT 347-1**
PROGRESS NOTES	Date: **09-2-04**

Anticoagulation Care Progress Note by Pharmacist

4:30 p.m.
S: No evidence of bleeding or skin discoloration.
O: Hgb = 14.1; Hct = 42; platelets = 350K; prothrombin time = 16; INR = 1.4; stool guaiac = (-)
A: The patient is an acceptable candidate for continuing warfarin therapy.
P: Dr. Rangert has determined the target INR goal range to be **2.0 – 3.0**. Begin warfarin at 4 mgs po qd

9/3/04 9:10 a.m.
SR is a 76 yo African American male who was referred to this service to initiate warfarin therapy for prophylaxis for atrial fibrillation
A: maintain warfarin 4 mgs po qd today. Obtain PT/INR this a.m.

Michael Jones

Pharmacist's Signature/phone extension or pager

Figure 10-10. Progress note prepared by pharmacist Michael Jones about Samuel Robinson's inpatient visit.

16. Daniels DE, Rene AA, Daniels VR. Race: An explanation of patient compliance—fact or fiction? *J Natl Med Assoc.* 1994; 86(1):20–5.

17. Dew MA, Roth LH, Thompson ME et al. Medical compliance and its predictors in the first year after heart transplantation. *J Heart Lung Transplant.* 1996; 15:631–45.

18. Lask B. Understanding and managing poor adherence in cystic fibrosis. *Pediatr Pulmonol Suppl.* 1997; 16:260–1.

19. Mason JS, Walker R. Management of steroid reducing regimens by patients. *Intl J Pharm Pract.* 1993; 2:77–81.

20. Hargrave R, Remler MP. Noncompliance—letter to the editor. *J Natl Med Assn.* 1988(1):7,11.

21. Hamilton RA, Briceland AA. Use of prescription-refill records to assess patient compliance. *Am J Hosp Pharm.* 1992; 49(7):1691–6.

22. Baily JE, Lee MD, Somes GW et al. Risk factors for antihypertensive medication refill failure by patients under Medicaid managed care. *Clin Ther.* 1996; 18(6):1252–62.

23. Frazier PA, Davis Ali SH, Dahl K. Correlates of noncompliance among renal transplant recipients. *Clin Transplantation.* 1994; 8:550–7.

33. Mcrea JB, Ranelli PL, Boyce EG et al. Preliminary study of autonomy as a factor influencing medication-taking by elderly patients. *Am J Hosp Pharm.* 1993; 50:296–8.

24. Parrilla JJ, Coll C, Bajo JM et al. Analysis of compliance with oral contraception in Spain. *The European Journal of Contraception and Reproductive Health Care.* 1996: 337–47.

25. Serfaty D. Medical aspects of oral contraceptive discontinuation. *Advances in Contraception.* 1992:8(suppl 1) 21–33.

26. Singh N, Squier C, Sivek C et al. Determinants of compliance with antiretroviiral therapy in patients with human immunodeficiency virus: prospective assessment with implications for enhancing compliance. *AIDS Care.* 1996; 8(3):261–9.

27. Myint T, Htoon MT, Win M et al. Risk factors among defaulters in the urban leprosy control centre of Thaketa Township in the city of Yangon, Myanmar, 1986. *Lepr Rev.* 1992; 63:345–9.

28. Monane M, Bohn RL, Gurwitz JH et al. Noncompliance with congestive heart failure therapy in the elderly. *Arch Intern Med.* 1994; 154:433–7.

29. Takaki S, Kurokawa T, Aoyama T. Monitoring drug noncompliance in epileptic patients: Assessing phenobarbital plasma levels. *Ther Drug Monit.* 1985; 7(1):87–91.

30. Conrad P. The meaning of medications: Another look at compliance. *Soc Sci Med.* 1985; (20)1:29–37.

31. Atwood JR, Aickin M, Giordano L et al. The effectiveness of adherence intervention in a colon cancer prevention field trial. *Prev Med.* 1992; Sep:21(5).

32. Patient barriers to compliance with cancer pain regimens. *Oncology News Intl.* 1998; 7(8):34–5.

34. Davidson AR, Kalmuss D, Cushman LF et al. Indictable contraceptive discontinuation and subsequent unintended pregnancy among low-income women. *Am J Public Health.* 1997; 87(9):1532–4.

35. Meyerson MD. Many cultures/more compassion. *J Clin Pharm Ther.* 1994; 19:215–8.

36. Johnson JA. Self-efficacy theory as a framework for community pharmacy-based diabetes education programs. *Diabetes Educator.* 1996; 22(3):237–41.

37. Brus H, Van de Laar M, Taal E et al. Compliance in rheumatoid arthritis and the role of formal patient education. *Semin Arthritis Rheum.* 1997; 26(4): 702–10.

38. Geest SD, Abraham I, Moons P et al. Late acute rejection and subclinical noncompliance with cyclosporine therapy in heart transplant recipients. *J Heart Lung Transplant.* 1998; 17:854–63.

39. Hamilton WR, Hopkins UK. Survey of unclaimed prescription in a community pharmacy. *J Am Pharm Assn.* 1997; 3:341–5.

40. Miller J. Parkinson's disease patients show poor compliance, knowledge. *AJHP.* 1994; 51:2554.

41. Morisky ED, Mabotte CK, Choi P et al. A patient education program to improve adherence rates with antituberculosis drug regimens. *Health Education Quarterly.* 1990; 17(3):253–67.

42. Hoover H. Compliance in hemodialysis patients: A review of the literature. *J Am Diet Assoc.* 1989; 89:957–9.

43. Leirer Vo, Morrow DG, Pariante GM et al. Elders' nonadherence, its assessment, and computer assisted instruction for medication recall training. *J Am Geriatr Soc.* 1988; 36:877–84.

44. Brooks CM, Richards JM, Kohler CL et al. Assessing adherence to asthma medication and inhaler regimens: A psychometric analysis of adult self-report scales. *Medical Care.* 1994; 32(3):298–307.

45. Berman RS, Epstein RS, Lydick E. Risk factors associated with women's compliance with estrogen replacement therapy. *J Women's Health.* 1997; 6(2):1997.

46. Kovacs M, Goldston D, Obrosky S et al. Prevalence and predictors of pervasive noncompliance with medical treatment among youths with insulin-dependent diabetes mellitus. *J Am Acad Child Adolesc Psychiatry.* 1992; 31(6):1112–9.

47. Okuno J, Yanagi H, Tomura S et al. Compliance and medication knowledge among elderly Japanese home-care recipients. *Eur J Clin Pharmacol.* 1999; 55:145–9.

Appendix 10-1

PATIENT FACT SHEET

20 Tips to Help Prevent Medical Errors

Medical errors are one of the Nation's leading causes of death and injury. A recent report by the Institute of Medicine estimates that as many as 44,000 to 98,000 people die in U.S. hospitals each year as the result of medical errors. This means that more people die from medical errors than from motor vehicle accidents, breast cancer, or AIDS.

Government agencies, purchasers of group health care, and health care providers are working together to make the U.S. health care system safer for patients and the public. This fact sheet tells what you can do.

What Are Medical Errors?

Medical errors happen when something that was planned as a part of medical care doesn't work out, or when the wrong plan was used in the first place. Medical errors can occur anywhere in the health care system:

- Hospitals.
- Clinics.
- Outpatient Surgery Centers.
- Doctors' Offices.
- Nursing Homes.
- Pharmacies.
- Patients' Homes.

Errors can involve:

- Medicines.
- Surgery.
- Diagnosis.
- Equipment.
- Lab reports.

They can happen during even the most routine tasks, such as when a hospital patient on a salt-free diet is given a high-salt meal.

Most errors result from problems created by today's complex health care system. But errors also happen when doctors and their patients have problems communicating. For example, a recent study supported by the Agency for Healthcare Research and Quality (AHRQ) found that doctors often do not do enough to help their patients make informed decisions. Uninvolved and uninformed patients are less likely to accept the doctor's choice of treatment and less likely to do what they need to do to make the treatment work.

What Can You Do? Be Involved in Your Health Care

1. The single most important way you can help to prevent errors is to be an active member of your health care team.

That means taking part in every decision about your health care. Research shows that patients who are more involved with their care tend to get better results. Some specific tips, based on the latest scientific evidence about what works best, follow.

MEDICINES

2. Make sure that all of your doctors know about everything you are taking. This includes prescription and over-the-counter medicines and dietary supplements such as vitamins and herbs.

At least once a year, bring all of your medicines and supplements with you to your doctor. "Brown bagging" your medicines can help you and your doctor talk about them and find out if there are any problems. It can also help your doctor keep your records up-to-date, which can help you get better quality care.

3. Make sure your doctor knows about any allergies and adverse reactions you have had to medicines.

This can help you avoid getting a medicine that can harm you.

4. When your doctor writes you a prescription, make sure you can read it.

If you can't read your doctor's handwriting, your pharmacist might not be able to either.

5. Ask for information about your medicines in terms you can understand—both when your medicines are prescribed and when you receive them.

- What is the medicine for?
- How am I supposed to take it, and for how long?
- What side effects are likely? What do I do if they occur?
- Is this medicine safe to take with other medicines or dietary supplements I am taking?
- What food, drink, or activities should I avoid while taking this medicine?

6. When you pick up your medicine from the pharmacy, ask: Is this the medicine that my doctor prescribed?

A study by the Massachusetts College of Pharmacy and Allied Health Sciences found that 88 percent of medicine errors involved the wrong drug or the wrong dose.

7. If you have any questions about the directions on your medicine labels, ask.

Medicine labels can be hard to understand. For example, ask if "four doses daily" means taking a dose every 6 hours around the clock or just during regular waking hours.

8. Ask your pharmacist for the best device to measure your liquid medicine. Also, ask questions if you're not sure how to use it.

Research shows that many people do not understand the right way to measure liquid medicines. For example, many use household teaspoons, which often do not hold a true teaspoon of liquid. Special devices, like marked syringes, help people to measure the right dose. Being told how to use the devices helps even more.

9. Ask for written information about the side effects your medicine could cause.

If you know what might happen, you will be better prepared if it does—or, if something unexpected happens instead. That way, you can report the problem right away and get help before it gets worse. A study found that written information about medicines can help patients recognize problem side effects and then give that information to their doctor or pharmacist.

HOSPITAL STAYS

10. If you have a choice, choose a hospital at which many patients have the procedure or surgery you need.

Research shows that patients tend to have better results when they are treated in hospitals that have a great deal of experience with their condition.

11. If you are in a hospital, consider asking all health care workers who have direct contact with you whether they have washed their hands.

Handwashing is an important way to prevent the spread of infections in hospitals. Yet, it is not done regularly or thoroughly enough. A recent study found that when patients checked whether health care workers washed their hands, the workers washed their hands more often and used more soap.

12. When you are being discharged from the hospital, ask your doctor to explain the treatment plan you will use at home.

This includes learning about your medicines and finding out when you can get back to your regular activities. Research shows that at discharge time, doctors think their patients understand more than they really do about what they should or should not do when they return home.

SURGERY

13. If you are having surgery, make sure that you, your doctor, and your surgeon all agree and are clear on exactly what will be done.

Doing surgery at the wrong site (for example, operating on the left knee instead of the right) is rare. But even once is too often. The good news is that wrong-site surgery is 100 percent preventable. The American Academy of Orthopaedic Surgeons urges its members to sign their initials directly on the site to be operated on before the surgery.

OTHER STEPS YOU CAN TAKE

14. Speak up if you have questions or concerns.

You have a right to question anyone who is involved with your care.

15. Make sure that someone, such as your personal doctor, is in charge of your care.

This is especially important if you have many health problems or are in a hospital.

16. Make sure that all health professionals involved in your care have important health information about you.

Do not assume that everyone knows everything they need to.

17. Ask a family member or friend to be there with you and to be your advocate (someone who can help get things done and speak up for you if you can't).

Even if you think you don't need help now, you might need it later.

18. Know that "more" is not always better.

It is a good idea to find out why a test or treatment is needed and how it can help you. You could be better off without it.

19. If you have a test, don't assume that no news is good news.

Ask about the results.

20. Learn about your condition and treatments by asking your doctor and nurse and by using other reliable sources.

For example, treatment recommendations based on the latest scientific evidence are available from the National Guidelines Clearinghouse at www. guideline.gov. Ask your doctor if your treatment is based on the latest evidence.

More Information

Select for more online information about medical errors. A Federal report on medical errors can be accessed online, and a print copy (Publication No. OM 00-0004) is available from the AHRQ Publications Clearinghouse: phone, 1-800-358-9295 (outside the United States, please call 410-381-3150) or E-mail: ahrqpubs@ahrq.gov.

AHRQ Publication No. 00-PO38
Current as of February 2000

Internet Citation:

20 Tips to Help Prevent Medical Errors. Patient Fact Sheet. AHRQ Publication No. 00-PO38, February 2000. Agency for Healthcare Research and Quality, Rockville, MD. www.ahrq.gov/consumer/20tips.htm

CHAPTER 11

Modifying the Care Plan through Patient Progress and Outcome Assessment

> "Nothing is more dangerous
> than an idea when it is the only
> one we have."
>
> Neal Whitman

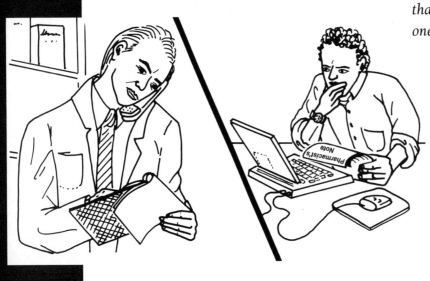

Chapter Outline:

- ❖ **Evaluate the Results and Outcomes from Implementation of the Care Plan**
  Assess Patient Status and Condition
  Assess Achievement of Desired Endpoints
  Assess the Reliability of Monitoring Data Collected from the Patient
- ❖ **Assess the Validity of Monitoring Data Collected from the Patient**
  Evaluate Reasons for Success or Failure in Achievement of Desired Endpoints
  Assess Need for Additional or Missing Information/Data

- ❖ **Document the Patient Progress and Outcomes in the Record**
- ❖ **Determine Changes to the Care Plan That You Would Recommend**
- ❖ **Document Recommended Changes to the Patient's Care Plan**
- ❖ **Implement the Revised Care Plan**

Objectives / To be able to understand:

1. the patient's overall health status and condition, and determine whether the desired endpoint or outcome for each monitoring parameter has been achieved;

2. the reliability of monitoring data collected from the patient;

3. the validity of monitoring data collected from the patient;

4. if a change in the care goals, care plan, implementation, or monitoring plan is needed;

5. a systematic approach to document your assessment and recommendations for changes in the care goals, care plan, implementation, or monitoring plan; and

6. the patient to design or modify the therapeutic regimen and overall care plan using the monitoring data available to you.

Purpose: In this chapter you will learn how to reassess the patient's response to the initial care plan implementation and revise the plan to continue to improve the patient's care.

Progress as well as outcomes assessment is needed with patients because responses are so individual. The effectiveness of medication that is optimally selected and used has the chance to produce positive results matching published studies designed to test the drug's effect. For most medication, however, an optimal response is observed in less than 100% of patients. Added to this fact is the knowledge that nonadherence is the most common problem associated with medication use. Prescription medicine misuse was identified by the National Council on Patient Information and Education (NCPIE) as "America's other drug problem" in 1997.[1] NCPIE outlines the vast use of prescription medications, with projections that the number of retail prescriptions will exceed 4 billion in 2004. The most common therapeutic service of physicians in office practice is prescribing, with 65.1% of the visits concluding with prescriptions being written. More than 36% end with two or more prescriptions being written, and 10% of visits end in four or more prescriptions being written.[2]

The fastest growing segment of the population will be 45–64 years of age by the year 2010. Healthy People 2010 is a set of objectives for the nation to achieve over the first decade of the new century. Two previous decades of reports were motivated by the U.S. surgeon generals (beginning in 1979). The Healthy People 2010 was developed through a broad consultation process built upon scientific knowledge and designed to measure programs over time.[3] The Healthy People 2010 goals have indicated that 95% of patients should receive verbal counseling from their prescribers and pharmacists on appropriate use and potential risks of medications.[3] This is an important social objective for our nation's health care.

But the lack of accurate knowledge that care providers possess about their patients' medication use is staggering. One research project determined that a 76% discrepancy rate exists between the medicines a patient actually takes (self-reported) from the medicines that were prescribed. Over half of these discrepancies were related to a lack of records with care providers about medication use by patients.[4]

In 14 years' time, sale of nonprescription or over-the-counter (OTC) medicines has increased by more than 60%. Expenditures on direct-to-consumer advertising have grown 50% per year since 1997, totaling $1.9 billion in 1999. In 1989, spending was just $12 million. Yet, prior to the introduction of the Medicare Improvement Act of 2003, one in three Medicare beneficiaries had no prescription drug coverage.[5]

Adverse drug reactions (ADRs) are estimated to be the fourth to sixth leading cause of death in the United States. Researchers found that in 1994, over 2.2 million hospitalized patients had serious ADRs, and 106,000 patients had fatal ADRs. Serious ADRs occurred in 6.7% of hospitalized patients.[6] These figures support the importance and relevance of the Healthy People 2010 goal.

When should a followup visit be scheduled with the patient? If followup is scheduled by you, then you will want to decide the earliest timeframe required to meet the first monitoring event in the care plan. For acute condition management, you may have cause to follow up the same day or within a 24-hour period, for example. On the other hand, multiple medication management, complex conditions, complex medication administration technologies, and chronic disease management approaches will require multiple followup visits to improve the patient's response to therapy through outcome assessment and redesign of the care plan.

EVALUATE THE RESULTS AND OUTCOMES FROM IMPLEMENTATION OF THE CARE PLAN

It is time for the patient to return for a visit. Alternatively, the patient places a followup phone call to tell you how things have gone. You discuss how he or she has responded to the care plan that you both developed. Did it work? This step seems straightforward and simple. But this is not necessarily the case. Between the time you and the patient developed a plan, much has often happened. The patient may not have decided to either fill or take the medication as planned. New problems may emerge that were not present at the last encounter. The patient's condition may change or drug therapy might be altered by a different provider. Likewise, when a medication is added, you may have to reconsider your assessment of several therapeutic issues. Finally, with time or additional information, your perception of the patient's situation or behavior may alter your previous assessment. Your perception of the information may change if the patient is diagnosed with a new medical problem or the severity of a medical problem changes. Because such modifications occur, you must regularly ascertain any changes using your metacognitive skills. **Figure 11-1** represents the dynamic nature of medication management and patient adherence.

Assess Patient Status and Condition

As new information emerges, you evaluate changes by comparing the baseline data from the various sources to current data. You should talk with the patient whenever it is practical to determine any changes. After completing this step, you should keep the general list of patient health needs up to date.

Assess Achievement of Desired Endpoints

Outcome success should be defined as responding as well as expected to the agreed upon treatment preferences of the patient. Assessing this response includes both interviewing and listening to the patient to determine the subjective and objective information needed to compare the expected monitoring endpoints to the original care plan goals. You should monitor adherence with the prescribed treatment at every patient visit. Following up outside of scheduled visits is appropriate. It is important to respect a patient's right to confidentiality when sharing medication-use experience with the patient's other health care providers, including nurses, pharmacists, physicians, and physician assistants. One method to assess patient adherence is using a monitoring form that can be incorporated into the patient's record you maintain. It is clear that implementation of systems to help you understand the patient's behavior will provide essential information to assist the patient in overcoming barriers and improving outcomes.

Assess the Reliability of Monitoring Data Collected from the Patient

Some monitoring data that you collect from the patient will be reliable (i.e., you can depend on the accuracy of that data each time you collect it). For example, you may have a patient that conducts home blood pressure monitoring using a cuff that keeps track of blood pressure readings and prints out a report or stores it for retrieval via computer. With proper education and training, the patient can use the device and obtain results that are repeatable over time, make sense, and reflect the experience of the patient. On the other hand, you may have a patient who is having more than one person take the blood pressure readings using a manual cuff. Variation in technique and skill can result in less reliable readings. Knowing the method and quality characteristics of the outcomes data being provided will help you assess

reliability. You have the expertise to advise the patient about how to achieve reliable monitoring data.

ASSESS THE VALIDITY OF MONITORING DATA COLLECTED FROM THE PATIENT

Validity relates to the appropriateness of the data being gathered to reflect what you want to measure or monitor in the first place. Some professionals suggest that monitoring refills of medications from the pharmacy are a valid measure of adherence. However, as we have learned in Chapter 10, there are many legitimate reasons why a person might not fill the prescription and then obtain the refill from the same pharmacy location. Someone may erroneously conclude that monitoring medication refills is always a valid measure of adherence. This is a measure that lacks specificity and is, therefore, not necessarily a valid reflection of adherence.

Evaluate Reasons for Success or Failure in Achievement of Desired Endpoints

Communication is the key to assessing success or failure in achievement of desired endpoints. Your skills in conducting an indepth interview of the patient to determine progress will be instrumental in the quality and accuracy of your evaluation. Healthy People 2010 emphasizes that the primary solution to improving the patient's use, and subsequent outcomes associated with medications, is to communicate about safe, effective medicine use. The "Medical Product Safety" objectives in Healthy People 2010 include the following:

- Increase the proportion of primary care providers, pharmacists, and other health care professionals who routinely review all new prescribed and OTC medicines with their patients aged 65 years and older and with patients who have chronic illnesses or disabilities.
- Increase the proportion of patients receiving information that meets guidelines for usefulness when their new prescriptions are dispensed.
- Increase the proportion of patients who receive verbal counseling from both prescribers and pharmacists on appropriate use and potential risks of medications.

A recent survey of older adults indicated that only 12% of respondents said they used "information sheets from pharmacists," and only 14% used "instructions from a doctor or nurse" to help them increase medicine compliance.[7] Today's new consumer is armed with health care information. However, your patients must tell you about all the medicines they're taking, and be truthful about their lifestyle and about their medicine compliance. It is this personal history and exchange that

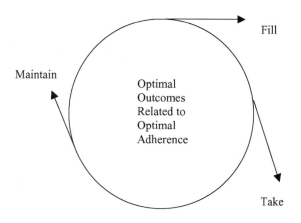

Figure 11-1. Adherence cycle studied—theoretical framework.

Fill

Maintain

Optimal
Outcomes
Related to
Optimal
Adherence

Take

will reveal much of what you really need to know. You, in turn, cannot depend upon written education to influence the patient's behavior alone. Your ongoing relationship, which involves promoting counseling and continuous communication, is essential.

Assess Need for Additional or Missing Information/Data

Your care plan should serve as a guide for determining the missing information or data you need to assess patient progress. For example, if the patient has diabetes, the plan should include identification of indicators such as fasting blood glucose, HgbA$_1$c, results of ophthalmologic exams, and other items identified for monitoring at followup visits. An increasing number of medical conditions have practice guidelines or standards of care that should be met by all care providers. Guidelines for asthma, diabetes, dyslipidemia, congestive heart failure, and other conditions have been developed. These guidelines provide recommended monitoring parameters to follow, and the timeframe and frequency with which to measure them. The return visits for monitoring are more focused on these important aspects of patient care and less on a global assessment of health. The return visit can be efficient and is used to provide patient feedback. This visit is not to suggest that you no longer pay attention to the patient's overall health needs. A balance should be achieved of these two aspects, with the focus adjusted to correspond with the status of the patient's health.

DOCUMENT THE PATIENT PROGRESS AND OUTCOMES IN THE RECORD

Documentation of progress and outcomes takes place following the same guidelines for preparing written progress notes presented earlier in the chapters. However, all of the information that comprehensively describes the progress and plan does not need to be repeated. Rather, documentation should reflect the impact of the therapeutic plan on the subjective and objective data included in your monitoring parameters. At this point, you are documenting progress to make decisions to either maintain or alter the plan.

DETERMINE CHANGES TO THE CARE PLAN THAT YOU WOULD RECOMMEND

Care plan changes emerge when your monitoring data indicate that the plan is not working in a desirable way. Changes are likely most of the time, as it often takes several visits involving assessment to determine what needs to be changed in order to achieve the desired outcomes. Changes are required when a patient experiences adverse effects or reactions, suboptimal therapeutic responses, treatments that are incompatible with lifestyle, or is nonadherent. You must evaluate each problem and how you will change the care plan. You must also anticipate what the impact will be on all other patient concerns when you decide the changes that you will recommend. Each change must be evaluated and its impact determined. In complex patient cases, you will find that you must systematically make changes in increments that allow you to determine the impact of the change by evaluating specific monitoring parameters at each point. It may take four or more visits with a patient to first conduct an initial comprehensive assessment and then implement incremental changes with monitoring parameters.

DOCUMENT RECOMMENDED CHANGES TO THE PATIENT'S CARE PLAN

Documentation requires expressing enough fundamental information in each note that you will be able to discern the importance of your observations without a comprehensive review of the chart. At a minimum, you should identify the problem that the note is addressing, the monitoring parameter, the outcome observed, and the revision to the plan. The revision should include a description of the modification to the treatment and the monitoring parameters that will be followed to assess response.

IMPLEMENT THE REVISED CARE PLAN

Revised care plans place a greater emphasis on monitoring. It is the "tweaking" stage of care. Or, in other words, tweaking implies that you are trying to modify rather than take large leaps in changing care. Your goal is to optimize the response that a patient has to treatment approaches rather than starting over with very different approaches. The monitoring plan developed should be reasonable for the patient, pharmacist, and primary care provider, when necessary. The checklist used to implement the care plan has been expanded to include the reassessment steps and is included here for your use (**Figure 11-2**).

SUMMARY

Progress and outcomes assessment is a critical component to achieving health improvements through use of pharmaceuticals and your supportive services to patients. Even in the ideal situation, not all patients experience the desired or expected outcomes from the medica-

CHECKLIST FOR PATIENT CARE PLAN REVISION AND FOLLOWUP

Check when completed	**Step in Care Plan Implementation**
	Evaluate the results and outcomes from implementation of the care plan • *Assess patient status and condition* • *Assess achievement of desired endpoints* • *Evaluate reasons for success or failure in achievement of desired endpoints* • *Assess need for additional or missing information/data.*
	Determine changes to the care plan you would recommend
	Recommend the care plan to the appropriate individuals • *Patient* • *Health care providers* • *Caretakers*
	Ensure that medication orders and/or prescriptions are written to facilitate care and monitoring of the patient
	Ensure patient receives medications and supportive technologies
	Conduct counseling relevant to the care plan • *Patient resources*
	Use methods of counseling to optimize patient adherence
	Document recommended changes to the patient's care plan • *Communicate with the primary health care provider*
	Document patient/caregiver response to care plan
	Document types of notes documented in the patient record
	Educate patients about how to contact you and other health professionals • *Business card*
	Ensure patient followup is scheduled

Figure 11-2. Expanded Checklist

tion and use plan. An individualized approach to understanding the patient's behavior is needed in order to assist him or her to achieve health improvement. No other care professional has access to both the product and the patient. Therefore, this situation creates a powerful opportunity for you to achieve success on behalf of the patient.

CASES

See pages 248–254 for cases.

Case 1: *Lauren Smith returns to the pharmacist's consultation and care visit for monitoring and followup with Nasir.*

Nasir: "It's great to see you, Lauren. Why don't we go through and see how you have been doing with this care plan?"

Lauren: "Good."

Nasir: "Have you had a return of any of your symptoms for the urinary tract infection?"

Lauren: "No. I have been drinking the water and haven't had any problems since."

Nasir: "Excellent. Tell me about the headaches."

Lauren: "Well, I have had three since I last saw you. I tried acetaminophen, and it seems to help. The headaches go away pretty quickly and are less intense. I haven't tried anything else."

Nasir: "Do you believe that acetaminophen is an adequate treatment for this problem for the time being?"

Lauren: "I think so. I would like to quit smoking first and see how it goes."

Nasir: (He takes Lauren's blood pressure while they sit and talk.) "How have you done with taking the hydrochlorothiazide?"

Lauren: "I have done very well. I have the medicine in the kitchen and, when I get my morning coffee, I take one."

Nasir: "Well, your blood pressure is lower…looks very good at 126/82. I think we have a good solution for this for the time being." (Lauren looks very pleased.) "You have done a good job, Lauren."

Lauren: "Thanks so much, Nasir. I really appreciate your support and feedback."

Nasir: "Now the really tough one. How is the stop smoking effort going?"

Lauren (beaming again): "I have not had a cigarette for 12 days straight. This is one of the toughest things I have done. I filled out the questionnaire for you."

Nasir: "This is great, Lauren. There is one trigger area to pay attention to—being around smoke."

[Nasir looks it over and finds a couple of trouble or trigger areas to pay attention to. He immediately counsels Lauren to pay attention to this and concentrate on avoiding it (**Figure 11-3**).]

Nasir: "The gum, if working properly, should eventually be tapered. Have you started the taper schedule?"

Lauren: "Yes. I haven't gone quite as quickly as is written on the instruction, but I am decreasing the quantity."

Nasir: "Terrific! As long as you are headed in the right direction, this should work!"

Nasir: "We really didn't finalize the birth control approach. What have you decided to do, Lauren?"

Lauren: "Well…I am not seeing anyone and finally decided that my break from the pill or patch would be much better for my health at this time. So …I stopped using them. We will see how it goes."

Nasir: "Well, it is a tough choice. I am pleased that you were able to come to a decision. Please remember that you need to use barrier protection at all times when sexually active; and there are some protections for you as well. As you are probably aware, using barrier protection helps to prevent AIDS transmission, herpes, and other sexually transmitted diseases. If you decide to restart the pill, make sure that you include barrier protection for at least one complete month after you start the pill again. But talk to me about this if you find you want to return to the pill" (**Figure 11-4**).

Nasir: "Here is my business card with my phone number and alternative emergency contact number. Let's check back again in another 4 weeks."

Lauren: "Thanks so much, Nasir. I will make an appointment for follow up with Joe at the check-out area again."

CASE 1: SPECIFIC QUESTIONS

1. Given Lauren's age and social circumstances, what might you anticipate changing in Lauren's situation to challenge her ability to quit smoking?

2. If acetaminophen did not provide acceptable relief, what other medicines should Nasir recommend to Lauren for self-treatment?

QUESTIONNAIRE: STOP SMOKING

For: *Lauren Smith*
Please return this questionnaire on your next visit!

Questions to Think About

Think about the following questions before you try to stop smoking. You may want to talk about your answers with your health care provider.

1. Why do you want to quit?
Lauren's response: *I don't like thinking I am making myself sick by smoking. I also don't like my appearance and having to cover up my breath.*

2. When you tried to quit in the past, what helped and what didn't?
Lauren's response: *I would chew gum and eat celery. These would help me. I would also try to relax - take a hot bath, do some sewing.*

3. What will be the most difficult situations for you after you quit? How will you plan to handle them?
Lauren's response: *Being around smoke. I will try to avoid it, but if I am going somewhere where there is smoke, I will take the chewing gum.*

4. Who can help you through the tough times? Your family? Friends? Health care provider?
Lauren's response: *I have a good girlfriend who doesn't smoke and has been on me to quit. I will contact Nasir if I am failing.*

5. What pleasures do you get from smoking? What ways can you still get pleasure if you quit?
Lauren's response: *I will try to expand my cooking and will also try to do my sewing hobby more.*

Here are some questions to ask your health care provider.

1. How can you help me to be successful at quitting?
2. What medication do you think would be best for me and how should I take it?
3. What should I do if I need more help?
4. What is smoking withdrawal like? How can I get information on withdrawal?

Quitting takes hard work and a lot of effort, but you can quit smoking.

Figure 11-3. Sample Smoking Questionnaire

Pharmacy Profile for:

Patient:	Smith, Lauren		New Patient	Print	Close Record

Demographic	OTC / Allergy		Insurance	Diagnosis	Contacts
General Health	Care Plans	Surveys	Account Status		Current Therapy
General Information	Illnesses	Systems Review	Vital Signs		Lab Values

Pharmacist's Progress Note - continued: Date: 02-10

S: Headaches decreased in frequency and intensity, but continue. Response to acetaminophen. Patient reports no smoking for 12 days. Chose to quit birth control pill and use the barrier method. Presently sexually inactive
O: BP #3 126/82.
A: Responsive to acetaminophen, not using Advil. Questionnaire reveals smoke exposure and environment where smoking takes place as triggers. Responsive to hydrochlorothiazide, no smoking for 12 days and lack of Advil use.
Plan:
#1 – UTI - Problem resolved – no return of signs or symptoms.
#2 – Headaches - Continue use of acetaminophen as needed.
#3 – Hypertension - Continue hydrochlorothiazide.
#4 - Smoking - Monitor for 4 weeks.
#5 – Method of birth control - Will follow up at next visit to determine if patient has continued with the choice.

Figure 11-4. Pharmacy Profile

Case 2: *Christine conducts a care visit for monitoring and followup with Mr. Montanez.*

Christine: "It is wonderful to see you, Mr. Montanez. We have several areas to assess regarding your progress and satisfaction. How do you feel about the visual correction?"

Mr. Montanez: "It is wonderful. I am pleased that I now have it." (The conversation continues through all of the issues in **Table 11-1**.)

Christine: "I am giving you a prescription for hydrochlorothiazide. This medicine is to help keep your blood pressure lower so that you do not have hypertension. The medicine is mild, and I am giving you a low dose."

Mr. Montanez: "Why do I need to take this?"

Christine: "This is medicine that will keep your blood pressure lower. Keeping it lower will reduce your risk of strokes or heart attacks. You will get to enjoy your family and loved ones longer."

Mr. Montanez: "You know…I can read the label. This is a change!"

Christine: "Good! I will give you more to read then!" (Mr. Montanez smiles. The visit concludes after the care plan modification discussion ends, and Christine provides her business card.)

Document the patient progress and outcomes in the record.

CASE 2: SPECIFIC QUESTIONS

1. Prepare a progress note using all of the available information displayed here among Christine, Mr. Montanez, and Maria.
2. Discuss your plan with others. Are there other considerations you might incorporate into the plan?

Case 3: *Luisa conducts patient counseling and followup 1 month later for Huong.*

Huong Tran returns with the social worker for a followup visit to determine how he is doing with his asthma control.

Luisa: "Hello, Huong. I am so happy to see you! I hope that your family is well."

Huong: "Yes, Luisa, they are very good."

Luisa: "I am pleased to know that. How has your breathing been?"

Huong: "Much better. I haven't had to come to the Emergency Room."

Luisa: "That is good, too."

[Luisa proceeds to ask a series of questions as a follow up that are provided by the National Asthma Education and Prevention Program (see page 252). Luisa then proceeds to provide education following the approach, as outlined in **Figure 11-5**. She directly observes and reinforces correct inhaler use behavior as shown in **Figure 11-6**. But Huong is an 8 year old. He may not be able to respond to all of these questions, as asked here in this manner. After asking a series of questions, Luisa determines that Huong's overall asthma status is improved and does not believe there is a need to change his medication.]

Luisa: "Please show me how you use your inhaler."

Huong: "Okay, Luisa." (He makes a few mistakes, and she assists him to correct this.)

Luisa: "You have done an excellent job of using your inhaler regularly, Huong. I am so pleased it has gone well. Please keep getting your prescriptions refilled with the help of the social worker and your family."

Huong: "I will, Luisa. Thank you."

CASE 3: SPECIFIC QUESTIONS

1. What did Luisa do well that supports her effectiveness in promoting Huong's compliance with his inhaler therapy?
2. Were any clues provided by Huong to suggest that a change was needed in his drug therapy?
3. Visit the questions provided for use by the National Heart, Lung and Blood Institute shown in Figure 11-1. How would you rephrase these questions in a way that an 8-year-old child is more likely to be able to understand?

Table 11-1. Problem Assessment

Problem	Status	Plan of Action
Vision	Not corrected	1. Assessed response to Mr. Montanez's visual correction. He is complying with wearing his glasses and finds this an improvement.
Diabetes	Poorly controlled	S: Maria states that he continues to use Cactus Flowers and Yucca. However, he is taking his Diabinese and his Tolinase every day as he is supposed to. O: Fasting Blood Sugar = 200 mg%. A: He is partially adherent to this regimen – taking his oral medication but also allowing his relatives to treat him. Overall, his blood sugar has improved but is not ideal. P: 1. Encourage continuing the oral medication and reinforce with Maria how good it is that his blood glucose has decreased. Keep up the good work. Do not work at reducing home treatments at this time. Continue to monitor for the potential for hypoglycemia as he gets closer to goal blood glucose. 2. Address alcohol use. This must be reduced to a drink a day. Work at this goal to improve glycemic control. 3. Monitor $HgbA_1c$ at next visit; expect lower value than 12.5 mg% 4. Monitor Fasting Blood Sugar; expect lower value than 200 g%.
Neuropathy – 2ndary to diabetes	Painful	1. Neuropathy not noticeably improved. 2. Consider pharmacologic therapy if no improvement in comfort once diabetes is controlled.
Nocturia	Long standing	1. Control diabetes 2. If not corrected with improved diabetes control, consider alternative causes.
Suspected hypertension		1. Patient blood pressure at 147/98 2. Initiate thiazide-type diuretic. Given his age and concurrent conditions – may be responsive to 12.5 mgs po qd for blood pressure control. Initiate prescription.
Immunization status		1. Interviewed Mr. Montanez about history. Reviewed medical charts available. Provided the following immunizations: Tetanus diphtheria; MMR; pneumoccal vaccine.
Dyslipidemia		1. Initiate statin therapy at low dose. 2. Schedule visit with dietitian for dyslipidemia, diabetes and hypertension. 3. Confirm patient is not adherent to aspirin. He is afraid it will cause a stomach bleed because this happened to a close friend. We decided not to continue the aspirin at this time; I want to gain more confidence in me and my intentions with the patient.

Assessment Questions	Information	Skills
	Recommendations for Initial Visit	
Focus on: • **Expectations of visit** • **Goals of treatment** • **Medications** • **Quality of life**	**Teach in simple language:**	**Teach or review and demonstrate:**
"What worries you most about your asthma?" "What do you want to accomplish at this visit?" "What do you want to be able to do that you can't do now because of your asthma?" "What do you expect from treatment?" "What medicines have you tried?" "What other questions do you have for me today?"	**What is asthma?** A chronic lung disease. The airways are very sensitive. They become inflamed and narrow; breathing becomes difficult. Asthma treatments; two types of medicine are needed: • Long-term control: medications that prevent symptoms, often by reducing inflammation • Quick relief: short-acting bronchodilator relaxes muscles around airways Bring all medications to every appointment. When to seek medical advice. Provide appropriate telephone number.	Inhaler (see Figure 11-6) and spacer/holding chamber use. Check performance. Self-monitoring skills that are tied to an action plan: • Recognize intensity and frequency of asthma symptoms • Review the signs of deterioration and the need to reevaluate therapy: • Waking at night with asthma • Increased medication use • Decreased activity tolerance Use of a simple, written self-management plan and action plan (see Table 11-1)
	Recommendations for First Followup Visit (2 to 4 weeks or sooner as needed)	
Focus on: • **Expectations of visit** • **Goals of treatment** • **Medications** • **Quality of life**	**Teach in simple language:**	**Teach or review and demonstrate:**
Ask relevant questions from previous visit and also ask: "What medications are you taking?" "How and when are you taking them?" "What problems have you had using your medications?" "Please show me how you use your inhaled medications."	Use of two types of medications. Remind patient to bring all medications and the peak flow meter to every appointment for review. Self-evaluation of progress in asthma control using symptoms and peak flow as a guide.	Use of a daily self-management plan. Review and adjust as needed. Use of an action plan. Review and adjust as needed. Peak flow monitoring and daily diary recording. Correct inhaler and spacer/holding chamber technique.

Figure 11-5. Delivery of asthma education by clinicians during patient care visits.

Please demonstrate your inhaler technique at every visit.

1.   Remove the cap and hold inhaler upright.
2.   Shake the inhaler.
3.   Tilt your head back slightly and breathe out slowly.
4.   Position the inhaler in one of the following ways (A or B is optimal, but C is acceptable for those who have difficulty with A or B. C is required for breath-activated inhalers):

 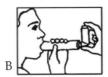

A   B   C   D

A. Open mouth with inhaler 1 to 2 inches away.
B. Use spacer/holding chamber (that is recommended especially for young children and for people using corticosteroids).

C. In the mouth. Do not use for corticosteroids.
D. NOTE: Inhaled dry powder capsules require a different inhalation technique. To use a dry powder inhaler, it is important to close the mouth tightly around the mouthpiece of the inhaler and to inhale rapidly.

5.   Press down on the inhaler to release medication as you start to breathe in slowly.
6.   Breathe in slowly (3 to 5 seconds).
7.   Hold your breath for 10 seconds to allow the medicine to reach deeply into your lungs.
8.   Repeat puff as directed. Waiting 1 minute between puffs may permit second puff to penetrate your lungs better.
9.   Spacers/holding chambers are useful for all patients. They are particularly recommended for young older children and adults and for use with inhaled steroids.

Avoid common inhaler mistakes. Follow these inhaler tips:
- Breathe out *before* pressing your inhaler.
- Inhale *slowly*.
- Breathe in through your mouth, not your nose.
- Press down on your inhaler at the *start* of inhalation (or within the first second of inhalation).
- Keep inhaling as you press down on inhaler.
- Press your inhaler only *once* while you are inhaling (one breath for each puff).
- Make sure you breathe in evenly and deeply.

NOTE: Other inhalers are becoming available in addition to those illustrated above. Different types of inhalers may require different techniques.

Figure 11-6. Steps for using your inhaler.

Case 4: *Michael Jones prepares Mr. Robinson for medication management post-discharge from the hospital.*

Michael Jones follows up the next morning and finds that Mr. Robinson's INR has risen to 1.7 (a good rise in response to the dose of warfarin being used). He looks over the remainder of the chart notes from others and decides that warfarin 4 mg orally every day is a good plan for discharge for Mr. Robinson (**Figure 11-7**).

Michael (enters Mr. Robinson's room): "Good morning, Mr. Robinson."

Mr. Robinson: "Good mornin'. I am pleased to see you today. I am ready to go home!"

Michael: "Well, it sounds like everyone around here thinks it's time for you to go home too. So this is good news. I know that a social worker is going to be by soon to discuss your at-home needs. I am here to talk about your warfarin—we sometimes refer to it as your blood thinner. We will go through this patient education sheet together. I will also get your prescriptions ready for you so, when you leave, you will be all set."

Mr. Robinson: "I am so pleased we are able to do this. This medicine really scares me, and I want to do it right."

Michael: "I know you will do well with this, Mr. Robinson. I also believe it is good if you let me educate your friends who have been visiting you regularly too. It is always better to have everyone around you informed about what your needs are and what the right things are that need to be done. They care about you a great deal and will probably feel some relief if they have the knowledge to do the right things."

Mr. Robinson: "Yes, son. I think you are right about that. I know that they would really appreciate it. Thank you for taking the time to do it."

[Michael Jones begins the counseling and completes a progress note afterward (**Figure 11-8**). Michael leaves his business card with Mr. Robinson for use at home and also leaves one for the social worker.]

GENERAL ASSESSMENT QUESTIONS

1. Why is it necessary to reassess the patient's general health and condition each time you visit with him or her to follow up on the care plan progress?
2. What are some things that following a monitoring parameter in a patient can inform you about?
3. What type of responses to a care plan would prompt a referral to the primary care provider?

ASSIGNMENT

1. Visit a pharmacist who maintains a clinical practice site. Shadow the pharmacist to observe how he or she reassesses the progress of the patients. Discuss the way in which the pharmacist monitors the patient and uses the information observed to alter the care plan. Does the pharmacist have conversations with the patients? Other health professionals? Family members or caretakers? What are the advantages and limitations with each type of relationship? How can you overcome the limitations?

REFERENCES

1. Anon. The other drug problem. New York Public Television Station WLIW; 1997.
2. National Ambulatory Medical Care Survey: 1998 Summary, Advance Data from Vital and Health Statistics. No. 315; July 19, 2000.
3. www.healthypeople.gov. Healthy People 2010; accessed March 2004.
4. Michael Hash. Health Care Financing Administration, Department of HHS, prepared statement, Subcommittee on Health and the Environment, House of Representatives, U.S. Congress; Sept. 28, 1999.
5. Bedell SE, Jabbour S, Goldberg R et. al. Discrepancies in the use of medications: their extent and predictors in an outpatient practice. *Arch Intern Med.* 2000; July 24 160(14):2129–34.
6. Lazarou J, Pomeranz B, Corey P. Incidence of adverse drug reactions in hospitalized patients. *JAMA.* 1998; 279(15):1200–5.
7. FCB Healthworks. New York, NY; 1999.

Patient Name:

_____

Date of Initial Instruction:

_____

	Initial Instruction Completed – no further instruction required	Patient Needs Additional Education	Repeat Education Provided	Patient Unable to Understand after Repeat Instruction	Comments	Initials
1. Previous anticoagulation Hx: None Yes Preexisting knowledge of AC: None Yes						
2. General information, ACS; diagnosis, expectations of therapy and patient obligations						
3. Explanation of warfarin with other medications. Discussed the risks and benefits of AC						
4. Need for regular blood tests						
5. Use of warfarin with other medications						
6. Symptoms to report to provider						
7. Pregnancy						
8. Missed pills/adherence						
9. Time of day to take pills						
10. Alcohol use						
11. Emergency department						
12. ID card and guidelines/book						
13. Calendar						
14. Call back/contacting care provider						
15. Activities of daily living						
16. Travel						
17. Diet (Vitamin K consistency/ETOH use/GI illness)						
18. Risk of bleeding, major and minor, and precautions (shaving/dentist visits/minor cuts, etc.)						
19. Patient comprehends all of the above information and is ready for AC outpatient therapy						

Pharmacist's Signature _____   Date: _____

Figure 11-7. Anticoagulation teaching checklist – inpatient service, Madison Hospitals and Health Systems.

Madison Hospitals and Health Systems	Patient Identification (Stamp)
	Name: **Samuel Robinson**
	Reg. No. **02946372**
PROGRESS NOTES	Location: **INPT 347-1**
	Date: **09-2-04**

Anticoagulation Care Progress Note by Pharmacist

9/4/04 10:30 a.m.
O: INR = 1.7 after 3 days of warfarin 4 mgs po qd.
A: Maintain warfarin 4 mgs po qd every day. Will verify PT/INR in a.m. Expect this dose to be the stable dose for discharge.
P: Provided discharge counseling program for warfarin and completed patient education sheet with Mr. Robinson. Provided educational brochures, manuals, medication tracking chart, and medication organizer for daily medication use. Have requested social work to assess in home assistance based on IADL's. Follow up appointment to check INR within 14 days of discharge.

Michael Jones, RPh
_____
Pharmacists Signature/phone extension or pager

Figure 11-8. Progress notes.

Appendices

APPENDIX A: GLOSSARY

Action Plan – a proactive document that describes your goals, what actions you will take, and when you will take them.

Acupuncture - an original Chinese practice of puncturing the body with needles at specific points to cure disease or relieve pain (as in surgery).

Adherence – the act, action, or quality of consistently behaving in a manner that is expected; used in the context of medication use or care plan steps.

Advocate – a person who pleads the cause of another.

Ambulatory Care Setting – care provided in outpatient and clinic environment(s).

Audit - an examination or review that establishes the extent to which a condition, process, or performance conforms to predetermined standards or criteria.

Auscultation – listening to the sounds made by various body structures and functions as a diagnostic method, usually with a stethoscope.

Biofeedback - the technique of manipulating unconscious or involuntary bodily processes (e.g., blood pressure) made perceptible to the senses (e.g., sphygmomanometer—blood pressure cuff) by conscious mental control.

Biomedical Model - the conceptual framework for the practice of Western medicine. The model describes disease in terms of symptoms and the pathology that, in part, is attributed to the cause of these symptoms. "Health" in this model is the absence of disease.

Care - assistive, supportive, or facilitative acts toward, or for, another individual or group with evident or anticipated needs to ameliorate or improve a human condition or life way.

Caring - direct and indirect nurturing and skillful activities, processes, and decisions related to assisting people in a manner that reflects behaviors that are empathetic, supportive, compassionate, protective, educational, *and others*; and dependent upon the needs, problems, values, and goals of the individual or group being assisted.

Centers for Disease Control and Prevention (CDC) – the lead federal agency for protecting the health and safety of people at home and abroad, providing credible information to enhance health decisions and promoting health through strong partnerships. CDC serves as the national focus for developing and applying disease prevention and control, environmental health, and health promotion and educational activities to improve the lives of people in the United States.

Chiropractic - a system of therapy using manipulation and specific adjustment of body structures such as the spinal column. It is based upon the premise that disease results from a lack of normal nerve function.

Clinical – relating to the direct observation of a patient to determine the course and symptoms of a disease or condition.

Clinical Guideline –an evidence-based, systematically developed statement to assist practitioners and patients in making appropriate decisions for specific clinical circumstances.

Clinical Performance – a method to monitor the extent to which the actions of a health care provider conform to clinical performance guidelines.

Clinical Reasoning/Clinical Problem Solving – terms used interchangeably to refer to the problem-solving process that clinicians employ with patient problems.

Clinical Research – patient-oriented research conducted with human subjects (or on material of human origin such as tissues, specimens, and cognitive phenomena) for which an investigator (or colleague) directly interacts with human subjects.

Clinician – the person encountering the patient in a professional relationship who evaluates the patient and recommends care.

Collaborative Practice Agreement - agreements by which practitioners of medicine, osteopathy, podiatry (or others), and pharmacists enter into voluntary, written agreements to improve outcomes for their mutual patients using drug therapies, laboratory tests, and medical devices. These agreements usually describe how one practitioner delegates authority to another to act within the scope of practice of another practitioner (e.g., pharmacist prescribing medication under a physician's delegated authority).

Compliance – see the term "adherence."

Computerized Physician (or Practitioner) Order Entry (CPOE) – a method of entering orders for patient care into a computerized system. It is intended to replace the use of paper.

Confidentiality - entrusted communication of information that is considered private and implies an ethical or legal principle.

Critical Literature Evaluation – a process of determining the overall credibility of an information resource, emphasizing an evaluation of the internal and external validity of a study.

Culture - a set of guidelines, both explicit and implicit, which individuals inherit as members of a particular society, and which tells them how to view the world and how to behave in relationship to other people.

Decentralized Practice – a professional practice in areas

other than the central pharmacy within a hospital or health system (e.g., on the patient care floor).

Delegated Authority - authority to prescribe medications, order tests, or perform procedures given from a practitioner with that power to another practitioner who normally does not have this authority under the law.

Department of Veterans Affairs (VA) – department established on March 15, 1989, succeeding the Veterans Administration, that it is responsible for providing federal benefits to veterans and their dependents. Headed by the Secretary of Veterans Affairs, VA is the second largest of the 15 Cabinet departments and operates nationwide programs for health care, financial assistance, and burial benefits.

Disease – any abnormal condition, affecting either the whole body or any of its parts, which impairs normal functioning.

Documentation – the process of recording relevant patient care information in a readily retrievable format.

Drug Information – the core knowledge that describes the characteristics of drug entities, their actual and potential uses, efficacy, effectiveness, and safety.

Drug of Choice – the pharmaceutical considered optimal, or the first one generally considered most appropriate, to be used for a particular diagnostic, treatment, or prevention.

Drug Utilization Review – review of a prescription, at the time of dispensing (concurrent) or after the fact (retrospective), for appropriateness based on a patient's medical condition, other medications the patient is already receiving, or patient-specific factors that might make the prescribed drug a poor choice. The term can also be applied to retrospective review of large numbers of prescriptions for appropriateness.

Empathy – intellectual and emotional awareness of another person's thoughts, feelings, and behavior, even those that are distressing and disturbing. Empathy emphasizes understanding the ability to sense the patient's experience and feelings accurately as well as communicate that understanding back to the patient.

Ethnocentricity – the interpretation of one culture using the norms of another culture, usually your own.

Evidence-based Practice – an approach to health care practice where the clinician is aware of the evidence in support of a particular practice, the strength of that evidence, and the appropriate application of that evidence to the practice.

Extended Care Setting – care provided in nursing homes, long-term care residences, assisted living, and other partially independent care arrangements.

Genuineness - the ability to be oneself in a relationship and not hide behind a role or façade.

Health – a state of well being that is mainly known and expressed in cultural meanings and ways, values, and beliefs. The concept of a state of well being varies greatly based upon the cultural and values-based context.

Health Literacy – the ability of a person to understand and process the health information available to him or her.

Heuristic - to find out; encouraging or promoting investigation; conducive to discovery.

HIPAA – abbreviation for the Health Insurance Portability and Accountability Act of 1996. The HIPAA regulates the use and disclosure of protected health information by covered entities.

Holistic - considers man as a functioning whole, or relating to the conception of man as a functioning whole. This term is related to holistic health.

Holistic Health - a system of preventive medicine that takes into account the whole individual, his own responsibility for well being and the total influences—social, psychological, environmental—that affect health, including nutrition, exercise, and mental relaxation.

Home Care Setting – care provided in one's home/residence.

Homeopathy - a system of medical practice that treats a disease, especially by the administration of minute doses of a remedy that would in healthy persons produce symptoms similar to those of the disease.

Hypothesis – descriptions of disease processes, pathologic processes, clinical entities or syndromes, etiologic or psychological processes, or social or economic factors that best explain the possible causes for a patient's problems. Initial hypotheses are working guides in clinical reasoning and change with accumulated knowledge.

ICD-9-CM (International Classification of Diseases) Code or Diagnostic Code– a system for assigning a disease label for the diagnosis assigned to a patient's medical problem

Ill-structured Problem – a problem that is characterized by inadequate information about the cause and lack of readily definable guidelines to approach solving it.

Illness – a term used by a patient to express a comprehensive view of not being well, feeling sick, or feeling unhealthy; a patient's personal experience of ill health.

Inspection – see the term "observation."

Malpractice – illegal or immoral conduct; practice contrary to established rules; specifically, the treatment of a case by a surgeon or physician in a manner which is contrary to accepted rules and productive of unfavorable results.

Manipulation – see the term "palpation."

Medical Chart - the permanent record of patient information that is used by health care providers to communicate and document the patient's progress in response to care. The medical chart may serve as a legal document.

Medicare - a benefit in the form of a health care service or supply that is paid by the federal government to qualified U.S. citizens.

Medication Order – a written order of a qualified physician for a medication to be used in the institutional setting. This is the equivalent of a prescription in the outpatient setting.

Metacognition – the continuous process of deliberation and reflection during problem solving.

Monitoring Parameter – a measurement, sign, symptom, or impression that represents the status of a patient in relationship to a specific outcome.

Monitoring Plan – the temporal use of outcome indicators to measure or observe a patient's response to care.

Naturopathy - a system of disease treatment that emphasizes the use of natural agents (such as water or sun exposure, and physical means like manipulation) rather than medications or surgery.

Normal Range – usually determined by applying statistical methods to results from a representative sample of the general population. The normal range represents the range of values where a large percentage (95%) of normal people (i.e., without the illness in question) fall. The average value plus or minus two standard deviations is usually taken as the normal range.

Observation – visual evaluation or assessment of the patient.

On-line Resource – an information resource found through connecting to other computer resources (e.g., Internet access to a web site via high speed cable).

Outcome – the resultant effect that a health care intervention or system change has on patients, systems, organizations, or communities. Outcomes are usually measurable and represent the clinical, economic, or humanistic domain. They represent a change in a patient's current and future health status that can be attributed to antecedent care.

Palpation – touching or feeling the patient with the hand to augment the data gathered through inspection.

Patient – a person who receives care and services from health care professionals.

Patient Encounter – the interchange between the pharmacist and patient during which the pharmacist gathers background information through conducting an interview and assessment to determine the patient's problems and develops a care approach. It is through the encounter that you develop and provide a therapeutic relationship with the patient.

Patient Interview – the communication component of the patient encounter during which you use questioning, listening, and observation skills to gather background information about the patient.

Patient Profile – a general term used to describe the documentation record maintained about the patient

database that is updated throughout the pharmaceutical care process by the pharmacist. It is common to see this term used in community and hospital pharmacy practice.

Percussion – striking of the body surface lightly but sharply to determine the position, size, and density of underlying structures as well as to detect fluid or air in a cavity.

Pharmaceutical Care - the direct, responsible provision of medication-related care for the purpose of achieving definite outcomes that improve a patient's quality of life.

Pharmacotherapeutic Regimen – the drug name, strength, dosage form, route of administration, duration of treatment, and schedule for use of a medication being taken by a patient.

Physical Assessment – the process of evaluating the health status of the patient through identification of the normal state and deviations from this state using the assessment techniques of inspection, palpation, percussion, and auscultation.

Pictogram – a symbol or icon that tells a story. The picture is used to replace written and verbal language that communicates a specific message.

Practitioner – one who exercises a profession.

Prescription - directions written for the preparation and administration of a drug.

Primary Resource – the publication that contains the original research or works, usually found in biomedical journals.

Problem List – a prioritized list of the patient's problems determined through clinical reasoning applied to the various sources of information that support the patient database. The problem list is the guide to care plan development and monitoring, and is updated as the pharmaceutical care process is applied.

Professional Care - cognitive and culturally learned behaviors, techniques and processes, or patterns that enable or assist an individual, family, or community to improve or maintain a favorable healthy condition or way of life.

Proxy Outcome – a measure that represents the likelihood of a particular outcome by virtue of its inherent relationship to that outcome.

Public Health – the science and art of preventing disease, prolonging life, and promoting **health** and efficiency through organized community effort.

Residency – a postgraduate program of organized training that meets the requirements of a residency-accreditation body.

Respect - the ability to accept the patient as a unique person as he or she is and to suspend critical judgment.

Secondary Resource – resources that index or abstract the primary resource literature found in biomedical journals.

Self Care - activities that individuals, families, and communities undertake with the intention of enhancing health, preventing disease, limiting illness, and restoring health.

Self-efficacy Theory - behavioral change facilitated by a personal sense of control. A person who believes in being able to cause an event can conduct a more active and self-determined life course.

Setting – the place where patient care occurs (e.g., community pharmacy, hospital, nursing home, outpatient clinic, emergency room).

Social Learning Theory – the likelihood of a behavior occurring in a given situation is a joint function of the individual's expectancy that the behavior will lead to a particular reinforcement and the extent to which the reinforcement is valued.

Systematic Review of the Literature – a structured literature review that summarizes a topic in a systematic fashion using preset criteria and guidelines for conduct.

Tertiary Resource – professional publications that contain a summary of information in full text, such as textbooks, review articles, compendium, handbooks, and electronic full-text references.

Therapeutic Monitoring – the process of assessing outcomes associated with a treatment to determine the need for modification for the purpose of optimizing the desired outcome.

Therapeutic Relationship – a relationship established between the patient and pharmacist that is characterized by trust, empathy, respect, authenticity, and responsiveness.

U.S. Food and Drug Administration – a scientific, regulatory, and public health agency that oversees items accounting for 25 cents of every dollar spent by consumers. Its jurisdiction encompasses most food products (other than meat and poultry), human and animal drugs, therapeutic agents of biological origin, medical devices, radiation-emitting products for consumer, medical, and occupational use, cosmetics, and animal feed.

Web Site – an electronic file system accessible through the World Wide Web. The address for a web site is called a URL (Universal Resource Locator).

World Health Organization – the United Nations specialized agency for health established on April 7, 1948 (www.who.int/en/).

APPENDIX B: LEARNING SKILLS BY CHAPTER

This table provides you with a high-level view of where the practice foundation knowledge content is organized within this book.

Practice Foundation Knowledge Covered in Each Chapter	Chapter Number										
	1	2	3	4	5	6	7	8	9	10	11
Understanding the patient's concepts of health	●										
Discerning between disease and illness	●										
Understanding the influence of culture on health perceptions	●										
Patient roles in health concepts of medication use	●										
Concepts of pharmaceutical care	●										
Patient–pharmacist relationship	●										
Professional philosophy of practice		●									
Professional culture of pharmacy		●									
Understanding the pharmacist's own personal concept of health and how it affects perceptions about patients		●									
Understanding patient-centered practice		●									
Professional and caring behaviors of pharmacists		●									
Clinical reasoning, empathy, moral reasoning, and metacognition		●									
Pharmacist's role as healer		●									
Pharmacist's roles as generalists and specialists		●									
Goal of expertise in the profession		●									
Social context of pharmacy practice			●								
Organizational context of pharmacy practice			●								
Practice settings of pharmacists			●								
Pharmaceuticals as treatments			●								
Fiscal aspects of pharmacy practice			●								
The pharmaceutical care process				●							
Integration of skills to provide patient care using the pharmaceutical care process				●							
Cognitive and behavioral actions of the pharmacist who provides pharmaceutical care				●							
Organizing the patient encounter interview					●						
Discerning relevant and important use of the mental status assessment in the patient encounter					●						
Questioning skills during the patient encounter					●						
Nonverbal communication during the patient encounter					●						
Physical assessment, problem identification, and drug therapy monitoring					●						
Use of the patient's medical chart						●					
Use of the patient's profile						●					
Determining the drug information and evidence needs							●				
Formulating a search strategy for retrieving information							●				
Retrieving drug information from appropriate sources							●				

continued

APPENDIX B: LEARNING SKILLS BY CHAPTER (CONT'D)

Practice Foundation Knowledge Covered in Each Chapter	Chapter Number										
	1	2	3	4	5	6	7	8	9	10	11
Evaluating the literature for quality							●				
Selecting useful drug information							●				
Assessing meaning from all information sources using evidence-based clinical reasoning								●			
Identifying the patient's health care needs and determining the problems to be addressed								●			
Determining patient care goals									●		
Designing the pharmacotherapeutic regimen									●		
Designing the monitoring plan									●		
Determining the pharmacist's care behaviors supportive of achieving the care goals for the patient									●		
Documenting the patient care plan									●		
Implementing the care plan										●	
Ensuring that medication orders and/or prescriptions are written to facilitate care and monitoring of the patient										●	
Ensuring the patient receives medications/supportive technologies										●	
Conducting counseling to optimize patient adherence										●	
Educating patients about how to contact you and ensure patient follow up is scheduled										●	
Reassessing patient's overall health status and condition, and if desired endpoint or outcome is achieved											●
Assessing the reliability and validity of monitoring data collected from the patient											●
Documenting your assessment and recommendations for changes in the care goals, implementation, or monitoring plan											●
Determining if a change in the care goals, implementation, or monitoring plan is required											●

APPENDIX C: GENERAL ASSESSMENT QUESTIONS ANSWER KEY

Chapter 1: The Patient

1. How do health professionals and patients differ in their concepts of health?

   Answer: Health professionals receive training that defines the concept of health. The most common training is a disease orientation founded in the traditional biomedical model that is central to the medical profession. In this model, health is the "absence of disease." Patients have a diverse set of concepts, ideas, and beliefs about what health is and what it means. They may choose multiple approaches and beliefs resulting in the pursuit of different forms of care and types of providers that best match these beliefs.

2. Distinguish between "illness" and "disease."

   Answer: The terms "illness" and "disease" are synonymous. However, illness represents the usual language used by a patient to express a comprehensive view of "not being well, feeling sick, or feeling unhealthy." Disease is a specific term used to describe the conditions that are recognized within the biomedical model of health and identified as areas requiring treatment or attention by the medical profession.

3. What is ethnocentricity? Why is it a problem in clinical care?

   Answer: Ethnocentricity is when we take our own cultural beliefs and norms and interpret the actions and intentions of other people as though they held these same cultural beliefs and norms. The central problem in ethnocentricity is that we can misinterpret meaning in communication and interactions with the patient by assuming the meaning based upon our own beliefs.

4. Why is it important to understand the patient's health values and beliefs?

   Answer: Understanding the patient's health values and beliefs provides you as a pharmacist with the ability to consciously adapt care for the patient in a way that is consistent with the patient's need from his or her context of the cultural framework.

Chapter 2: The Pharmacist

1. Distinguish among disease-centered, pharmaceutical-centered, and patient-centered pharmacy practice.

   Answer: A patient-centered practice places the care plan development around the patient's concerns and needs. This orientation provides the pharmacist with the framework to accommodate and modify the care plan to optimally match the patient's concerns and needs. A disease-centered practice focuses on the care and outcomes associated with the disease, and not necessarily on the patient's comprehensive health needs. Similarly, pharmaceutical-centered practice focuses on the care and outcomes associated with the pharmaceuticals that are used to treat the disease or conditions identified.

2. Describe the care aspect of pharmaceutical care, as perceived by a patient.

   Answer: Patients perceive caring through interpersonal communication and the behaviors demonstrated by the pharmacist. It is represented to the patient as behavior that results in a more satisfactory experience because the behavior is directed at the right things from the patient's point of view.

3. What distinguishes a generalist practice from a specialist practice?

   Answer: A generalist pharmacist has a broad knowledge base about pharmaceuticals and treatments, and must be able to draw upon a substantial memory of information rapidly on demand. Use of a broad, readily retrievable body of expertise and adeptness at use of information sources when needed quickly characterizes the generalist. A specialist, on the other hand, has great depth in a narrower area of pharmaceuticals and treatments that are associated with a high degree of complex needs. These complexities may be in the clinical reasoning, product preparation, and delivery or administration.

4. Describe the characteristics of a pharmacist that separate the novice from the expert.

   Answer: Experts perform complex tasks more accurately than novices, know more about their area, and demonstrate higher performance at perception of patterns among the cues when gathering data needed to do their work. The expert has a practical form of knowledge that is built upon both experience and a process of reflection beyond that taught in professional programs.

Chapter 3: Comprehensive Pharmaceutical Care

1. Why do some organizations waver in their support of pharmacists in the provision of patient-centered pharmaceutical care?

    Answer: Organizations must have pharmaceutical care in their philosophy in order to expect pharmacists to perform these duties. Excessive workload and organizational downsizing may cause an organization to waver and modify its expectations of professionals.

2. What can the physical layout of a pharmacy or health care facility suggest to a patient?

    Answer: The setting that the pharmacist works in implies a set of expectations in the mind of the patient and the boundaries on the goals with which the pharmacist can respond. The ability to create a private environment is important to the pharmacist's ability to work in a confidential and respectful manner with the patient. A waiting area that is comfortable and oriented toward patient education and communication could promote patient relationship building. There are many examples that can be generated here in discussion to imagine how to create the environment to facilitate the patient–pharmacist relationship.

3. What barriers to the delivery of patient-centered pharmaceutical care can you identify? List them. What strategies might be considered to overcome them?

    Answer: Barriers might include 1) lack of organizational philosophy to support this form of practice, 2) professional competency, 3) individual commitment to patient-centered care, 4) attitude of a supervisor, 5) characteristics of a practice setting you work in such as workload and method of remuneration for services, and 6) others. Strategies to overcome barriers should be developed to match a response to the barrier. It is important to identify the strategies most likely to succeed and implement them. For example, the pharmacist can enhance professional competency by making a personal commitment to lifelong learning and an individual commitment to practice patient-centered care whenever possible to practically do so. The pharmacist can also make recommendations to the organization and administrators that are consistent with improving the work environment to enhance practicing in this way.

4. If your workload is too demanding for you to see all patients, what criteria should you consider when making a choice?

    Answer: The pharmacist might consider this approach: 1) take care of those patients who first seek your care, 2) identify the elderly patients who have a critical need because of the high medication use common to the population, 3) consider those who are in critical care need of service, 4) respond to formal consultations, and 5) in high-demand areas, consider identifying those who might benefit the most by finding patients who have a higher likelihood of adverse drug event experiences or have conditions known to be associated with these problems.

Chapter 4: Overview of Pharmaceutical Care Plan Development and Implementation

1. What are the therapeutic core qualities of a clinician? Why are they so important to patient care?

    Answer: The therapeutic core qualities of a clinician have been identified by psychologist Carl Rogers and include respect, genuineness, and empathy. Patients perceive these qualities immediately upon the first encounter with the pharmacist. It is critical that the patient perceive these qualities in order for the trust relationship to begin.

2. When do you obtain expert opinions in the delivery of patient care?

    Answer: It is appropriate to seek expert opinion when you are unable to find the information you need to proceed with care planning decisions or, alternatively, the information is not known in the published literature and resides in the expert knowledge of others more experienced in the specific area than you. Once you have exhausted your readily available resources within the time frame and urgency of care needs for your patient, you should seek the expert opinion of others.

3. Describe the reasons why you should document care provision in writing.

    Answer: Documentation of care in writing provides useful information about the approach to care that has been taken and the progress being made by the patient, provides data that can then be used to construct a logical association when untoward events occur, provides a record of therapeutic preferences expressed by patients, and provides a legal record. There are many reasons why documentation is a positive action when caring for the patient. More can emerge through a discussion on this subject, especially with experienced practitioners.

4. What is the purpose of a S.O.A.P. note?

    Answer: The S.O.A.P. note is a method for documenting information that occurs in the patient encounter in an organized fashion readily retrievable for the pharmacist to track progress as well as other health professionals who may be involved in caring for the patient.

5. What circumstances warrant redesigning a patient's care plan?

   Answer: A care plan should be considered for redesign when the patient's needs are not being met. Reconsideration is part of the reflective process and monitoring activity in providing care.

Chapter 5: The Patient–Pharmacist Encounter: A Primary Source of Information

1. Describe the optimal environment for conducting a patient interview.

   Answer: The ideal environment provides privacy and is relatively quiet in order to optimize communication between the pharmacist and patient. The ability to communicate at eye level and without physical barriers separating you will further enhance your opportunity to communicate in a meaningful way.

2. What should you communicate to the patient when you first meet him or her?

   Answer: You should greet the person, introduce yourself, and briefly explain your purpose for communication. You should ensure that the information gathered will remain confidential.

3. What will you evaluate about the patient when you have your initial interaction?

   Answer: You should pay attention to details about the patient's characteristics that are likely to reveal the cultural context, social, socioeconomic, spiritual, and/or family background that might influence your interaction. The patient's gender, age, sensory, or communication difficulties should be initially assessed.

4. Describe ways to enhance your communication with a visually impaired patient.

   Answer: Auditory forms of communication become more important to the visually impaired patient. Speaking up clearly so the patient can understand you and confirming that the person *does* understand is important. Use of large print labels, magnifying glasses, and other visual aids and teaching tools can be useful. The poorer the vision, the less useful these aids and tools become.

5. Describe ways to enhance your communication with a hearing impaired patient.

   Answer: Use visual forms of communication with a hearing impaired patient. Reduce background noise as much as possible. Use of gestures and placing yourself directly in front of the patient so he or she has a clear view of your face when you are speaking is necessary. Speak clearly, in short sentences, and at a reasonable pace for the patient to assimilate what you are saying. Sign language interpretation may be useful for some patients. This resource is more likely available in organized health-system settings.

6. What key points should you communicate to the patient when you close the patient encounter?

   Answer: In general, you should review what you view as important findings, and tell the patient back what you have identified as the list of problems or concerns and the priority for responding to them. You should secure agreement on a plan of action and determine what your responsibilities are and what the patient's responsibilities are, if possible.

Chapter 6: The Patient's Record: A Primary Source of Information

1. Describe five common uses for the medical chart.

   Answer: 1) organizing and remembering information for patient care use, 2) primary communication mode between health professionals who are caring for the patient, 3) a record for the patient him- or herself to enhance self-care and maintain continuity of health records longitudinally, 4) administrative uses, 5) research uses, 6) public health use for epidemiologic questions, 7) legal use, 8) educational use for training professionals, and 9) audit use for quality-assurance purposes.

2. Describe the differences between subjective and objective information.

   Answer: Subjective data are open to individual interpretation and often is the information reported to you by the patient. Objective data are easily duplicated or quantified, and is generally information directly observed by you or collected through a systematic approach (e.g., use of a blood pressure cuff and recording of the BP data within your own setting).

3. How does the Privacy Act protect a patient's confidentiality?

   Answer: The Privacy Act preserves the individual's right to privacy by requiring that he or she give consent for the use of data collected for any purpose other than the intended purpose, such as providing health care. The patient has the right to indicate what information will be made available and to whom.

4. What action should you take as a pharmacist when a patient's medication order or prescription is difficult to read or unclear in its intent?

   Answer: Pharmacists should contact the prescriber when any aspect of an order is unclear.

5. If you wanted to audit several medical charts for patients to gather data about a pharmacy program's effectiveness (you do not intend to publish this), would you need to seek each patient's consent before you did it?

   Answer: No, as long as it is not possible for someone to identify individuals and their data from the reports and documents that describe the program and its effectiveness.

Chapter 7: Gathering Drug Information and Evidence

1. Why is it important to "classify" the subject matter of a drug information question?

   Answer: Classifying the subject matter from a drug information question will help you to determine the information sources from which you need to gather data, including the published literature.

2. Once you have classified the question, what is the correct searching strategy? Describe the types of references and order of searching that is generally pursued.

   Answer: References are generally distinguished into tertiary, secondary, or primary, and then further as general or specialty references within each. References are most correctly searched by identifying the general references first then moving to specialty references, starting with tertiary, then secondary, and finally primary. Using this systematic approach will result in you being more likely to find the information in the most relevant resources.

3. What is the purpose of a clinical practice guideline? By what process is it usually developed?

   Answer: Clinical practice guidelines are a published source of information that provide steps to diagnosing or managing clinical problems by integrating evidence from the published literature with the expertise gained through clinical experience.

Therefore, these guidelines are generally produced using a consensus approach of experts assembled at the direction of professional associations or organizations with an interest in having the guideline produced.

4. What advantages do drug information sources offer when made available on handheld devices?

   Answer: Increasingly, drug information, including primary literature sources and graphical information from secondary sources, can be received and used immediately at the point of care. This can substantially shorten the amount of time, or even enhance the available information when needed.

5. What is the nature of reliable drug information?

   Answer: Reliable information is valid, truthful, and without bias, or the biases are made transparent in the context of the information source itself.

6. Explain why experts hold a unique body of knowledge.

   Answer: Not all information you will need to practice is available through published sources. Experts have gained tacit knowledge that is often not found anywhere in the published world yet useful to specific situations in patient care you may encounter. This knowledge is gained through experience.

Chapter 8: Application of Clinical Reasoning

1. Can someone have sound clinical reasoning skills without having content expertise in the subject matter of concern? Explain the rationale for your answer.

   Answer: If you have sound clinical reasoning skills, then you would include content expertise as part of the essential knowledge required to make a sound clinical judgment. Content expertise is interpreted in the context of the patient's needs and concerns and, thus, is given meaning in part through this way. Alternatively, if one has content expertise but does not use reasoning skills, the use of the content expertise may be suboptimal in the patient's care. Content expertise is part of sound clinical reasoning skills.

2. Differentiate the characteristics of empathy from sympathy.

   Answer: Empathy is a reflexive understanding of both yourself and the patient, leading to an understanding of what exactly is being told to you by the patient through all forms of communication. Sympathy is an emotional reaction you might experience in response to the patient.

Chapter 9: Designing the Patient Care Plan

1. Why is it important to write a care plan and document it?

   Answer: This written document provides you with the necessary history to assess how the patient is progressing, provides needed information to other health professionals, and documents evidence of care and outcomes experienced by the patient.

2. What is the name of the section of the care plan that describes your evaluation of the patient's condition and the rationale for this evaluation?

   Answer: This is commonly called "assessment."

3. Describe how to prioritize the patient's problems.

   Answer: Use your clinical reasoning skills to first address matters of urgency. Next you should express to the patient and other team members (if applicable) what you would determine to be the next most important areas to address, ranking them from most immediate to least immediate priorities. Once you have reached agreement, you have a prioritized list of problems to guide your care planning.

Chapter 10: Implementing the Patient Care Plan

1. There are many reasons why a patient may be non-adherent to a medication plan. Interview a close friend, neighbor, relative, or another classmate who has had the need to take medications. Question this individual about his or her medication-taking behavior. What were challenges to adhering for this individual? How do these match what you have learned in this chapter?

   Answer: To address this answer, first document the problem list that is revealed in your interview. Then use Table 10-1 and compare what you learn from the interview with the factors listed. Identify as many as possible that match your interviewee's situation.

2. What are tools you might use with a patient to assist the individual with carrying out the care plan you develop?

   Answer: Encourage the patient and teach him or her to ask questions. This will help the patient clarify information and learn correct actions when what is expected might not be clear. Use written support materials such as counseling sheets, calendars, brochures and leaflets, books, lists of relevant web sites, videos and CDs, and access to specialized classes as tools for which you can be a primary resource provider.

Chapter 11: Modifying the Care Plan through Patient Progress and Outcome Assessment

1. Why is it necessary to reassess the patient's general health and condition each time you visit with him or her to follow up on the care plan progress?

   Answer: Much has usually happened between the initial time you assessed a patient and the followup opportunity. The patient may not have adhered to all aspects of the plan, new problems may have emerged that need to be taken into consideration, or the patient's underlying problems may have changed.

2. What are some of the possible things that following a monitoring parameter in a patient can inform you about?

   Answer: A monitoring parameter may inform you about the adherence behavior of a patient, the difficulty the patient may be having with the selected approach to care, an actual change in the patient's underlying condition, and the extent of success that the treatment approach actually achieves.

3. What type of responses to a care plan would prompt a referral to the primary care provider?

   Answer: A failure to respond after optimizing behavior or an unsafe or adverse reaction should prompt immediate referral. If a patient was not successful in response to the care plan and you employed all options within your scope of practice, a referral to someone who had alternative approaches through specialized expertise would also be a reason for referral.

INDEX

D

E

X–Z